Copyright © 2024 by Parker Nelson

All rights reserved. No part of this publication may be reproduced, distributed, or transmitted in any form or by any means, including photocopying, recording, or other electronic or mechanical methods, without the prior written permission of the publisher, except in the case of brief quotations embodied in critical reviews and certain other noncommercial uses permitted by copyright law.

ISBN: 979-8-3303-7194-5 (IngramSpark)

ISBN: 979-8-3405-7928-7 (KDP)

Cover design by Miracle Manor.

Printed by IngramSpark.

First printing edition 2024.

Nutrition Nonsense

How Social and Psychological Biases Sabotage Our Eating Habits

Parker Nelson, MS, RD

For Phyllis, Steve, Heather, Alexis, Collin and Maxwell

CONTENTS

INTRODUCTION..4
CHAPTER 1: PANACEA...............................14
CHAPTER 2: ORIGINS................................43
CHAPTER 3: MARKETING..........................66
CHAPTER 4: EXPERTISE............................96
CHAPTER 5: SCIENCE...............................121
CHAPTER 6: DUALITY...............................148
CHAPTER 7: CONVERSATION....................175
CHAPTER 8: UNIQUE.................................199
CHAPTER 9: FUNDAMENTALS....................226
CHAPTER 10: FORWARD...........................256
REFERENCES..272
ACKNOWLEDGEMENTS.............................340

INTRODUCTION

Food is one of life's greatest pleasures. It provides nourishment, fosters community, and is often tied to cherished memories. Food has a remarkable ability to heal, but it can also be a source of tension. We've all been there—you're sitting around the table at Thanksgiving and Aunt Sue won't touch the stuffing because she thinks bread makes her fat, and she's letting everyone know. Or how about the nutrition advice we are bombarded with on social media and the wild "anti-aging" claims we are now seeing on health products. These experiences, and many more, can taint our love for food and are what I like to call "nutrition nonsense."

I define "nutrition nonsense" as the culmination of all the myths, misinformation, and misguided perspectives that steer people away from healthy eating habits. It is the collective noise that drowns out simple, reliable nutritional advice, making it harder for people to navigate their relationship with food. As a dietitian, I hear about this nonsense all the time from my patients and clients. Whether it's chasing after extreme diets or the promise of a cure-all detox, so many are drowning in this overwhelming sea of myths and misconceptions.

This isn't a small problem, either. Nutrition nonsense is everywhere—from restrictive diets disguised as "lifestyles" to the marketing madness that bombards us online and in grocery stores. From false health claims on packaging to over exaggerating the benefit of trendy superfoods, nutrition nonsense convinces us that our bodies are never good enough and shames us for not eating "healthily" enough. These myths leave us disoriented, infuriated, and depressed. The spread of these harmful health trends and misleading advice is more rampant than ever, and there is no clear end in sight.

But despite this growing tide of confusion, I believe there's hope. By exploring the deep-seated fallacies and biases that have taken root in our understanding of food and health, we can start to make sense of these misunderstandings surrounding the nonsense and reclaim our right to enjoy healthy food with confidence. In this book, we will journey together through the maze of nutrition myths, uncover the truth of healthy eating habits, and empower ourselves to approach food with the joy and freedom it deserves.

My commitment to solving the problem of nutrition nonsense is deeply personal, and it fuels my determination to find the answers we all need to live happier, healthier lives. The desire to address all of this nonsense began with two pivotal experiences in my life: my mother's battle with cancer and my own (sometimes challenging) health journey. These personal experiences revealed the ingrained misconceptions and prejudices that plague our understanding of food and wellness, sparking my commitment to helping others navigate through the confusion.

MY MOM

In 2013, my mom was diagnosed with adrenal cancer. It wasn't until years later as the disease advanced, that I truly began to grasp the gravity of her situation. Around the same time, my growing interest in health prompted me to explore a new career path—nutrition. Fueled by a desire to help, I started offering my mom nutritional remedies that I hoped might give her a fighting chance against cancer. Although I had just started a nutrition certification program, I was eager to make a difference. I concocted smoothies and dishes packed with every superfood I could find—berries, cruciferous vegetables, and powders made from beets, mushrooms, flaxseed, and spirulina. I believed I had created the healthiest smoothie known to man, pairing it with the purest and cleanest protein-packed recipes I could create. Although I had only made these smoothies a few times (and she could barely tolerate the dreadful taste) I clung to the hope that even a few sips of my "magical elixirs" might cure her.

But it didn't. On August 25, 2020, my sweet mother passed away. As my family navigated the painful process of grief, I was consumed by anger. I was angry that I hadn't progressed further in my nutrition studies in time to save her and frustrated with the health and nutrition sources that had filled my head with the idea that food alone could save her. This was my first real confrontation with nutrition nonsense, and it is the first myth I want to put an end to. My ultimate realization wasn't about the power of food. In fact, I still believe in the profound impact diet has on our health and how important it is to make good choices. But I began to see that much of what we hear and believe about nutrition, from diets to detoxes, is complete and utter nonsense.

MY GROCERY STORE CONFRONTATION

My mother's battle with cancer left me with deep questions about the promises of nutrition. But it wasn't until a bizarre encounter at the grocery store a year later that I fully grasped just how pervasive and harmful nutrition misinformation can be. This strange moment, which initially left

INTRODUCTION

me puzzled, ultimately set me on a path that would shape my career and passion for helping others navigate the confusing world of food and health.

One afternoon, while browsing the aisles of Trader Joe's, I stopped at one of my favorite sections, the peanut butter aisle. Peanut butter had always been a staple in my diet, so I picked up a jar and began to read the label. But as I scrolled through the nutrition facts, I put the peanut butter back and swapped it for a jar of almond butter, which I'd recently started using instead after reading on social media that it would be a healthier option.

As I stood there, focused on the almond butter label, a man, about 35 years old, suddenly appeared behind me. He peered over my shoulder like he was copying answers from a test before he decided to grab my attention. With a display of confidence, I've rarely seen since, he said, "Ah! Almond butter. Now that's a great choice. You know why, right? Because it's so much better for you than that peanut butter right there. Our bodies can't actually digest peanuts properly, which leads to all kinds of health and gut issues. Trust me, stick with the almond butter and don't fall for that peanut butter scam." He continued to rant about how his friend had lost 40 pounds by switching to almond butter and how peanut butter was nothing more than "toxic sludge."

This bizarre and almost surreal encounter happened so quickly that it left me speechless. I didn't have a chance to respond before the man slipped away, vanishing as quickly as he had appeared. It was a bewildering experience, especially as I was just beginning to immerse myself in nutrition. I felt so confused as I wondered, "Is peanut butter really that bad for you?" The man had been so certain about the benefits of almond butter and was so convincing. He even offered an emotional story about his friend who had supposedly lost 40 pounds! And yet, my naturally skeptical side kicked into gear. How could he be sure it was the almond butter that led to his friend's weight loss? Knowing that the nutrition labels on both jars are nearly identical and having never had any issues with peanut butter myself, how could I separate this man's claims from my own experience?

Well, after a few days, I returned to the same grocery store, and in a twist of fate, Trader Joe's was out of almond butter, forcing me to reconsider peanut butter as my only option. But this time, something had changed. I felt a twinge of nervousness about buying peanut butter again. It was unbelievable. A single encounter with a random stranger had made me question a food I'd enjoyed for years. By now, I had lost a little bit of weight and was focused on healthier food choices, so the thought of jeopardizing my progress made me anxious. What if the man was right? What if peanut butter really could ruin my health?

That initial fear soon gave way to something else: frustration. I was furious that a stranger's unsolicited advice had shaken my confidence in my favorite food choices. Determined to prove him wrong, I bought the peanut butter and used it liberally on everything. I paid close attention to how I felt and even tracked my weight over the next two weeks. And guess what? Nothing changed. While I wasn't able to compare eating peanut butter to almond butter at the time, I felt that I had "proved" that the former wasn't the demonic or toxic food that the grocery store fiend had claimed. Although I was thrilled to have "proven" that stranger wrong, I wasn't entirely satisfied. I still didn't have the certainty I was looking for in making good food choices. I would soon come to find out that I was not the only one wrapped up in this problem—almost everyone I know has faced some level of nutrition nonsense.

WHY THIS MATTERS

In a world awash with dietary advice and nutrition theories, it can be challenging to discern fact from fiction. The intention of this book isn't just to be another guide to what's right and wrong in nutrition; it is a deep dive into the psychology behind our dietary choices and beliefs. It explores why these things matter and how you can adopt a better perspective. If you're here seeking validation for your diet as the most "superior one," this is definitely not the book for you. Instead, I want to challenge your own biases and social tendencies in order to uncover why you believe what you do about food and health.

The journey to understanding nutrition begins with mastering the basics. I wrote this book because I was once confused, annoyed, sad, and misled about nutrition. My aim is to help you find clarity and freedom from the nonsense that pervades this field. You don't need to obsess over trivial health tips; you need a reminder to focus on the fundamentals. Many people overcomplicate nutrition with dramatic and unnecessary practices, and ignore the simple, consistent habits that lead to better health.

Ultimately, I want to help you avoid wasting anymore time, money, or resources on bad decisions that can harm your health. Debunking nutrition myths and helping you understand the topic better might not seem like life and death—but it could be.

THE TOLL ON MENTAL HEALTH

This widespread confusion around nutrition can have serious consequences for our health and well-being. From a mental health perspective, misleading nutrition information can exacerbate existing eating disorders, which already affect nearly 30 million Americans over their lifetimes. These disorders are most prevalent among adolescents and continue to rise.[1,2] Shockingly, eating disorders have the second highest mortality rate of any mental health condition, surpassed only by opioid addiction.[3] While eating disorders are complex, and not solely caused by conflicting nutrition advice, the barrage of misinformation likely plays a significant role. Even for those without an eating disorder, the frustration and confusion of navigating fad diets and attempting to eat healthier in a challenging food landscape can take a serious toll on mental health.

THE TOLL ON PHYSICAL HEALTH

The physical health implications of nutrition misinformation are equally staggering. Countless problems, from heartburn to constipation, have proven nutritional solutions that are often obscured by a sea of false claims and scam diets. Perhaps most critically, chronic diseases like cancer, heart disease, and type 2 diabetes, which are the leading causes of disability and death in the United States, demand genuine nutritional interventions.[4] These three alone are responsible for much of the $4.1 trillion spent annually on healthcare in America. The magnitude of these numbers is difficult to fully grasp, but the personal impact is undeniable. Many of us have faced the struggle and heartache of battling a chronic illness, or have watched a loved one wrestle with an eating disorder.

Eliminating nutrition nonsense won't solve these problems entirely, but it can make a profound difference. By reducing confusion and promoting accurate information, we can save lives. If even one person finds clarity in the complex world of nutrition because of this book, then every word will have been worth it.

EXTREME SCENARIOS

Sometimes statistics alone fail to convey just how tragic this problem truly is and some stories can help us see this problem in a more meaningful light. In 2023, Zhanna Samsonova, known to her millions of social media followers as Zhanna D'Art, tragically passed away, likely due to malnutrition and related infections.[5] The Russian influencer had built a large online presence across TikTok, Instagram, and Facebook, where she promoted an extremely restrictive diet consisting almost entirely of fruit, while avoiding oil, salt, and protein.[6] This dangerously unbalanced diet appears to have led to her death.

Despite her public claims that the diet improved her mood, mental clarity, and energy levels, Zhanna's story is a heartbreaking reminder that feeling good doesn't always equate to being healthy. Her case represents an extreme form of an eating disorder, one that severely limited not just her food intake, but also water, ultimately contributing to her demise. As news of her death spread across social media, it became a battleground for opposing nutrition groups, each using her story to push their own agendas. In the midst of this, Zhanna's grieving mother made a desperate plea: "She is already dead, she is no more. Please stop writing bad things, it hurts me a lot. She chose this path. I fought for many years [but] she did not listen to her mother."

To those close to her, it was clear that Zhanna needed to stop her restrictive diet. However, her unwavering belief in the fruitarian lifestyle likely drowned out any warnings from her loved ones. What could drive someone to such extreme dietary practices? It's difficult to pinpoint her exact motivations, but they likely included a combination of maintaining her social media persona, idealizing a false ideology, and falling prey to misinformation from unreliable sources.

As I read through the comments on an article about her death (a dangerous place to seek rational discourse), I was stunned by the level of nutritional misinformation and unhelpful chaos on display. Here are a few comments that perfectly encapsulate the current chaos in the world of nutrition:

- "Our ancient ancestors were strict fruit eaters for millions of years while in the tropical forest."
- "Ironically, eating vegetables raw is the worst way to eat vegetables." Followed by: "Seriously? Why do I always hear conflicting points about cooking vegetables? Does this vary by person? I never have had a problem with raw veggies. Do you think fermenting veggies is a good idea?"
- "The best way to prepare vegetables is with animal fats—true butter, a bit of animal lard. That makes the vitamins which are fat-soluble more absorbable. Weston Price foundation. None of the awful vegetable oils which are causing a huge rise in autoimmune disorders and inflammations."

INTRODUCTION

- "I don't eat meat, but I eat plenty of nuts. Cottage cheese is also good."

If you needed more evidence that the comment section is one of the worst places to seek nutrition advice, now you have some. Amid the few humorous or nonsensical remarks, these comments are a stark reminder of how deeply people are entrenched in misinformation and how urgently we need a reset in our approach to nutrition.

This isn't an isolated issue unfortunately. It's not just a handful of influencers promoting dangerous diets. There are thousands of equally troubling stories. With the rise of social media, false health claims can spread like wildfire, often with devastating consequences.

The tragic story of Zhanna Samsonova is a clear example that the consequences of misguided nutrition beliefs extend beyond individual tragedies. I recently heard about a dietitian who was treating a severely malnourished baby in the hospital. The baby's parents had put their child on a strict carnivore diet, leading to such critical nutrition deficiencies that the healthcare team considered contacting social services. While the parents may have had good intentions, this extreme approach to nutrition highlights a harsh reality: neglecting proper nutrition can be a form of child abuse.

Or we can take the infamous case of Belle Gibson, a celebrity nutrition figure who gained fame by claiming she cured her malignant brain cancer with a sugar-free and gluten-free diet. Her story inspired many until it was revealed she never had cancer at all. Gibson fabricated her diagnosis and recovery, exploiting the trust and hopes of vulnerable people for personal gain.

Equally alarming is the ongoing case of Barbara O'Neill, an Australian wellness guru who was banned from practicing her wellness coaching after promoting dangerously false health advice. She claimed raw goat's milk could replace breast milk for infants and that cancer is a fungus treatable with baking soda.[7]

These are just a few of the many cases we'll explore in this book, highlighting the widespread and sometimes lethal impact of nutrition misinformation. Stories like these underscores the urgent need for clear, science-based guidance in today's increasingly confusing food landscape.

WHY IS THIS HAPPENING?

Here's the hard truth: many of the myths and misconceptions we believe about nutrition aren't just random misunderstandings. They stem from a complex web of *social and psychological biases*. From the subtle influence of the placebo and Dunning-Kruger effects to the more insidious forces of corporate greed, celebrity worship, and the powerful sway of social media algorithms, these factors shape our beliefs and behaviors around food in ways we often fail to recognize. The wildest part is, most of us assume it's someone else who's falling for nutrition myths. We don't even realize we've been caught in these nutrition scams ourselves. Chances are, you've been misinformed without even knowing it.

One reason we often fall for nutrition myths and develop a distorted view of health is that we unconsciously prioritize the wrong things. As David Foster Wallace famously noted in his "This is Water" speech, humans are wired to worship something—whether it's money, possessions, fame, our bodies, achievements, or self-righteousness. When these misplaced priorities dominate, they skew our perception of what true holistic health means.

It's important to recognize that these pursuits aren't inherently negative however. Striving to eat better, following influential voices, or setting goals for our bodies can all be positive steps. However, when we chase these goals without self-awareness or balance, we risk becoming trapped by the very myths we're trying to escape. This book aims to help you break free from these automatic behaviors and reclaim your ability to make conscious, intentional choices about your health and well-being.

FIGHTING BIAS WITH A REALITY CHECK

The Greek philosopher, Plato, illustrated the power of revealing truth through a parable known as the allegory of the cave. In this parable, he paints a picture of a group of prisoners chained up inside a dark cave, able to see only shadows on a wall. These shadows are cast by objects they can't perceive, and represent a facsimile of reality. We face a similar experience in regard to modern nutrition advice. Much of what we hear seems real, and might be based on a kernel of truth, but by the time it makes it to us, it is nothing but a warped representation.

As Plato's story continues, one prisoner is freed and stumbles out of the cave into the blinding sunlight. At first, he's overwhelmed, but as he adjusts, he begins to see the world as it truly is. He realizes that the shadows were mere reflections of a much larger, more complex reality. When he tries to return to the cave to share his newfound knowledge, he struggles to readjust to the darkness, knowing that those still chained would likely reject or misunderstand the truth he's seen.

Just as I fell for nutrition myths during my mother's battle with cancer and my own efforts to improve my health, many of us are trapped in a narrow perspective, our understanding of health shaped by biases, dogmatic beliefs, and external influences like celebrities, corporations, and even family. Like the prisoners in the cave, we cling to familiar shadows, unaware of the larger truths waiting to be discovered.

I once felt the same way, until I was fortunate enough to encounter people dedicated to exposing the myths and lies surrounding nutrition. These hard truths were difficult to face, but they were essential in transforming my approach to health. Once I saw through the nutrition nonsense, there was no going back. This journey is not easy, and we all need help uncovering these truths, which is exactly why I wrote this book—to help pass on just some of the wisdom that I was lucky enough to finally work towards.

My hope for this book is to inspire you to step out of the cave, to become a curious and investigative learner willing to look beyond the shadows you encounter every day. Seeking truth in health and nutrition can be painful because it requires confronting our own habits, biases, and misconceptions. You don't have to abandon everything you believe, but by being open to exploring where your ideas come from, you might just discover a healthier, more fulfilling approach to nutrition—one that frees you from the chains of misinformation and leads you toward a more vibrant life. As a nutrition professional who empowers individuals every day with solutions to this problem, I want to offer this book as an opportunity to help you separate fact from fiction in the world of nutrition.

CHAPTER 1: PANACEA

"Better a cruel truth than a comfortable delusion."

— **Edward Abbey**

American culture is overrun by a pervasive demand for instant gratification, especially when it comes to matters of nutrition and health. This "quick fix" obsession, evident in trendy detoxes and extreme diets, can ultimately undermine your well-being. Instead of investing in sustainable health practices, people chase after miraculous solutions that promise hassle-free happiness. This mentality neglects the necessary effort for genuine health and diverts attention away from the fundamental pillars of wellness. The burgeoning detox industry, forecasted to reach $75 billion by 2026, epitomizes the popular desire for a miracle cure.[1] Rather than cleansing their bodies, people are actually detoxing their wallets. The constant influx of health fads perpetuates a cycle of false hope, which squanders time, money, and health.

This first chapter is all about breaking down the tempting appeal of nutrition panaceas we all face and encourages a smarter use of our resources to build long-term well-being.

WHAT IS A PANACEA?

A panacea (pan-uh-see-uh) is a term used to describe any cure-all elixir, typically related to health. The term is taken directly from the name of the Greek goddess of universal remedy, Panacea. According to Greek mythology, Panacea possessed a miracle tonic with which she could heal any human malady. Just about every diet or supplement we see now, from keto to colostrum, promises a similar but more subtle promise of curing all of our ailments.

It's not surprising that so many of us are looking for a nutritional panacea, as the constant struggle to maintain healthy habits can be massively discouraging. Not to mention, we are getting very little help from the disappointing healthcare system.[2,3] Over time, this dissatisfaction begins to corrode people's sense of control, prompting people to seek solace in a quintessential American pursuit—consumption. Most people have a single strategy to cope with a loss of control of their health which is to consume

CHAPTER 1: PANACEA

as much stuff as possible. In the U.S., it's believed that the more we consume, the more we can control. Whether it's shopping for the latest and greatest supplement or trying out a fancy new protocol, there's the ever-prevalent hope that we can *buy* our way back to good health. As a result, marketing teams everywhere are salivating over this collective desperation for control.

Janey Chrzan, a nutritional anthropologist, says this type of consumerist approach is actually what makes fad diets so alluring. She writes, "We suspect that buying things to solve problems creates a sense of agency among dieters: purchasing special foods makes them feel more efficacious than if they just ate a little bit less all the time."[4]

Although the intention to reclaim agency over health is commendable, many make the mistake of directing their efforts toward interventions that lack merit. While a few of these approaches can provide some value worthy of individual consideration, none of them are magic bullets that can act alone in reclaiming health.

Rather than getting stuck on the never-ending chase of the elusive panacea, it's imperative that you prioritize sustainable habits, even if it means putting in the extra effort. Among the many quick fixes that promise to solve your health and nutrition struggles, perhaps none is as popular or as misleading as the juice cleanse.

THE JUICE CLEANSE

Promising an array of remedies for every ailment from acne to cancer, the juice cleanse is an attempt to "reset" our bodies—as if we were machines that could return to factory settings. Cleansing efforts often exclude all foods and beverages for days or weeks at a time, while relying solely on a juice made up of an arbitrary list of fruits, vegetables, and whatever exotic ingredient is currently trending. As if all it took was acai, goji berries, and raw organic bee pollen to make you young again.

Typically, people turn to these cleanses in hopes of tackling persistent health challenges that have become overbearing, such as weight loss efforts or dealing with chronic fatigue. Tackling these issues is not easy, so falling for the promise of a juice cleanse is not at all shameful. However, such complex health issues are often rooted in multifaceted underlying causes that require legitimate solutions, not Hail Mary's. But as the idiom goes, desperate times call for desperate measures, and no one capitalizes on desperation quite as well as the juice-cleansing market.

CHAPTER 1: PANACEA

CAPITALIZING ON OUR PAIN

Unfortunately, the organizations and influencers that sell detox juices and cleansing protocols capitalize on discouragement – which comes from so many failed attempts to lose weight or solve a chronic health problem. They do this remarkably cleverly, tapping into your momentary state of vulnerability and uncertainty.

Marketing experts often exploit your vulnerabilities first, specifically targeting your lingering health struggles that you can't seem to overcome. They craft messages that feign genuine concern, using catchy phrases like "discover the secret to health" or "refresh and recharge your body." When you're feeling emotionally drained from failed attempts at improving your nutrition, it's easy to believe you've missed some elusive answer that only detox programs can provide. As a result, you become convinced that without signing up for the latest 5-day detox, you might miss out on a life-changing solution. And, of course, for a "limited time," these detoxes are conveniently 25% off—discounted from an inflated price that marketing teams arbitrarily assign.

Every attempt to sell the value of these short-term fixes' preys on the idea that your health is a reflection of your morality. You're led to believe that poor health equates to being a "bad" person and that the only way to become pure and whole again is by somehow cleansing your body. Unfortunately, the harsh reality is that starving yourself with low-protein, low-fiber, and calorie-deficient detoxes can cause more harm than good. Not only can these approaches lead to long-term health issues, but they also drain your already low energy levels during fasting. While some people may experience a brief surge of energy, this is often due to an adrenaline rush or because they removed unhealthy habits that were working against them.

Rather than falling into this unhelpful cycle, the best way to genuinely support your health is to prioritize sustainable habits that prevent these slumps in the first place. It might not be fast or glamorous, but consistently eating more fruits and vegetables, along with daily physical activity, is far more effective for long-term wellness than the absurd quick-fix promises we are shown in advertising campaigns.

And yes, while the body does need to detoxify harmful substances, this is how juice cleanses promoters also capitalize on the average person's uncertainty about how human physiology actually works.

CHAPTER 1: PANACEA

Most people were never taught basic physiology (or didn't pay attention in class), which led to widespread misunderstanding. This knowledge gap allows detox marketers to imply that without using their products, toxins will keep accumulating in our bodies. But here's the real issue: this premise simply isn't true, nor does it make any physiological sense.

Although you may have heard a confident pitch about the certainty that toxins are building up in your body, this is almost always a myth. While there are some extreme cases, almost everyone does not experience this buildup. This is because the body has intrinsic detoxification mechanisms, facilitated by the lungs, skin, digestive tract, kidneys, and liver, that do all the cleansing of the toxins we do come in contact with.[5]

Contrary to popular belief, it is not a juice cleanse that can purge the body of all unwanted toxins; it's the body's intricate systems that do this work for us. The best way to support these systems is through healthy lifestyle habits like sleep, exercise, and proper nutrition. Juice cleanse companies, however, are banking on your uncertainty about these facts and your distrust in your own body's natural abilities. The collective ignorance about how the body works opens the door for companies to sell products based on fear of the unknown.

But what happens in cases where you are exposed to a heavy dose of toxins that is too much for your body to handle? To understand these cases, let's take a look at an example of how your body processes a common toxin: alcohol.

When you drink alcoholic beverages, you are consuming ethanol, a toxin that is broken down by the liver. The result of liver breakdown is acetaldehyde, a carcinogenic metabolite or byproduct that is then turned into acetic acid.[6] This is then converted into carbon dioxide and water, which leave the body through breathing and urination, no longer posing a threat to your health.[7] Your organs are so attuned to the danger of this toxin that they prioritize its metabolism over the breakdown of carbohydrates, protein, and fat. In cases where the liver cannot handle the consumed amount of alcohol, whether due to acute overconsumption or chronic exposure, you would experience severe health complications.

If your liver or kidneys fail to remove toxins, like during a binge-drinking episode, you wouldn't just feel fatigued; you could experience vomiting or blacking out. If you had a significantly harmful buildup of toxins in your body, it would require medical attention, not a homemade juice blend with some spinach and pineapple. Unfortunately, the juice cleanse fad has continually found ways to override the reasonable logic of prioritizing healthy habits, all in an effort to push more products and protocols.

POTENTIAL FOR HARM

So why call out juice cleanses and detox protocols, especially when some claim to experience positive results from them? Because they waste precious time and resources and can even mislead those with serious health issues who need proper medical solutions! Model Irena Stoynova nearly died while trying to cure her cancer using a popular podcaster's "cancer-curing" juice methods. She eventually shifted to conventional care and went into remission (and admitted that the side effects from chemotherapy were far easier to manage than those caused by her initial juicing regimen).[8] That's a striking statement, considering the notoriously harsh side effects of chemotherapy.

Similarly, Australian wellness influencer Jessica Ainscough tragically passed away in 2015 following Gerson therapy, which involves coffee enemas (injecting room temperature coffee into the rectum) and other cleansing protocols.[9] Considering detoxes and cleanses as magical cure-all solutions, capable of replacing proven healthy habits or medical treatments, is a dangerous and distorted approach to health.

You might believe that enduring these extreme cleanses (that some might compare to the taste of sewage water) earns you a badge of honor, but this is not an effective way to support detoxification or develop long-term healthy habits. While trying out every kind of remedy when you become desperate is tempting, there is no scientific evidence that juice cleanses effectively eliminate toxins.[10] Instead, you would be far better off investing your time and money into improving your dietary habits with the help of a nutrition professional. After all, eating a balanced diet that nourishes your body's natural detoxifying organs is a much safer and more sustainable way to support your health.

DIETING

To some, juice detoxes may seem like an obvious myth, but there are countless other diets that present more legitimate-sounding solutions. While I can't cover the hundreds of diets out there, insight into a few popular ones may help you better assess the legitimacy of any diet you come across in the future.

CHAPTER 1: PANACEA

KETO

The ketogenic diet, which has surged in popularity in recent times, appeals to those looking for rapid weight loss. Originally proposed by Dr. Wilder at the Mayo Clinic in 1921, the keto diet was actually intended as a treatment for epilepsy, offering the benefits of fasting without the need to abstain from food in the long term.

Wilder's ketogenic diet restricts carbohydrates and emphasizes fat-rich foods. Without carbs as the body's primary energy source, it switches to ketosis, using ketones for fuel. To achieve ketosis, carb intake must be limited to 10-15 grams per day (about one slice of bread), protein to 1 gram per kilogram of body weight, and the remaining calories must come from fat.[11] Peterman's research showed that 95% of 37 young epileptic patients had improved seizure control while on this diet, a remarkable achievement.[12] The keto diet remains a clinical option for epilepsy patients who don't respond to medication.

The popularity of fat-centric diets grew further with the introduction of the Atkins diet in the 1960s. Despite initial ridicule, its success stories gained national attention.[13] Though the Atkins diet eventually waned in popularity, it was rebranded using many of the same ketogenic principles.

Today, the keto diet is often promoted as the ultimate weight-loss solution, claiming efficient fat-burning mechanisms. However, when compared to other diets, it does not seem to be superior. While keto can lead to rapid weight loss, 61% of this weight loss is typically from water, not fat.

In contrast, a study comparing keto with a mixed-macronutrient diet found that 59.5% of weight loss in the mixed diet group was from fat loss, compared to just 37% in keto participants.[14] This difference is explained by carbohydrate storage, which retains water. So, when you stop the keto diet, much of the initial weight loss returns as water weight.

Some keto dieters aren't concerned by this, citing higher fat-burning rates on the diet. While true that on a low-carb, high-fat diet, the body does burn more fat, it doesn't necessarily lead to fat loss. If the energy from this fat isn't needed, the body restores the fatty acids as fat. Simply put, keto increases fat breakdown, but it also increases fat storage if calorie needs are met from the high fat intake. In layman's terms, keto helps you *burn* fat, but it'll also make sure you store more fat. Like any diet, fat loss on keto still depends on maintaining a calorie deficit.

Reliable evidence shows that those on low-carb diets lose or maintain weight at the same rate as those on low-to moderate-fat diets.[15] In fact, Laurence Kinsell and his team, back in 1964, demonstrated this in a study where subjects maintained constant calorie intake but varied macronutrient composition, ranging from 12% to 83% of calories from fat, and 3% to 64% from carbs. Physical activity was consistent across groups.[16] The researchers concluded that "the first law of thermodynamics applies to the human machine quite as predictably as it does to inanimate objects."

While calling people "human machines" feels a bit off-putting, their study does highlight a fundamental truth: calorie balance, not macronutrient composition, determines weight loss. This conclusion has been echoed in more recent studies, such as Kevin Hall's 2017 review, which found no significant differences in weight loss across diets with varying fat and carb ratios when calories and protein were matched.[17]

Fat loss isn't the only reason to try a diet, though. Take bodybuilder Mark Taylor as an example of keto's limitations for working out. After years of success using the keto diet, Taylor saw new gains after dramatically increasing his carb intake—he would eat potatoes 6 times a day at the age of 42.[18] Now, while most of us don't need to eat six potatoes every day, Taylor's experience is a reminder that carb-limiting diets like keto may restrict muscle growth and athletic performance, and while the keto diet can be beneficial for certain groups, it's far from a one-size-fits-all solution for most people.

ALKALINE

The alkaline, or pH, diet remains a persistent trend in the media. This is largely thanks to Robert Young, author of the best-selling book "The pH Miracle." This diet's popularity has sparked products like alkaline water, which claim to boost health by altering your body's pH. But there are major flaws in this concept. Alkaline water is often made by adding sodium bicarbonate (baking soda) or another base to raise its pH, with the idea that it will shift your body's concentration of hydrogen. But here's what happens when you drink alkaline water: when it reaches the stomach, it's neutralized by highly acidic hydrochloric acid. The body adjusts the pH level of what you consume, rendering the alkaline water's benefits moot. In fact, your digestive system uses buffers to maintain an acid-base balance, and your blood pH stays tightly regulated between 7.35 and 7.45.

Fortunately, alkaline products don't change the pH of your blood, as even slight alterations could lead to severe medical conditions or death. While there's no reason to fear alkaline water, there's also no evidence it offers any real benefit.

So, when it comes to an alkaline diet, the notion that basing your food choices on their pH can improve health, has no scientific backing.[19,20,21] Like many fad diets, it wastes time and energy, and in extreme cases, it can be harmful. In 2015, a San Diego jury awarded $105 million to a cancer patient who, based on the advice of the diet's creator, opted against chemotherapy in favor of an alkaline-based treatment, which allowed the cancer to progress to stage IV.[22]

AUTOIMMUNE PROTOCOL (AIP)

The Autoimmune Protocol (AIP) diet has gained popularity for a good reason: people with autoimmune diseases constantly struggle with their health and want relief. The diet avoids typical culprits like alcohol, sugar, oils, coffee, and processed foods, but it also eliminates grains, legumes, dairy, eggs, and nightshade vegetables during its elimination phase, with the possibility of reintroducing them later.[23]

The drawback of this diet is that it offers a one-size-fits-all approach, suggesting benefits for nearly 80 different autoimmune diseases, which is far too broad.[24] Autoimmune conditions vary greatly, and applying a generalized diet to all of them ignores the unique nutritional needs of individuals. Additionally, the AIP diet's blanket restrictions, especially for legumes, dairy, and whole grains, are arbitrary and contradict evidence that shows these foods can actually benefit certain autoimmune conditions, such as multiple sclerosis.[25]

Working with a nutrition professional to identify problematic foods can be helpful. But the highly restrictive AIP diet often leads to confusion and unnecessary fear around health-promoting foods. It may even result in undereating, fatigue, and worsened autoimmune symptoms because the temporary relief some experience from AIP diets is often due to cutting out ultra-processed foods and additives that can aggravate symptoms.

Diets like the AIP diet or another trendy option like the carnivore diet aim to eliminate a large range of foods, but this can actually backfire as it almost serves the purpose of an antibiotic, starving off both good and bad gut microbes.

There are much healthier ways to shift your gut microbiome and keep the healthy bacteria that do not sacrifice the diversity of gut microbes or limit the intake of nutrient-rich food choices. Cutting out many foods at once can prevent you from identifying the true cause of your autoimmune flare-ups.

Ultimately, the AIP diet oversimplifies complex autoimmune conditions, and those with such issues need personalized, systematic dietary plans developed with the help of a qualified nutrition professional.

INTERMITTENT FASTING

Intermittent fasting is refraining from eating for a specific period. There are many variations: some people alternate days of eating with 24-hour fasting windows, while others stick to a daily fasting window of 12–16 hours. With so many methods, knowing which one might work best can be confusing. The basic idea behind fasting is that by skipping food intake for extended periods, your body will react in ways that are beneficial.

One of the main attractions of intermittent fasting is its potential for weight loss. In recent years, research on alternate-day fasting and time-restricted eating has shown notable weight reductions, along with improvements in cholesterol, blood sugar levels, and triglycerides.[26] This isn't surprising. After all, eating less will naturally lead to weight loss, which, in turn, can improve metabolic health. But what if you don't want to explore intermittent fasting? Will you miss out on these benefits?

As it turns out, well-controlled studies comparing intermittent fasting with regular calorie restriction (portion control) show no difference in weight loss or health outcomes.[27,28] Studies where participants ate the same amount of protein and calories, whether through fasting or just portion control, found no differences in cardiometabolic risk factors, blood lipids, fat loss, or autophagy.[29,30,31] This makes sense, because whether you eat in a 12-hour window or an 8-hour window, the energy balance is the same if the total food intake is the same. This is why fat burning isn't superior on a fasting diet. If you make up the energy difference during eating windows, you'll replace the energy burned during the fast, including the fat.

Drs. Krista Varady and Vanessa Oddo, nutrition researchers at the University of Illinois, emphasize that fasting diets work for weight loss because they help people eat less. "The popularity of time-restricted eating is likely due to its simplicity, as it doesn't require counting calories."[32] In essence, like any other diet, fasting works if it helps you control overeating habits. The real question is what method works best for you in the long run, as this consistency will have the greatest impact on your health.

BUT, AUTOPHAGY!

Autophagy, the process by which cells break down and recycle their components for maintenance and survival, is getting a lot of attention lately. This process is constantly happening in the body, and it increases when it is low on energy or under stress, such as during fasting. However, autophagy doesn't turn "on" or "off." It simply fluctuates between higher or lower levels.[33] Many things, including intense exercise, can increase autophagy, not just fasting.

So, should the goal be to maximize autophagy? Well, much like the immune system, more isn't always better. Autophagy needs to be balanced. Both too much and too little have been linked to health risks like tumor formation or cancer. The key is balance, which you achieve by eating enough (but not too much) and exercising regularly. Most people fast naturally while sleeping, providing enough time for maintenance processes.

In the end, fasting can be a useful tool for some people. If an eating window helps you control food intake, it's worth continuing. But the misconception about intermittent fasting is the belief that it's more powerful or offers unique benefits compared to other diet approaches.[34]

SUPPLEMENTS

The dietary supplement market in America is a monster. In total, the U.S. population spends over $50 billion collectively on vitamins and dietary supplements, which is almost 10% of the out-of-pocket healthcare spending fees.[35] The average supplement user in the U.S. spends between $40 and $70 per month on supplements. This conservatively amounts to over $500 per year and $30,000 over a lifetime.[36,37,38] With all of this spending, did you ever wonder if they actually do anything?

BIG PHARMA VS. BIG HERBA

A common theme among heavy supplement users is the desire to restore or optimize health using "natural" alternatives to pharmaceutical drugs. This stems from widespread frustration with the pharmaceutical industry, or "Big Pharma," known for its greed and influence, which has led

CHAPTER 1: PANACEA

Americans to spend twice as much on medications as people in other comparably affluent countries.[39] Many agree that a pill-dependent society feels like a dystopian concept, and while medications certainly have their place, many people try to avoid them, turning instead to supplements. But replacing medications with supplements isn't as ideal as it seems. In fact, most users are unaware that many popular supplement brands are owned by the same major corporations that produce pharmaceutical drugs.

WHO OWNS YOUR SUPPLEMENT?

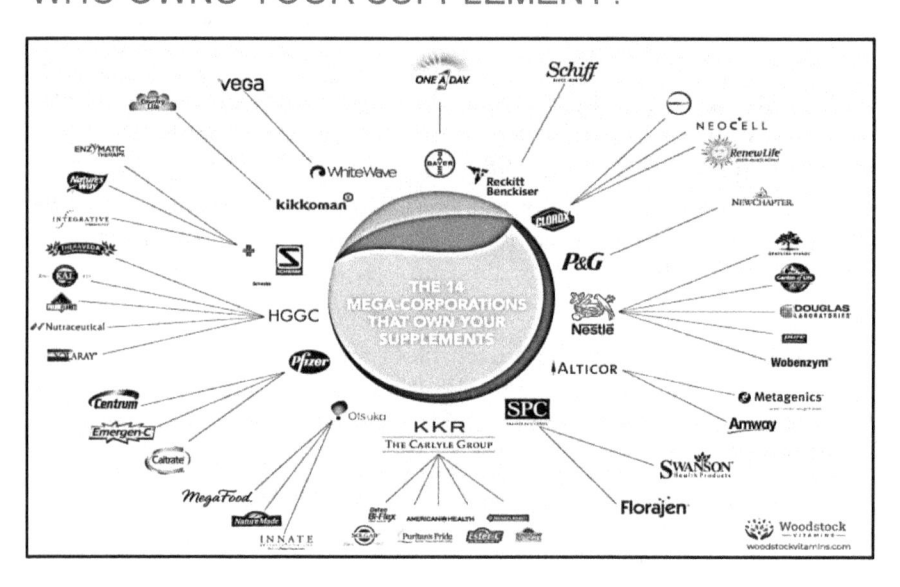

Even if you think your supplement is a "trustworthy" or "natural" choice, you might still be engaging with products that are far from a healthier alternative to pharmaceutical drugs. In reality, "Big Pharma" and what some now call "Big Herba" are more alike than people want to admit. In fact, many of the supplements you use are owned by these big companies you were trying to avoid. And while the global pharmaceutical industry is worth $1.6 trillion, the global wellness industry, which heavily includes nutrition supplements, is worth $5.6 trillion.[40,41,42] Though wellness involves more than just supplements, it's clear that the supplement industry, too, profits from the endless pursuit of better health. Both medications and supplements can be useful, but they should be approached with the same healthy skepticism.

24

HEALTHY SKEPTICISM

While supplements are often considered inherently good for health, there's reason to be much more skeptical. According to the "Natural Medicines Comprehensive Database," only about one-third of the 54,000+ dietary supplements on the market have any scientific backing for safety and effectiveness. Not only that, a significant number of supplement ingredients available in stores or online pose risks to the liver and kidneys, with 12% of studied supplements linked to safety concerns or quality problems.[43]

Believe it or not, many supplements don't even contain what's listed on the label at all. Bottles of Walmart-brand echinacea, for example, were found to contain none of the herbs, while GNC-brand St. John's Wort, sold as a depression remedy, contained rice, garlic, and even a tropical houseplant but no actual St. John's wort.

But it doesn't stop there. DNA testing of store-brand supplements found that 80% didn't contain advertised herbs but were packed with cheap fillers like rice or beans.[44] Third-party testing is crucial for ensuring supplement quality, but that doesn't mean you need to overspend. Just be aware of what you're getting and approach supplements with a dose of skepticism.[45]

REAL TOXINS

As previously mentioned, the body's natural detoxification systems work best when you avoid toxic exposure. Ironically, however, supplements can be a significant source of toxicity. In the U.S., 20% of cases of hepatotoxicity (liver damage) are related to herbal and dietary supplements, the main culprits being anabolic steroids, green tea extract, and multi-ingredient supplements.[46] Other potentially harmful herbal supplements include aloe vera, black cohosh, cascara, chaparral, comfrey, kava, and ephedra, which, depending on the dosage, can pose liver risks.[47]

Even vitamins and minerals can be toxic when taken at high doses. That's why it's important to understand the upper limits of each nutrient when taking supplements. Many products exceed these limits, especially fat-soluble vitamins like A and D, which can accumulate in tissues and become dangerous. Though supplements *are* regulated by the FDA (a common misconception), they are not typically reviewed *before* hitting the market, meaning you could be unwittingly consuming toxic substances.[48]

When you use supplements, you're often a guinea pig for big companies and their products that may not have undergone thorough testing. Although herbal options may pose the highest risk for toxicity, vitamin and mineral supplements can also be toxic at high doses. You may have seen nutrient percentages as high as 5,000% of the RDA on some bottles, which is likely concerning, especially for fat-soluble vitamins, as they can build up in tissues more easily. Despite this, many vitamins and minerals on the market unfortunately exceed these upper limits—ignoring the purpose of these regulations.[49]

MULTIVITAMINS

Multivitamins are one of the most popular supplements available because they can be a convenient means of covering nutrient gaps. Data shows that multivitamin users can often avoid common deficiencies, except for iron, calcium, and magnesium.[50] Multivitamins may benefit older adults, in particular, who often struggle with changing eating patterns and nutrient absorption. These older adults could improve their intake of folate, iodine, selenium, and vitamins B6, B12, and D through supplementation.[51]

Other groups, like pregnant women, children, or those with specific conditions that require extra micronutrients, can also benefit from taking multivitamins. However, while multivitamins can address deficiencies, large-scale studies show they don't reduce the risk of cancer, cardiovascular disease, or overall mortality.[52,53] Instead, they help fill nutrient gaps but don't significantly improve long-term health outcomes.[54]

Oftentimes, populations with sufficient and diverse food intake (who are often wealthier) are the ones that take these supplements but are the ones *least* in need of them, so using them will provide no meaningful benefit.

VITAMIN C

The daily recommended vitamin C intake for adults is just 75–90 mg, which you can get easily just by eating half a large red bell pepper.[55] Despite this, many supplements contain 1,000 mg or more of vitamin C. Yet, while vitamin C supplements are relatively harmless, they have a very low storage capacity in the body, making these mega-doses unnecessary. Since vitamin C is water-soluble, excess amounts are excreted by the body, which has led to the adoption of the term "expensive urine."

CHAPTER 1: PANACEA

As for vitamin C's role in common cold prevention, unfortunately for those who routinely catch the winter bug, the evidence is pretty weak. More than likely, it doesn't prevent or reduce the duration of colds, though it may benefit those under extreme physical stress or the elderly by easing respiratory symptoms.[56,57]

BOOSTING IMMUNITY?

A recent study of the 30 most-purchased immune-boosting supplements on Amazon found that 17 had inaccurate labels, 13 were misbranded, and nine contained unlisted ingredients.[58] Even if they were correctly labeled, the idea of "boosting" the immune system is flawed. Dr. Suzanne Cassel, an immunologist at Cedars-Sinai, explains, "You don't want your immune system to be stronger; you want it to be balanced... Too much of an immune response is just as bad as too little."[59]

Supplements marketed to "boost" immunity often have little to no effect anyway, and focusing on lifestyle habits like rest and nutrition will do far more for your immune health than any supplement can provide.

PROBIOTICS

Probiotics are beneficial microorganisms found in fermented foods and supplements, and they're often promoted for gut health. Fermented dairy products like kefir and yogurt can improve lactose malabsorption and aid in H. Pylori eradication.[60] However, while probiotics are often advertised as a cure-all for gut health solutions, they work best for specific conditions such as IBS, IBD, and C. Diff infections.[61,62]

In supplement form, probiotics are also poorly regulated, and doses are often far too low to impact the 40 trillion microbes in your gut. Even products with 100 billion bacteria amounts to only 0.25% of your gut microbiome, meaning they may not have lasting effects. Probiotic supplements often end up as "expensive poop."

But what about using probiotics after a course of antibiotics? While it's a great idea to try reducing long-term complications from antibiotics, more recent findings question the effectiveness of probiotics after taking antibiotics. Using probiotics after antibiotics is a common practice, but it may actually slow the recovery of native gut microbes.[63]

With fairly high rates of antibiotic usage in the U.S. and roughly 30%

of those prescriptions being unnecessary, it's important to know that probiotic supplements may not be your best bet for recovery.[64] To return to a healthy gut focus instead on eating *prebiotic* foods like garlic, onions, fruits, vegetables, and whole grains to support healthy bacteria. There are also some benefits from fermented foods with active cultures, like yogurt with Lactobacillus, Bifidobacterium, and Saccharomyces, which can also be beneficial for certain conditions.[65]

Even though we all have very distinct microbial populations in our intestinal tract, generic probiotic products are being promoted as positive for everyone, but this is often not the case.

IV DRIPS

IV therapy was once reserved for critical hospital care; now, it has become a concerning health trend. While IVs are essential for patients with severe hydration or absorption issues, they're now marketed as a quick fix for nutrition. In some cases, people even skip meals in favor of IV therapy, which is both unsafe and unnecessary.

Recently, a Texas mother of four died after receiving IV therapy that included a TPN electrolyte solution, which requires a prescription and is known to cause complications.[66,67] In another case, influencer Bea Amma contracted a bacterial infection from IV therapy, leading to festering skin lesions, millions in medical debt, and lifelong health complications.[68] Although an IV spa seemed like a harmless treatment, Bea had to deal with this new infection that caused her body to literally eat itself alive.

Unless medically necessary, IV therapy is risky and should not be used as a substitute for food-based nutrition.

LACTATION COOKIES

Having embarked on fatherhood recently, my exposure to pregnancy, infant, and toddler nutrition has increased dramatically. It's a really intriguing area of nutrition, but it can also come with a lot of misconceptions and frustrations for those involved.

One product that I find particularly misleading is lactation cookies, marketed to boost milk supply. However, a recent trial with 176 breastfeeding mothers found that foods containing galactagogues, ingredients believed to enhance milk production, had no effect on milk production, perceived insufficient milk, or breastfeeding confidence.[69] Lactation cookies often just deliver false hope then to a vulnerable population, leading to unnecessary purchases.

MEASURING UP

There are many tools used to measure our nutrition efforts, but the accuracy of these methods is often overstated or, in some cases, downright misleading.

CALORIE COUNTING

Did you know the FDA allows nutrition labels to be up to 20% inaccurate?[70] This means if a label shows 100 calories, it could actually contain anywhere from 80 to 120 calories. It's also more common for labels to under-report calories than overestimate them. While calorie counting and label reading can provide general guidance, tracking calories is not always precise.

Food tracking apps add another layer of inconsistency because they rely on different databases for nutrient and calorie analysis, making it difficult to get accurate information. Not only that, but fitness apps designed to track calories burned during workouts are notoriously inaccurate. One study found these apps were off by as much as 93%.[71,72]

For example, those who eat almond butter absorb more calories than those who eat whole or chopped almonds.[73] Blending foods, like smoothies, can also change how the body responds by providing an easier and faster intake of calories and a lower level of satiety. When you skip chewing—a critical fullness cue for the brain—it may lead to faster eating and delayed fullness. Additionally, blending food reduces the energy your body would otherwise expend breaking down the food itself, a process known as the "thermic effect of food." While these effects are marginal, how you prepare and consume food can add up in a way that influences total energy balance.

For some, calorie tracking provides motivation and structure, helping them make better food choices. But for others, it can become a frustrating and unhealthy habit, leading to negative physical and mental health outcomes. Either way, you should not rely solely on calorie counting, as it can detach you from your body's natural hunger cues. Long-term weight changes are dictated by total energy balance, but tracking calories can lead to disordered eating that neglects other healthy habits.

CHAPTER 1: PANACEA

FOOD SENSITIVITY TESTS

Generic food sensitivity tests, especially those you can buy online, will not solve your nutrition problems either. Most of these tests measure IgG antibodies, which indicate *general food exposure*, not a true sensitivity. Essentially, the foods labeled as "sensitivities" are just those you eat regularly. Cutting out foods you enjoy can lead to unnecessary dietary restrictions without solving the real issue.

To better understand food sensitivity, it's important to distinguish it from a food *allergy* or food *intolerance*:

Food Allergy – An immune response where the body abnormally reacts to a food protein, typically through IgE antibodies. Common examples include peanut or egg allergies, which should be strictly avoided.

Food Intolerance – Not immune-mediated, food intolerance arises from improper digestion (e.g., lactose intolerance due to a lack of lactase enzyme) or other factors like IBS.

Food Sensitivity – A less defined and often confused term with the above categories. Sensitivities may present as stomach pain or other negative symptoms but without the immune response or digestive issues seen in allergies or intolerances.

While it is helpful to know these differences, it is not helpful to use an IgG test for any of these as they do not accurately detect food sensitivities, allergies, or intolerances. According to the European Academy of Allergy and Clinical Immunology, these tests are "irrelevant" for food-related complaints and shouldn't be used for diagnosis.[74]

In fact, every major allergy organization worldwide agrees that IgG-based tests are ineffective for diagnosing food allergies.[75] So the next time you see an ad for a food sensitivity test you can take at home, just realize it will not provide you with the information you hope for.

NO SENSITIVITY ON VACATION?

Many at-home food sensitivity tests are not useful for diagnosing allergies or sensitivities, but problematic reactions to certain foods are still real and seem to be very common. The problem with these sensitivity tests is that they often instill a "food-fearing" mindset, which can lead to an unhealthy relationship with food. This fear can result in unnecessary dietary restrictions and a mental association between specific foods and negative symptoms, and this restrictive mindset often fades when we go on vacation.

Interestingly, many people I work with notice that these reactions often disappear while traveling to another location or country. Some attribute this change to higher-quality food, but I think a shift in mindset and lifestyle likely plays a much bigger role.

A common example is people who are sensitive to bread when they're in the U.S. but not when they eat it in Europe. Some think the difference is due to strains of wheat unique to the U.S., but the European Union (EU) imports about 1.1 million tons of wheat from the U.S. each year.[76] So, if you've eaten grain products in Europe, you likely consumed the same wheat as in the U.S. The difference, then, is often psychological—less fear and restriction, leading to better physical outcomes.

When people travel, they also tend to walk more, stress less, and engage in mindful eating practices. These lifestyle changes can promote better digestion and overall well-being. *How* we eat, and the way we perceive food is just as important as *what* we eat. A relaxed mindset may improve gastrointestinal issues without needing expensive, unproven tests.[77]

CONTINUOUS GLUCOSE MONITORS

Continuous glucose monitors (CGMs) have become popular outside their intended use for diabetics, offering real-time data that can help with decision-making. But do these devices override your natural ability to recognize hunger and health cues?

CGMs measure blood sugar levels, which is critical for those with diabetes, as their bodies don't regulate blood sugar effectively. However, for non-diabetics, short-term fluctuations in blood sugar are normal and are not a cause for concern. A 2020 study on healthy individuals found that different CGM brands produced drastically different readings, leading researchers to warn that CGMs might lead to "poor dietary choices" based on misleading data.[78]

The fear of brief blood sugar spikes has become a persistent myth, but as long as blood sugar normalizes within two hours after a meal, your body responds well to insulin.[79] Yet, people now use CGMs to scrutinize their blood sugar within minutes of eating, causing them to fear natural glucose responses to healthy foods like fruits.

For example, one cup of grapes has more sugar than three Oreos, which could cause a higher blood sugar spike. That doesn't mean Oreos are healthier than grapes, which are rich in polyphenols that lower cardiovascular risk.[80, 81, 82, 83] You honestly shouldn't need a CGM to tell you which of those items was healthier on a regular basis. But if you focus solely on glucose levels, like some well-known influencers do, you can absolutely distort your understanding of nutrition.

While some argue that glucose spikes increase hunger, research shows that even high doses of glucose don't impact appetite or fullness.[84,85] Similarly, weight loss is not hindered by glucose spikes. One fitness trainer proved this as he lost 12 pounds in 30 days while following a diet that spiked his blood sugar.[86] Ultimately, energy balance, not glucose fluctuations, dictates weight outcomes.

To promote insulin sensitivity and healthy glucose levels, prioritize regular exercise, especially resistance training, and limit hypercaloric foods. High-calorie intake over time can impair your cells' response to insulin, which can increase the risk of type 2 diabetes.

If you're looking for a better solution, getting regular A1c tests would be a far more reliable measure of long-term insulin sensitivity than a CGM. Rather than fearing short-term glucose spikes, remember they're a normal part of your body's energy regulation. The goal should be long-term blood sugar balance, not short-term worrying.

GUT TESTING

For those experiencing gut issues, it's tempting to turn to gut health tests to find a solution. While gut microbiota composition is crucial to health, many gut tests on the market are not validated and could even be considered scams that take advantage of those looking for actual support. While the basics of good gut health are known, there are a lot of unknowns at this point, so rest assured, anyone claiming to know everything about the gut is probably lying. Even the world's best experts have yet to decipher what a healthy gut microbiome resembles in detail.[87,88] Something that is well established is the fact that an unhealthy gut has low microbe diversity, providing yet another reason why you should ignore restrictive diets. Stool analysis, commonly used for these tests, doesn't provide a full picture of your gut microbiome either, as it only shows what's excreted, not what's inside.[89,90]

As with other nutrition trends, gut testing is more about profit than health improvement. Plus, even if the gut health tests, like GI maps, were accurate, you would need to know your own personal microbial baseline from previous years. Because without a personalized baseline for your gut microbiome, these tests are meaningless.

Many companies claim their results are tailored, but when everyone gets the same advice, it's the opposite of personalized care. Like other health fads, gut testing often sells confidence with little or no actual evidence, leaving consumers unaware of its limitations.

WHERE DID THIS NONSENSE COME FROM?

Knowing *which* nutrition fads fall short is certainly helpful, but knowing *why* they continue to trick us is even more beneficial, as it sets you up to recognize a false promise for yourself in the future. That's why at the end of each chapter I lay out just a few of the social and psychological biases that prevent us from making more rational health choices. So why exactly do we keep falling for these nutritional panaceas?

THE PLACEBO EFFECT

The placebo effect is a fascinating phenomenon that often leads people to mistakenly attribute real therapeutic value to ineffective treatments. It's one of the key reasons why people sometimes fall prey to nutrition myths and pseudoscientific claims.

So, what is the placebo effect? The placebo effect is when a person experiences a beneficial effect after taking medicine or a supplement that does not have a therapeutic benefit and therefore this benefit was a result of their belief in that treatment. Because of this, many assume that if a treatment is based on the placebo effect, it must be ineffective, but the truth is more nuanced. The placebo effect actually does exert *significant* and *tangible* benefits on both the brain and body, but these are driven purely by the power of belief and perception, not due to underlying mechanisms from the specific intervention in question.

See, when it's believed a treatment will work, your brain can actually initiate physiological changes that mimic the expected benefits. For instance, taking a placebo pill can release endorphins, the body's natural painkillers, and even alter neurotransmitter levels, affecting mood and pain perception. This ability of the mind to influence the body's chemistry is a testament to the power of belief.

A great example of the placebo effect comes from a classic golf study, where one group of players were told that they were using a "lucky" ball. Those who believed they had a special advantage performed significantly better than those who didn't, even though the balls were identical. This boost in performance was purely psychological, a result of their belief in the power of the "lucky" ball."[91] This is why nutrition interventions, like juice cleanses, supplements, and fad diets, have such a stranglehold on us all. They don't just offer some minor benefits; they can actually improve mental and physical health, which validates people's belief in them even more. The placebo effect, while powerful, is not the ultimate panacea you may be hoping for, however.

The placebo effect, while powerful, is not the ultimate panacea you may be hoping for, however as it does have significant downsides. These include:

1. **Temporary Nature** – The placebo effect tends to diminish over time. Initially, the belief in a treatment's efficacy can produce noticeable improvements, but as the novelty fades or as symptoms persist, the effect often wanes. This makes it unreliable for chronic conditions or long-term health management.

2. **Lack of Consistency** – The placebo effect is unpredictable. Unlike genuine health interventions such as balanced nutrition or regular exercise, which have consistent and well-documented effects on the body, the placebo effect varies from person to person and situation to situation. This makes it an unreliable basis for making health decisions.

3. **No Actual Cure** – While the placebo effect can alleviate symptoms, it does not address the underlying cause of a health issue. For example, a placebo might temporarily reduce physical pain, but it won't heal a broken bone or treat an infection. Therefore, relying on placebos instead of proven medical treatments can lead to delayed care and worsening of conditions.

4. **Ethical Concerns** – The use of placebos raises ethical issues, especially when patients are misled into believing they are receiving an effective treatment. This can reduce trust in healthcare providers and evoke broader skepticism about medical science.

5. **Dependence on Belief** – The placebo effect relies heavily on the patient's belief in the treatment. If a person is skeptical or discovers that the treatment is not based on scientific evidence, the placebo effect can be nullified entirely. In contrast, real treatments work regardless of whether the patient believes in them or not.

MAGIC TRICKS

The marketers behind the juice cleanse and detox efforts discussed earlier often publicize fake results as reassurance that they are worthwhile. But here's the thing: these results are more like a magic trick—they're a manipulative way of making you think your health is improving.

CHAPTER 1: PANACEA

PARASITES

One example of deceptive detox practice is when products are marketed as "detoxifying foot pads." These foot pads do nothing to pull toxins from your body. Instead, you just think they did because the "detoxifying foot pads" contain a chemical that turns black when it comes into contact with sweat. Naturally, you think that the black residues on the pad are toxins when, in reality, you just have sweaty feet.

A common nutrition detox method is using colon cleanse tablets that contain substances that bind to your stool and change the consistency of your poop so that you end up seeing long, gray ropes in the toilet, intended to look like parasites. They are actually just harmless polymers.[92]

Other products that claim to help remove parasites and worms actually just shed fragments of mucous membrane from your gut lining that resemble worms.[93] These results may look very convincing, but it's just a trick to make you think your body is constantly filled with parasites, worms, and toxins to get you to buy more stuff.

FATIGUE AND WEIGHT LOSS

A lot of these protocols will point to low energy levels as a necessary part of the detox process. But the truth is that fatigue isn't part of getting healthier; it's just a negative side effect of an improper diet that consists exclusively of fruit and vegetable juices. The same goes for weight loss claims. Losing weight does not always equate to better health. It depends on the person and how they are losing weight.

A byproduct of extreme weight loss may be missing necessary nutrients, which is counterproductive to your body's innate detoxification efforts. Plus, these cleansing diets are often associated with rebounding weight gain in the future, which is a negative and undesirable outcome for long-term health goals.[94,95]

THE RESET MYTH

So many people are looking for ways to "reset" their body or their gut in the hopes that they can start over and wipe the slate clean. But these juices, powders, and pills can't reset your body. You really can't reset something like your gut unless you use antibiotics, which can have negative consequences for long-term gut health.[96,97] Any other proposed way of "resetting" the gut is either inaccurate or potentially damaging to future microbiota status. So, trying to reset your body is not even a smart goal. Instead, you should aim to shift your gut microbiome health with good food choices, not band-aid detoxes.

BATHROOM BINGE

Finally, please do not mistake your juice cleanse-induced diarrhea for a detox. Some protocols include actual laxatives, while others will just create a laxative effect thanks to the change in diet. In either case, by going to the bathroom more, you are not removing more toxins; you are just limiting nutrient absorption potential while also passing a lot of water. That can lead to dehydration, malnutrition, and electrolyte imbalances. Even temporary acute cases can be bad for the gut microbiome.[98]

AMBIGUOUS LANGUAGE

The overly generic phrases I often see with juice cleanses, like "boosting metabolism," "optimizing health," or "removing toxins," are a sneaky way of pretending to provide benefits. Of course, detox plans never actually specify *which* toxins they are removing because if they did, we could just run a blood test before and after to see if these toxins were removed. By quantifying the results, the efficacy of these detoxes could be disproved. But this is exactly why you'll see a lot of vague terminology used—to make sure you don't find out the truth about the sham nature of these products and protocols.

This terrible tactic allows any person or business to profit from your inexperience with the human body. And when they don't provide an actual explanation of how it all might work, you are left with the mysterious claims that it can cure every one of your health issues. It's this mysteriousness that draws people in too. Robyn A. Osborn, RD, Ph.D. points out that many nutrition scams work because "people are very much intrigued by those things that seem to demystify the whole thing, whether it's some magic hormone, or there's something in your blood type, or you have to eat certain foods together because of how they're metabolized."[99]

Instead of realizing there's a deficit in our health habits that requires putting in work or seeking out professional guidance, many of us are so drawn to the thrilling and puzzling nature of the quick-fix detox that can rescue us instead.

SUNK COST FALLACY

The sunk cost fallacy is a mental habit that compels people to keep investing in a particular course of action because they have already committed significant time, money, or effort to it. They do this to avoid feeling like their past investment was wasted, leading people to persist with decisions that may no longer be rational. After spending considerable money and time on these misguided nutrition interventions, we often feel pressured to continue, hoping that the next purchase will finally deliver the promised results. This emotional investment makes us overlook the reality that these products may not be effective, and we might be throwing away good money for bad products. Yet, rather than acknowledging the losses and moving on, the sunk cost fallacy keeps us trapped in a cycle of spending, driven by the hope that our past investments will eventually pay off. It's this cycle that prevents us from recognizing the extent of our losses and the false promises that led us into the situation. To overcome this fallacy, take a step back and rationally consider your situation from an outsider's perspective. This mindful perspective is exactly what this book is here to offer—a new path forward so that you can avoid falling for these health traps.

REGRESSION TO THE MEAN

The phrase "time is a great healer" captures the natural tendency of many health conditions to improve over time, often leading people to mistakenly credit their recovery to the latest diet or wellness trend they've tried. This misunderstanding is rooted in a concept known as "regression to the mean," which refers to the statistical principle that extreme conditions or outcomes are likely to return to a more average state over time. For example, if you experience a particularly bad bout of fatigue or severe acne, these symptoms will likely lessen over time, even without direct intervention. However, suppose you coincidentally begin a juice cleanse, extreme diet, or probiotic during this period. In that case, you might mistakenly believe that these were responsible for your clean skin or increase in energy when, in fact, it was just a natural return to baseline health. This is a regression to the mean at work.

Fluctuations, whether in health or other areas, often normalize over time. This can lead people to misattribute improvements to actions that may not have had a significant impact.

SELECTION BIAS

There are different types of selection bias, and three of them seem to play a big role in our misconceptions about cure-all nutrition interventions.

NON-RESPONSE BIAS

Non-response bias occurs when only a small, vocal minority of participants share their experiences. This creates a skewed perception of success. Imagine 1,000 people trying a juice detox. If only 25 of them experience positive results, those 25 are far more likely to share their success stories, whether through social media, testimonials, or word of mouth. On the other hand, the other 975 people, who saw no benefit or felt disappointed in the results, might stay silent, either out of shame, indifference, or simply because they have nothing positive to report. This selective reporting can lead people to believe that the detox is far more effective than it actually is. Why? Because the majority of neutral or negative experiences are ignored, it gives a distorted view of its true efficacy.

VOLUNTEER BIAS

Volunteer bias occurs when the people who choose to participate in a study or take a particular action are considered inherently different from those who do not. For example, people who decide to take supplements are often already invested in their health. They may exercise regularly, eat a balanced diet, and be more proactive about their well-being. This is similar to the "healthy-user bias," where the act of taking supplements is more common among those who are already leading healthy lifestyles. As a result, studies that overlook this bias might overestimate the benefits of supplements, mistakenly attributing the supplements to positive health outcomes instead of recognizing that the overall healthy behaviors of the participants are the real cause.[100] In reality, those who might benefit most from supplements, such as those with poor diets or limited access to nutritious food, are the ones least likely to use them.

SURVIVORSHIP BIAS

Survivorship bias occurs when the focus is on only those who have succeeded in a particular endeavor while ignoring those who failed or dropped out along the way.

Consider a study where 100 participants are asked to follow an extremely restrictive diet. If 80 of them drop out because the diet is too difficult to maintain, the remaining 20 may complete the study, with 10 reporting positive outcomes. On the surface, it may seem like the diet has a 50% success rate. But this is only because it ignores the 80 participants who couldn't stick with the program, most of whom likely experienced no benefit or even negative effects. As a result, the diet's true effectiveness is vastly overstated. This bias also manifests in anecdotal evidence, where only those who successfully complete extreme diet challenges tend to share their stories, leading to a skewed presentation of the diet's effectiveness. The reality is that the majority may not achieve the same results or even be able to complete the regimen.

HOW TO AVOID THE FALSE PANACEA

So, now that you understand the perils of the quick fix, to avoid any more wasted time and resources, you need to focus on tangible ways that you can avoid these psychological fallacies and implement better nutrition behaviors. In that case, here are some practical ways forward:

1. **Be More Skeptical of Cure-alls** — Move away from the belief that any diet, detox, protocol, supplement, or any other remedy can miraculously fix your health. Practicing a healthy dose of *skepticism* and forward thinking can help you avoid the pain of another failed diet or detox.

2. **Put Reliable Nutrition Habits First** — Take a food first approach to getting your micronutrients rather than relying on supplements. The use of supplements should be based on what can't be delivered with food first. Extra considerations should be given for ages and stages of life with increased needs, such as young children, pregnancy, older age, or if you have high activity levels or eating challenges. Also, remember, IV therapy is a life-saving intervention, not a spa day treatment.

3. **Ditch Detoxes and Diets** — Detoxes and cleanses won't clear toxins on their own. Instead, eating a range of fruits and vegetables can provide nutrition support that helps your body do its job, which includes detoxification. So instead of trying out a restrictive detox protocol from time to time, just consume colorful produce in the way you enjoy it most. This can have the effect of a permanent detox method. Fasting, keto, and many other diets can be great tools to use to control how much you eat but they are not magical or superior. For others, simply removing excess snacking throughout the day or improving portion control at mealtimes

with the help of more home cooking and the inclusion of more nutrient-dense foods can help.

4. **Empower Yourself** — Whether it's supplements, cleanses, fad diets, lactation cookies, fasting, or anything else, you should not blame yourself for the clever marketing tactics used to reel people in. Instead, use it as an opportunity to practice *critical thinking* as it takes time to learn about your body and to separate fact from fiction. And while many factors are to blame, there's always some responsibility that we have ourselves to put in consistent effort. Progress should be the ultimate goal, not perfection.

5. **Understand There are No Shortcuts** — Eating more fruits and vegetables over a lifetime without restrictive cleanses is a more holistic model of health. Engaging in consistent, boring behaviors may be far less appealing, but avoiding these will only delay progress. Instead of randomly throwing probiotics into your system, most people are better off eating foods containing prebiotics and initiating other good gut habits like stress management and exercise that create a lovely home for beneficial bacteria.

Understanding how to avoid quick fixes is just the first step—next, we'll explore the myths surrounding the origins of human nutrition to uncover how misconceptions about our dietary past continue to influence modern health trends.

CHAPTER 2: ORIGINS

"We can learn from history, but we can also deceive ourselves when we selectively take evidence from the past to justify what we have already made up our minds to do."

— **Margaret MacMillan**

It's undeniable that we are currently bombarded with a wide array of health trends. One of these movements that has surged to prominence is the "ancestral lifestyle." This approach to living is most recognizable through the paleo diet. Its principles are based on the assertion that eating like our ancient ancestors can optimize your health as it aligns best with your genetics. This compelling premise has spurred many to adopt ancestral nutrition as a guiding ethos, promising profound insights into modern-day wellness. With such a growing cultural fascination it has created a global paleo food market that is currently valued at a staggering $11.2 billion.[1] But is this massive investment worth the hype?

This chapter explores the origins of human nutrition, with a focus on the foundational tenets of the paleo diet, as it can reveal much more about a wellness lifestyle that values the ideals of ancient living. The most enlightening revelation will be centered around the paleo diet's misguided assumptions and obvious flaws. We will also continue to discover just how many different faces diet culture can take on.

WHAT DOES PALEO EVEN MEAN?

Whether you're a dedicated follower of the paleo diet or just beginning to explore this popular trend, let's break down the basics. The term "paleo" is short for "paleolithic," referring to a period in history that began roughly 2.5 million years ago, marked by the invention of stone tools and humanity's earliest technological leap. During this era, our ancestors were nomadic hunter-gatherers, relying on hunting, fishing, and foraging for food. This way of life persisted until around 10,000 BC, when the advent of agriculture enabled the formation of settled communities.[2] Although the paleolithic era ended approximately 12,000 years ago, interest in the "paleo" lifestyle and dietary habits remains remarkably strong today.

At the core of the paleo diet is the belief that the human body has not fully adapted to the rapid changes in modern food production and consumption, which has led to the rise of chronic diseases. In particular, the Western diet's shift from home-cooked meals to processed, fast food is considered a major contributor to health issues. To counteract these problems, paleo advocates suggest returning to a diet similar to that of our ancient ancestors, which they believe can help combat modern health challenges. This approach resonates with many people who are seeking solutions to their struggles with nutrition and health in the 21st century.

So, where did the modern paleo diet originate? The idea of a "caveman" diet first gained traction with gastroenterologist Walter L. Voegtlin's 1975 book, *The Stone Age Diet*. Voegtlin advocated for a meat-heavy diet, with limited vegetables and starchy foods, arguing that early humans were primarily meat-eaters until agriculture reshaped their diets around 12,000 years ago.[3]

While Voegtlin's ideas sparked interest, the paleo movement truly surged in popularity with the release of Loren Cordain's *The Paleo Diet* in 2002.[4] Cordain, who holds a Ph.D. in physical education, is considered the driving force behind the modern paleo movement. He not only coined the term "Paleo Diet" but also established the dietary guidelines that have become central to the community and created hope that these principles can ward off all modern chronic diseases.[5]

THE PALEO RULES

To understand the nutritional components of the paleo diet, let's review the guidelines provided by the official "Paleo Diet" website. Two of the key nutrition rules are:

1. "Enjoy nutrient-dense foods like vegetables, fruit, meat, fish, eggs, nuts, and certain oils."

2. "Avoid grains, legumes, dairy, added salt and sugar, and processed foods."[6]

At first glance, these rules look legitimate to the average consumer. But are they truly an accurate representation of what our paleo ancestors consumed? To answer that, let's explore the historical accuracy of these foods among hunter-gatherer cultures, beginning with those deemed "paleo-approved."

HUNTER

Let's start with the most obvious food source for any hunter-gatherer: meat. Paleo advocates often emphasize meat because it is relatively easy to substantiate as a food from the paleo era. Archaeological sites have revealed animal remains that show evidence of meat processing for consumption, indicating that it was indeed part of the paleo people's diet.[7] Eggs, likely tied to animal tracking and hunting, were also almost certainly consumed.

Paleo society wasn't just limited to consuming land animals. Coastal paleo communities would have made use of their environment and gathered shellfish and caught smaller fish.[4] Because of this, seafood falls into a crossover category between hunting and gathering. While both land and sea animals are emphasized in modern paleo circles, it's important to recognize that their actual role in the diet varied significantly depending on regional and seasonal availability. Unlike modern paleo dieters, who have access to these foods year-round, ancient populations' diets fluctuated with the seasons and geography.

Another subtle discrepancy in modern paleo diet advertising is the focus on fatty cuts of meat. Even Loren Cordain, who has led the paleo movement, acknowledged that it wasn't fatty cuts that our ancestors ate. They primarily consumed lean meat, as the animals of that era weren't raised in the controlled environments of farms. Meat, in general, was a highly prized resource.

GATHERER

When examining the accuracy of "gathered" foods in the paleo diet, there is little debate that nuts, olive oil, fresh vegetables, and fruits were staples.[8] Top paleontologists agree that these foods made significant contributions to the diets of paleolithic communities.[4]

However, a notable omission from the approved paleo list includes insects, seeds, flowers, root vegetables, and honey, all of which were likely integral to ancestral diets. Despite their abundance and nutritional value, these items are absent from the modern list, probably because they lack cultural appeal today. In other words, some foods simply aren't "cool" enough for contemporary paleo enthusiasts, so they get ignored. Despite these discrepancies, most of the foods on the official paleo-approved list appear to have solid historical justification.

THE PALEO BLACKLIST

Now, let's turn to the "blacklist," the foods that modern paleo promoters deem unacceptable. As with any fad diet, misconceptions abound. According to paleo guidelines, grains, legumes, dairy, added salt and sugar, and processed foods should all be avoided. Yet, this exclusion is based on questionable evidence and presents a rather inaccurate portrayal of the foods ancient people might have consumed.

LEGUMES

Let's begin with legumes, an intriguing food group that includes over 16,000 species.[9] Among these are many familiar varieties, such as:

- Peas
- Peanuts
- Broad Beans
- Chickpeas
- Lentils
- Soybeans
- Lima Beans

These species, and many more, have long been part of human diets, even if modern paleo proponents advise against them. It turns out that various types of legumes were almost certainly consumed by Paleolithic people on a regular basis, despite popular belief to the contrary. Pulses, the edible seeds from legume plants, were likely eaten as far back as 40,000 to 60,000 years ago.[10]

Evidence of legume consumption comes from the discovery of microfossils in the dental calculus of Neanderthal skeletons, which provides valuable insights into ancient dietary habits.[11] In addition to these microfossils, legumes were uncovered at Middle Paleolithic sites, such as the Kebara Cave on Mount Carmel in the Near East, where preserved plant remains from the legume (Papilionaceae) family were found among Neanderthal remains.[12]

But don't think these legumes weren't confined to a single region. In fact, they were a staple food in nearly every major civilization, both modern and pre-modern. Historical combinations like barley and lentils, corn and beans, and rice and soybeans have nourished people across the globe for thousands of years. Radiocarbon dating from the Shanidar archaeological site in Northern Iraq suggests that legumes, along with other plant matter, were part of the diet in this region at least 44,000 years ago,[11] and in Morocco, around 15,000 years ago, archaeobotanical remains indicate the consumption of acorns, pine nuts, and legumes.[13]

The domestication of legumes shows their importance and historical usage. Lentils, for instance, began to be domesticated around 11,000 BC.[14] Shortly thereafter, chickpeas received the same treatment around 10,000 BC in the Fertile Crescent.[15] The domestication of crops like these indicates that legumes had long been an essential part of the diet. After all, ancient people would have needed to cultivate these crops as a food source and to provide energy, even without understanding modern concepts like calories or health benefits. Given the overwhelming evidence of legume consumption during the paleolithic era, it seems illogical to reject this significant food group, which has sustained human populations for tens of thousands of years. The decision to avoid legumes in the modern paleo diet is, therefore, a questionable one, especially considering their historical importance to human nutrition.

GRAINS

Another food group on the modern paleo blacklist is grains. While staple grains such as wheat, barley, and ryegrass rose to prominence during the agricultural revolution (which directly followed the paleolithic era), evidence shows that humans were consuming grains long before this period.[4,16] For example, oats were likely ground into flour for meal preparation as far back as 30,000 BC in Italian regions.[17,18] Similarly, around 75,000 years ago in Western Asia, both topographical and fossil remnants suggest grains were part of people's diet.[19] In fact, the oldest known instance of grain consumption comes from starch granules discovered on stone tools, dating back 105,000 years. It's clear, therefore, that early humans relied on grass seeds and grains, such as sorghum, to meet their nutritional needs.[20]

Although many of the grains consumed during the Paleolithic period were wild, they were often eaten, similar to how we consume grains today. Wheat grains, for example, were ground into flour to make bread, while rice was steamed and eaten either hot or cold. Oats were mashed with water or other liquids to create a type of oatmeal, and barley was used to make one of the oldest known manufactured beverages: beer.[19] Despite the historical presence of grains in the diet, the paleo diet inaccurately labels grains as a modern dietary error, ignoring their significant role in prehistoric cultures' diets. These cultures not only consumed grains but also benefited from their nutritional value in ways similar to how we do today.[4,17,1]

DAIRY

Dairy is another food group excluded from the paleo diet, but this exclusion seems more grounded in historical accuracy. Human dairy consumption appears to have begun roughly 8,500 years ago, after the Paleolithic period ended.[21] While prehistoric humans likely didn't consume dairy products, the consumption of milk and other dairy products has been practiced for long enough to prompt significant evolutionary adaptations in certain populations, allowing them to benefit from dairy nutrition.

One of the primary reasons for excluding dairy is the prevalence of lactose intolerance. This occurs when someone does not produce enough lactase, the enzyme required to digest lactose or the sugar found in milk. Without enough lactase, undigested lactose ferments in the gut, leading to gas, bloating, and stomach cramps. It's estimated that up to 70% of the global population experiences some level of lactose intolerance.[22] However, even people without the lactase-producing gene can typically tolerate up to 12 grams of lactose (about one cup of milk) in a single sitting, and up to 24 grams across an entire day.[23] This is why about six billion people around the world are still able to consume milk or other dairy products regularly without side effects.[24]

So, how did certain populations develop the ability to digest lactose? It began during the spread of farming into Southeastern Europe; a genetic mutation arose that allowed people to continue producing lactase into adulthood, which gave them a survival advantage because of milk's nutritional benefits.[25] Over time, natural selection increased the prevalence of this mutation, especially throughout Northern Europe, where today, up to 90% of people can digest dairy without issue.

Interestingly, lactose tolerance isn't limited to European populations. Recent discoveries in Africa, particularly Kenya and Sudan, have revealed that humans there have been consuming milk and milk-based foods for at least 6,000 years. Milk-specific proteins found in dental calculus suggest these populations were consuming dairy long before they had the biological capacity to fully digest it.[26] This indicates that dairy played a crucial role in their diets, even before lactose tolerance had become widespread. While excluding dairy from a strict paleo diet might be a historically accurate choice, it shouldn't put off more modern-minded individuals from consuming dairy. After all, multiple cultures have successfully adapted to make dairy a key part of their nutrition.

SALT AND SUGAR

Now, let's look at both salt and sugar. These are two substances that are widely consumed today but definitely were not part of the Paleolithic diet in their isolated forms.

The earliest evidence of salt extraction dates back about 6,000 years. Communities in Romania and China began boiling naturally occurring salt water or collecting salt from evaporated salty spring water.[27,28]

A little later, in ancient Egypt, at around 2,000 BC, the use of salt in food preservation became particularly important.[29] This is because salt works by drawing out moisture from food, which prevents bacterial growth and helps preserve the food for longer. This technique was crucial before the invention of refrigeration. But during the Paleolithic era, early humans hadn't caught on to the idea, meaning they likely consumed far lower amounts of salt.

One area where paleolithic diets had an advantage over modern diets, however, was the higher ratio of potassium to sodium. This is a balance that is difficult to achieve in our food habits today.[30]

Sugar in its isolated form was not extracted from sugarcane until around 4,000 BC.[31] But even then, the manufacturing of cane sugar granules from sugarcane juices began about 2,000 years ago in India.

So, while sugar and the minerals that comprise salt (sodium and chloride) naturally occur in whole foods, the concentrated forms we consume today are relatively modern innovations. Avoiding these highly processed substances in the paleo diet makes sense, as they are not really reflective of what humans ate during the Paleolithic period. Not only that, but the much more recent and widespread use of refined salt and sugar is a departure from the dietary practices of our ancestors.

So overall, while the paleo diet aims to replicate the eating habits of our hunter-gatherer ancestors, it actually often overlooks or misrepresents the historical consumption of key food groups like legumes and grains. The exclusion of these foods, alongside the nuanced approach to dairy, salt, and sugar, demonstrates that modern interpretations of the paleo diet may not fully align with the true dietary patterns of the Paleolithic era.

PROCESSED FOODS

Now, for the most important yet tricky aspect of assessing paleo diets: processed foods. This *appears* to be straightforward, but part of the problem is getting the language right, as there is a lot of ambiguity in terminology.

Here's the issue—processing food is a very vague term that can include anything from home cooking to industrial transformation methods. In other words, there's a big difference between coring an apple and creating an apple-flavored pop tart. Here's why it matters: every type of processing can change the nutritional value of food, both positively and negatively, which is why more specific guidelines around food processing need to be set. This way, everyone can understand how to engage with them more appropriately. For example, a basic paleo principle was discovering the use of fire and stone tools, which allowed them to cook and process foods to increase their nutritional bioavailability. That means that, although processing food has always been a practice, the degree and manner in which people are exposed to processed foods now is drastically different. Because of this, we can recognize that the current use of processed foods is problematic and yet, processing can't just be eliminated altogether. So where should the line be drawn, then?

One helpful perspective on processed food comes to us from the NOVA classification system. First proposed in 2009 by a team of researchers from the University of São Paulo, Brazil,[32] their aim was to create a framework that reviews the extent and purpose of food processing. While this system is far from perfect when representing how nutritious each food really can be, it has been one of the few tools used to inform nutrition research and policy. NOVA classifies food into four groups based on their degree of processing. These are:

1. Unprocessed or minimally processed foods
2. Processed culinary ingredients
3. Processed foods
4. Ultra-processed foods [33]

Group 1 Unprocessed or Minimally Processed Foods	Group 2 Processed Culinary Ingredients	Group 3 Processed Foods	Group 4 Ultra-Processed Foods
Fresh, dry, or frozen vegetables or fruit, grains, legumes, meat, fish, eggs, nuts and seeds.	Plant oils (e.g., olive oil, coconut oil), animal fats (e.g., cream, butter, lard), maple syrup, sugar, honey, and salt.	Canned/pickled vegetables, meat, fish, or fruit, artisanal bread, cheese, salted meats, wine, beer, and cider.	Sugar sweetened beverages, sweet and savory packaged snacks, reconstituted meat products, pre-prepared frozen dishes, canned/instant soups, chicken nuggets, ice cream.
Processing includes removal of inedible/unwanted parts. Does not add substances to the original food.	Substances derived from Group 1 foods or from nature by processes including pressing, refining, grinding, milling, and drying.	Processing of foods from Group 1 or 2 with the addition of oil, salt, or sugar by means of canning, pickling, smoking, curing, or fermentation.	Formulations made from a series of processes including extraction and chemical modification. Includes very little intact Group 1 foods.

Increasing Level of Processing →

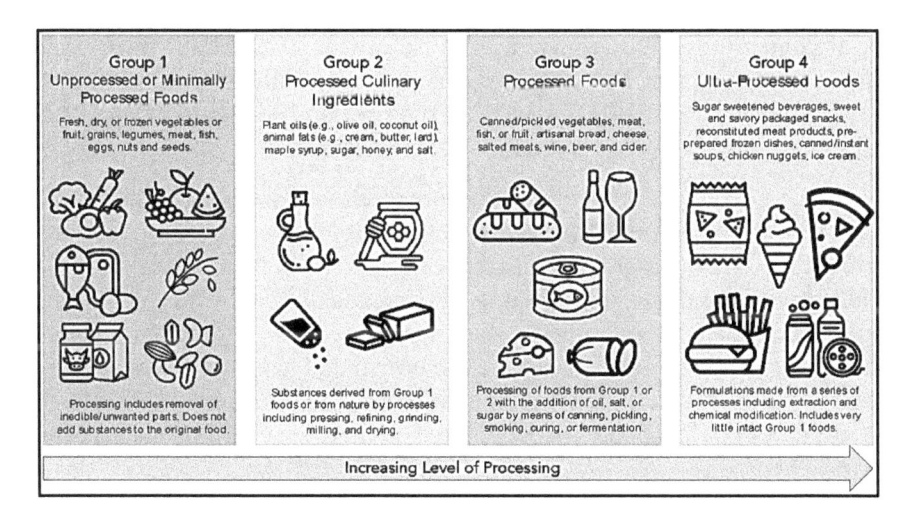

This graphic on processing is a good example that most people generally understand the importance of emphasizing foods on the far left (unprocessed) vs. those on the far right (ultra-processed). Group 1 is clearly the only match for the paleo diet, but it doesn't mean it's the only one that can provide nutritional value. This is where we need a better system for assessing food because many of these choices are actually out of place in terms of their effect on our health. Take protein isolate (the most basic form of protein powder), for example. It's in the same group as carbonated soft drinks, which you can imagine have very different implications for people's health. In fact, protein isolates have been shown to provide positive nutrition outcomes.[34,35]

Meanwhile, sugar-sweetened beverages are associated with a much higher risk of metabolic syndrome, type 2 Diabetes, and other chronic diseases.[36] But due to the degree to which they are transformed, both are considered ultra-processed food. So, while the NOVA degree of processing classification gives us a good starting point and general direction of understanding how healthy different processed foods can be, we really need a lot more specificity to understand how different processed foods affect our health.

A very useful way to evaluate the health benefits of processed food is to consider what has been *added* or *removed* from the original source. Concerning early human diets, most foods would have kept their natural nutritional components with very few additions. This is important for health because processed foods often contain non-nutrient compounds like antioxidants and polyphenols, as well as micronutrients, fiber, and protein.

CHAPTER 2: ORIGINS

Now, as food processing technologies advanced, many of these beneficial compounds were removed. Because of this, the overall nutritional quality was lowered. But as noted earlier, while isolated protein might have a positive health effect, removing the fiber and adding high levels of salt, sugar, and fat are often bad for people's health.

That's why, whether cooking at home or choosing store-bought products, it's helpful to prioritize nutrients that are often removed in modern processing, like fiber, protein, and omega-3 fats. At the same time, it's crucial to limit ingredients like added salt, sugar, and unhealthy fats. Although these aren't the only ingredients affected by processing, they are among the most significant that can reduce the nutritional value of foods. In this regard, the paleo diet's focus on reducing processed foods is beneficial, as ultra-processed foods have been linked to many nutrition-related diseases.[37,38]

It's crucial to remember, though, that no single food choice causes or prevents health problems. Instead, it's the cumulative effect of many choices over time that determines the quality of your overall health. While moderation is certainly possible, ultra-processed foods are designed to be hyperpalatable, making them easy to overconsume, and their high caloric density further contributes to this problem. And overconsumption can be one of the most difficult obstacles to maintaining a balanced diet. While indulgent foods can certainly be part of a healthy lifestyle, many people struggle to moderate their intake. This only leads to an unhealthy imbalance.

But to be clear, although food processing is having a largely problematic effect on our food environment, not all processed foods are harmful, and many can even help you meet nutrition goals specific to your own needs. By being mindful of how processing has altered the components of these foods, you can better understand what their positive or negative impact might be on your health.

PALEO PANCAKES?

Now that we've delved into the topic of processed foods, it's become clear that modern "paleo" products have reached a level of absurdity. While the paleo diet might be popular, many of the products marketed as "paleo" today are far from anything that our paleolithic ancestors would have eaten. Just consider the following examples of so-called paleo products I recently encountered:

- Paleo chocolate-covered almonds – (chocolate wasn't created until the 1900s)
- Paleo Mayonnaise – (mayonnaise first appeared in the 1700s)
- Paleo Pancake Mix – (pancakes were invented around 600 BC)
- Paleo Marshmallows – (marshmallows didn't exist until 2000 BC)

Clearly, none of these products were part of any ancestral diet, and our early ancestors certainly weren't engineering such concoctions. While that doesn't mean you can't enjoy these foods, it highlights how far the "paleo" trend has diverged from its intended principles. The marketing hype surrounding paleo products is often disconnected from the true values of the diet, creating inconsistencies and confusion. With all of these modern "paleo" products lining store shelves, it begs the question: what truly represents the eating patterns of paleolithic humans?

THE REAL PALEO DIET

One of the most valuable lessons that can be learned from paleolithic evidence is that there was not one *singular*, definitive paleo diet. There were actually *numerous* dietary patterns varying across time and geography. Just consider how difficult it would be to define a modern diet. Would you point to the typical diet in America or Japan? What about Greece, or perhaps India?

Even within countries like the U.S., dietary habits are very different between regions like California and Mississippi. If there's no singular "modern diet," why should it be expected that there was a single paleo diet?

As Leslie Aiello, president of the Wenner-Gren Foundation for Anthropological Research, said, "We didn't have just one caveman diet… the human diet goes back at least two million years. We had a lot of cavemen out there." Aiello and biological anthropologist William Leonard emphasize that the hallmark of being human wasn't the consumption of meat, but mankind's adaptability to thrive on a wide variety of foods across different habitats.[39]

Paleoanthropologist Daniel Lieberman agreed, referencing recent research conducted on 12 hunter-gatherer tribes from around the world. These tribes, all with substantial dietary data, showed incredible variation in their diets. As Lieberman puts it, "none of them match the paleo diet. Not a single one."[40] This suggests that the modern, more restrictive version of the paleo diet fails to reflect the diverse, adaptable diets of our ancestors.

But why did ancient humans have such variations in diet? It's because it was largely determined by *geography*. Evolutionary biologist Herman Pontzer believes that the ratio of plant to animal foods consumed depended heavily on climate and location.[41] After all, Paleo humans in warmer climates ate more plants, while those living in colder regions—above 50 degrees latitude—relied more heavily on animal products. In other words, geography dictated what food sources were available, and because of this, most societies likely consumed a balanced mix of plants and animals. This balanced diet helped early humans survive. But should we avoid certain food groups today because they no longer match our physiology? Did the transition from the paleo era to modern life alter our bodies to the point that we should now reject either plants or animals from our diets?

VEGAN VS. CARNIVORE

Despite popular claims in documentaries or blog posts, humans are not physiologically maladapted to consuming either plants or animals. In fact, our bodies possess numerous traits that demonstrate that we have an omnivorous nature. Let's work out how.

Cooking with fire and the use of stone tools were pivotal in human evolution, enabling significant changes in both brain size and digestive tract function. Early humans faced unpredictable climates and landscapes, which made securing enough energy (calories) challenging. Meat provided a dense source of calories and fat, helping early humans survive.[42] This shift also led to a shortening of the digestive tract, favoring the consumption of meat. But because humans originally relied on plants, our digestive system remains sufficiently long to process plant materials, including the fermentation of fiber in the large intestine. This fermentation is beneficial, as it supports a diverse gut microbiota, which contributes to positive health outcomes.[43]

Our teeth also illustrate our omnivorous nature. Molars, which are well-suited for grinding plant material, are complemented by incisors, which are effective for eating meat.[44] In addition, our salivary enzymes are adept at breaking down carbohydrates found in plant foods.

Taken together, these traits reveal that humans are well-equipped to consume both plants and animals, making us omnivores by design. This adaptability has been crucial to our survival as opportunistic feeders.

While individual choices about diet, whether for ethical, environmental, or health reasons, may lead some to focus more on plant-based or animal-based foods, it's clear that from a physiological standpoint, we are capable of consuming both.

STILL MANY GAPS IN KNOWLEDGE

While anthropological evidence has provided fascinating insights into the dietary patterns of paleolithic humans, much remains uncertain. Big gaps in our knowledge make it difficult to draw definitive conclusions about what the paleo diet really consisted of. As Marion Nestle, a molecular biologist and public health advocate, points out, "The diets of early humans are still circumstantial, incomplete, and debatable, and there is insufficient data to identify the composition of a genetically determined optimal diet."[45]

Part of the problem is that the Paleolithic era predates written records. So, in other words, there are no detailed diet recalls or health assessments from this time period, which makes it difficult to determine exactly what foods were consumed. According to Nestle, anthropologists can still work out, however, what diets once consisted of by looking at fossilized bones, teeth, shell mounds, tools, and the topography of archaeological sites. Not only that, but chemical analyses of bones, teeth, and plant remains, as well as rare samples of fecal remains and stomach contents, offer some direct evidence of ancient diets.[45]

These methods, along with comparisons to modern hunter-gatherer tribes give researchers a way to make general assumptions about paleolithic diets. But despite this, a lot of today's paleo diet guidelines are based on flawed or outdated data. For instance, early advocates of the paleo diet mistakenly leaned on the Ethnographic Atlas, an index of 20th-century ethnographic data, to figure out what early humans ate. The problem is that the atlas included societies that weren't exclusively hunter-gatherers or had already shifted to farming.[46]

So, while the concept of the paleo diet may seem appealing, bear in mind that it's based on incomplete and often inaccurate ideas of early human diets. One thing that's clear is that our ancestors ate a wide variety of foods, and modern dietary adaptations continue to shape what we can and should eat today.

CHAPTER 2: ORIGINS

WHERE DID THIS NONSENSE COME FROM?

While modern paleo diet guidelines aim to replicate the diet of our ancestors, they often rely on inaccurate anthropological records and biased assumptions. These issues, along with certain psychological fallacies, have contributed to the creation of paleo diet myths.

Below are some of the key reasons why the paleo diet, along with other fad diets, emerged and continue to be popular to this day.

REDUCTIONISM

Reductionism is a common mistake in nutrition. It's where complex health issues get oversimplified by blaming a single nutrient or food group for all health issues. The paleo community is no exception. Although, there's a tendency to zero in on specific compounds or nutrients to argue that certain foods aren't fit for humans. This kind of narrow thinking ignores the complexity of foods and the variety of nutrients they contain. Here are a few examples of the overly simplistic claims often made by paleo supporters.

Typical Paleo Claim #1: Legumes, grains, and dairy are not nutrient-dense food choices.[47,48,49]

The Reality:

- **Legumes** – In just one cup of peas, you'll find 7 grams of fiber, 8 grams of protein, 96% of your daily vitamin C needs, 11% of your daily iron, and 12% of your daily magnesium.[50]

- **Dairy** – One cup of milk contains 8 grams of protein, 25% of daily calcium needs, 50% of daily vitamin B12, and high amounts of vitamins A and D.[51]

- **Grains** – Half a cup of oats delivers 4 grams of fiber, 5 grams of protein, 27% of daily zinc needs, 28% of daily magnesium needs, and 31% of daily thiamin (vitamin B1) needs.[52] Furthermore, both legumes and grains contain diverse fibers that provide prebiotics, benefiting gut health.[53]

Typical Paleo Claim #2: Legumes and grains are unhealthy because they contain anti-nutrients.[48,49]

The Reality:

Legumes and grains do contain compounds referred to as "anti-nutrients" (phytates, lectins, and saponins), which can prevent some vitamins and minerals from being absorbed.[54] But these anti-nutrients don't entirely eliminate the benefits of the foods.

Research shows that the evidence behind these claims often comes from animal studies using high doses of these compounds, which don't accurately reflect human experiences.[55]

Moreover, these so-called anti-nutrients also possess antioxidant, cholesterol-lowering, and anticancer properties that can contribute to long-term health benefits, which are conveniently not mentioned in paleo circles.[56] But instead of focusing on a reductionist view, a more holistic approach to nutrition looks at the actual results of what happens when you eat these food groups. The overwhelming majority of evidence reveals:

- Eating legumes, such as chickpeas, can help prevent and manage diabetes, cardiovascular disease, digestive issues, and certain cancers.[57,58]

- Oats can improve blood lipid profiles and lower cholesterol.[59,60]

- Whole grains can reduce systemic inflammation by lowering levels of inflammatory markers like hs-CRP and IL-6.[61]

- Whole grains also reduce the risk of diabetes, stroke, heart disease, colorectal cancer, and mortality from all causes.[62,63,64,65]

- Pulses, consumed at about one serving per day (½ cup), significantly reduce cardiometabolic risk factors such as HbA1c, LDL cholesterol, body weight, and blood pressure.[66]

Clearly, the nutritional benefits of grains and legumes far outweigh any potential drawbacks. So, instead of reducing food to isolated components, it's essential to consider the complete nutritional value when making food choices.

HALF-TRUTHS

Building on reductionism, the paleo diet ideals also suffer from the half-truth fallacy. This occurs when someone presents only part of the evidence to support their ideas, omitting key details that provide a fuller picture.[67] Paleo advocates often focus on the potential downsides of grains and legumes but ignore their well-documented benefits. Similarly, they tend to skip over the potential health risks of paleo-approved foods.

What about red meat and eggs? Well, paleo-approved foods like red meat and eggs are high in choline, which can lead to the production of trimethylamine N-oxide (TMAO) in the gut. Elevated TMAO levels have been linked to an increased risk of cardiovascular disease in multiple studies.[68,69,70] But banning these foods outright would be an overreaction. Both meat and eggs offer valuable nutritional benefits, and their inclusion in a balanced diet can be beneficial. So, instead of falling for the half-truths that underpin paleo ideology, consider the complete picture and understand that no food is wholly good or bad.

STRAW MAN FALLACY

The *straw man fallacy* occurs when someone distorts an argument to make it easier to attack. In the context of debating nutrition principles, this fallacy is often employed to justify the paleo diet.

Let's take a look at a couple of examples.

Typical Paleo Claim #3: Dairy is inflammatory and bad for bone health.[47]

The Reality:

While some people, such as those with milk allergies, may experience inflammation from dairy, that doesn't mean dairy is inherently bad for everyone. Take, for example, a systematic review of 16 studies involving both healthy and metabolically abnormal participants that found no inflammatory effects from dairy consumption. In fact, a reduction in inflammation was even observed in some cases.[71]

Similarly, the claim that dairy is harmful to bone health is misguided. Dairy provides calcium, vitamin D, phosphorus, and protein, all of which support bone formation. Bone health depends on a range of dietary and lifestyle factors, including exercise. In fact, large studies have shown that consistent dairy intake lowers the risk of hip fractures and increases bone mineral density.[72,73,74,75] To claim that dairy is universally bad for bones or inflammatory ignores its numerous health benefits.

Typical Paleo Claim #4: Beans are toxic when eaten uncooked.[49]

The Reality:

Raw beans contain toxins like phytohaemagglutinin, which can cause gastroenteritis. Thankfully, people really don't eat raw beans.[76] Cooking beans for as little as 10 minutes deactivates these toxins. Even canned beans are cooked, rendering this argument irrelevant for modern consumers who only eat beans that have been cooked.

Typical Paleo Claim #5: Grains cannot provide enough nutrition on their own.

The Reality:

The official paleo website claims that "Trying to survive solely on grains is a losing proposition," but I don't know anyone who advocates for a grain-only diet.[48] This argument is irrelevant; no single food group provides optimal nutrition by itself. While the overreliance on grains during the agricultural revolution did cause malnutrition in some populations, today's well-rounded diets incorporate a wide variety of foods, including grains, to meet nutritional needs.[77] The real issue is not grain consumption but the widespread availability of ultra-processed grains lacking nutritional value. In their whole form, grains offer significant health benefits.

HAVE YOUR CAKE AND EAT IT, TOO

Paleo enthusiasts often overlook the value of modern technology while mixing foods from different regions, which would have been impossible for our ancestors. Archaeological scientist Christina Warriner highlights this contradiction when she assessed a paleo cookbook: "It looks like a delicious and nutritious breakfast, but a Paleolithic person wouldn't have had access to it. The blueberries are from New England, the avocados from Mexico, and the eggs from China. This would have never appeared on any Paleolithic plate."[78]

While we benefit from global food trade today, paleo guidelines tend to ignore this modern reality. Paleo advocates can't fully embrace both ancient eating habits and modern conveniences without contradicting the diet's original premise.

AMERICAN OBSESSION

The paleo diet seems particularly popular in the U.S., but it's impractical and nutritionally unsustainable for much of the world. Billions of people worldwide rely on foods like grains, legumes, and dairy for their daily sustenance, with many living longer and healthier lives.[79] From rice and beans to cheese and yogurt, these foods are staples in populations with some of the longest life expectancies on earth and the lowest rates of chronic diseases. If these foods were inherently harmful, widespread health issues would be expected in these populations. Yet, the opposite is true.

ROSY RETROSPECTION BIAS

Have you ever watched a movie that you loved as a child again as an adult but thought to yourself, "I remembered this being a lot better than it is." I believe if we were to travel back in time and be forced to survive on the conditions and dietary experiences of our paleo ancestors, we would be saying something very similar. Yet, many of us seem to hold onto this view that diets were somehow perfect back then. This idealistic perception of previous experiences or time periods is an example of the rosy retrospection bias. This probably happens because, in the present, we must engage with both positive and negative experiences. But when we think about the past, there's no need to confront the negative, as the emotions tied to them are gone. As a result, many of us view the past in an overly positive light.

It was often not very glamorous either. "Everybody thinks you wander out into the savanna, and there are antelopes everywhere, just waiting for you to bonk them on the head," said Paleoanthropologist Alison Brooks.[39] Truthfully, our ancestors often didn't get their first choice as they scavenged for less glamorous food sources—bugs, termites, insects, leaves, and tubers—while waiting for opportunities to catch meat. Harsh environments controlled their eating habits, making their diets less idyllic. Our ancestors, despite what you may have heard, were not perfectly suited to their environment, and their resulting diets were not perfect either. They faced significant health challenges, too, but they were just different from the ones we experience now. But this is something we need to realize. The world our ancestors lived in was very different from what we have today. We can't just map every ancestral habit and dietary choice over our lives now and expect it to fix all of our problems. Each time period and environment require unique solutions based on the specific challenges at hand.

CHAPTER 2: ORIGINS

Dr. Lee Goldman captures these distinctions along with a more realistic perspective of different time periods in a paper where he outlines three public health challenges across human history.[80] During the paleo period, for example, survival was more about avoiding starvation, disease, and violence. Optimal long-term nutrition wasn't the goal; survival was. And survival depended on managing starvation, infectious diseases, and even violence, so needless to say, the focus wasn't on perfect nutrition or superfoods or specific diet plans. Especially considering the average life expectancy was only about 33 years.

Three Global Public Health Encounters			
	First Encounter	Second Encounter	Third Encounter
Starting date	200 000 BCE	About 1850	Late 20th century
Era	Natural environment	Industrial era	Leisure era
No. of human generations	8000	7	3
Human life expectancy, y	33	43–65	> 80
Public health challenges	Basic survival	Pollution and man-made hazards	Genetic mismatch and indifference
Leading public health challenges	Infectious diseases; starvation; dehydration; maternal/fetal mortality; murder; accidents	Air pollution; sewage/water pollution; industrial toxins; smoking; motor vehicle accidents	Obesity; diabetes; hypertension; anxiety/depression/suicide; myocardial infarction/stroke; degenerative diseases
Solution(s)	Rising standard of living	Legislation/regulation	Modern medicine Legislation/regulation Behavior change

Now, as we currently live in what Goldman describes as the "third encounter," a surge in technology has improved our quality of life but has also introduced new challenges. In just 100 years, the average human lifespan has nearly doubled, thanks largely to sanitation and medical advancements that are now taken for granted. But this longer lifespan has come with new health concerns. Modern lifestyles have introduced many chronic diseases, including obesity, diabetes, and mental health challenges. In developed countries, food abundance is often in the form of highly processed foods. While it's easy to focus on the problems of overeating and unhealthy diets, it's important to remember that many people worldwide face the opposite issue: malnutrition and food insecurity. In fact, the ongoing challenge of providing sufficient nutrition to all is arguably the more pressing global health threat.

So, a major takeaway we should all learn about the reality of the past is this: although valuable lessons can be learned from previous generations, romanticizing the past will not always solve the problems we face today. Instead, solutions that are tailored to the current environment must be developed, addressing both the overconsumption in wealthy areas and the undernutrition in poorer regions.

One great example of a solution that's needed today but wasn't needed in the same way for previous generations is the concept of structured exercise. In the past, movement was integral to survival—hunting, gathering, farming, and daily tasks required physical exertion. However, a modern, sedentary lifestyle has eliminated regular movement, even though it's needed to stay healthy. Nowadays, exercise has become a deliberate practice to make up for the physical activity that's no longer part of our daily routines.

Just as exercise meets an old human need in a modern way, our approach to nutrition should do the same. We can adopt good habits from the past, like eating in moderation and choosing seasonal, unprocessed foods, without following outdated or unrealistic diets like the paleo diet. Foods that promote health should be embraced as long as they contribute to our well-being. Instead of holding onto an idealized vision of the past, we should develop a balanced approach that allows us to thrive in the present. A more holistic perspective on food and health will help us address today's challenges more effectively than simply trying to copy what worked for our ancestors.

HOW TO REALISTICALLY APPLY THE ORIGINS OF HUMAN NUTRITION

Seeing through the nonsense is an important step in promoting better nutrition habits moving forward. But to really apply some of the key lessons from the origins of the human diet and insights from this chapter, here are some things to consider:

1. **Aim for Diversity and Flexibility** – While variations should be considered, most people can handle a variety of foods, which is key to a true paleolithic diet. Cutting out entire food groups can lead to nutrient deficiencies, so it's best to include as many as possible or consult a nutrition expert to plan your diet.

2. **Know Your Processing** – Whether we like it or not, processed foods are a broad category that is here to stay as it continues to feed a global community. This reality brings unique challenges that require us to adjust accordingly. The key is understanding what has been added or removed. Ultra-processed foods, often high in added sugars, fats, and sodium, offer little nutritional value and should be minimized. Instead, focus on whole or minimally processed foods that keep most of their inherent nutritional components. This approach follows the best principles of many diets, including paleo, without extreme restrictions. Modern environments require us to create healthier food options since willpower isn't always enough. We don't need to eliminate all processed foods; we just need to manage them wisely.

3. **Avoid Arbitrary Food Restrictions** – Whether it's paleo-approved or not, all food groups can provide nutritional benefits. For whole grains, consider eating a bulk of them and with smaller amounts of additional fat, sugar, and salt. For those who are lactose intolerant, you can still enjoy up to 1 cup (or more) of dairy products per day. And for legumes, please cook them.

4. **Take a Holistic and Realistic Approach** – The health value of a food shouldn't be judged just on a single nutrient or compound but on the sum of its parts. Foods are complex, and their benefits or risks depend on a variety of factors, including their nutrient profile, sustainability, and long-term ability to stick with dietary changes. Rather than adopting a narrow view, consider how a balanced, enjoyable diet impacts your overall well-being. If your nutrition choices are too restrictive or unsustainable, you risk falling into a cycle of yo-yo dieting, which is detrimental to both physical and mental health.

5. **Understand Your Own Personal Needs** – Although food groups like legumes will benefit a vast majority of people, there are always outliers and reasons a person may actually need to avoid a specific food. Dietary choices must be individualized, as not all grains, dairy, or other foods affect people the same way. Plus, not every food within a food group is the same, so we must not overgeneralize when it comes to individualized decision-making. Ultimately, you have unique needs based on allergies,

environment, and preferences that are your own. If you find success with a paleo diet or any other diet, then by all means, make that choice. My only hope is that you make such an important health decision based on all of the information provided and not based on potential biases and misguided assumptions.

Even with a clear understanding of the origins of human nutrition, marketing can cleverly exploit our misconceptions, steering us toward unhealthy habits—next, we'll uncover how these tactics shape our choices and how to navigate them wisely.

CHAPTER 3: MARKETING

"Advertising is legalized lying."
— **H.G. Wells**

Nutrition marketing is a confusing and often deceptive landscape. We are constantly inundated with mixed messages about what we should eat, from big food corporations to social media influencers and sensationalized headlines. This overwhelming amount of information can make navigating the complexities of nutrition and wellness incredibly difficult. It gets even worse when celebrities and influencers who lack formal nutrition training endorse fad diets and questionable health products. Their influence creates a merry-go-round of bad advice fueled by pseudo-scientific claims that undermine our ability to make informed, long-term health decisions.

Nutrition marketing often focuses on two extremes: body image and indulgence, both of which can be detrimental to our mental and physical health. Companies spend an astounding $14 billion annually on food advertising, while the CDC's budget for preventing chronic diseases is just $1 billion.[1] This disparity helps explain why, despite increasing awareness of health and wellness, we struggle for better public health. Unqualified TikTok influencers, misleading food packaging claims, and the pervasive culture of dieting all contribute to a toxic health environment, and it's time to hold companies and content creators accountable. Let's take a look at just how distorted nutrition can seem through the lens of both media and marketing.

WHAT COUNTS AS NUTRITION MARKETING?

Marketing is the strategic promotion and selling of products or services. In the world of nutrition, it takes many forms and is designed to influence consumer choices. However, these methods are not always focused on promoting genuine health benefits. Some common types of nutrition marketing include:

- **Health Claims on Food Labels** – Eye-catching claims on packaging that highlight supposed health benefits, often without robust evidence.

- **Targeted Ads for Ultra-Processed Foods** – Commercials directed at children in between their favorite TV shows, promoting snacks high in sugar, fat, and salt.
- **Social Media** – Both individuals and businesses use platforms like Instagram and TikTok to share skewed information about diets and health products, often without scientific backing.
- **Influencers and Endorsements** – Social media personalities who mix questionable advice with endorsements for their expensive services and specific dietary protocols.
- **Traditional Media Coverage** – Articles, blogs, newspapers, and even shows that provide updates on trending nutrition stories are often driven by clickbait headlines that lack depth or accuracy.

While some marketing may offer useful information, it's often driven by financial incentives that lead to biased messaging. These incentives may not always be harmful, but they contribute to the spread of myths and misinformation about nutrition.

Most nutrition marketing is to maximize profits or increase views rather than to promote genuine health and wellness. A clear example can be seen in grocery stores, where product placement and promotions are more about sales than nutritional value. Ultimately, marketing strategies focus on pushing what sells instead of what benefits consumers' health, leading to a distorted understanding of healthy choices.

FOOD MARKETING

Food companies often appeal to consumers' desires for improved health and happiness through marketing strategies that frequently rely on buzzwords and bold claims that can be misleading. This steers consumers toward purchasing decisions based on perception rather than factual nutritional information. Certainly, some marketing terms provide relevant insights; however, they can also create confusion. This can lead customers to focus on individual nutrients or health benefits instead of thinking about the overall dietary impact of the food.

BUZZWORDS

Many consumers are swayed by food packaging that's designed to evoke positivity. These buzzwords may hint at health benefits. Yet, they often conceal the product's true nutritional value.

Let's take a closer look at some common buzzwords used in food marketing:

- **Natural** – Products labeled "natural" might avoid artificial ingredients, but this says nothing about their overall nutrition profile. The term plays into the "naturalistic fallacy," where consumers equate natural with better, even when that may not be the case.

- **Organic** – Organic sugar is still sugar. And organic donuts are likely still high in fat, sugar, and calories, making them no healthier than conventional options.

- **Low-Fat** – This label might indicate reduced fat content, but it often neglects to mention what ingredients have replaced the fat, which is often added sugar.

- **Low-Carb** – While popular in certain diet circles, low-carb products often fail to clarify whether the fats used are healthier unsaturated fats or not and neglect the bigger issue of calorie density and lack of health-promoting ingredients.

- **Gluten-Free** – Essential for individuals with celiac disease, gluten-free labels don't necessarily mean a product is healthier for the general population. These foods may lack essential nutrients and offer worse overall nutrition quality.

- **Non-GMO** – Some products, such as salt, have been labeled as "non-GMO," even though they can't be genetically modified. In other cases, the label is applied to foods where no GMO version exists, like popcorn in the U.S. This really goes to show the misleading nature of this label. I myself once fell for this and bought popcorn with the non-GMO label (costing me more money), only to realize that there has never been (nor is there currently) any GMO popcorn for sale in the U.S.[2]

- **Multigrain** – The term "multigrain" simply means the product contains more than one type of grain. However, this doesn't necessarily mean these are *whole* grains. It's important to check whether these grains are refined, as refining removes fiber and valuable nutritional components.

- **Made with Real Fruit/Wholesome Ingredients** – A product may claim to contain "real fruit" or other wholesome ingredients, but the amount is often negligible and lacks any meaningful nutritional benefit.

- **Light** – "Light" or "Lite" can refer to reduced calories or fat content, but it's often in comparison to the regular version of the same product. This reduction may result in added sugar or other unwanted ingredients to enhance flavor.[3]

HEALTHWASHING

While some food labels provide helpful information, many rely on overhyped phrases that sound great but lack real substance. These terms contribute to the psychological phenomenon called the *halo effect*. This is where consumers perceive products as healthy based on a single positive attribute. This causes the customer to overestimate the product's health benefits. This, of course, can result in poor dietary choices.

Examples of these overhyped phrases include:
- Anti-inflammatory
- Superfood
- Clean
- Simple
- Gut-friendly
- Boosts immunity/metabolism
- Chemical-free
- Hormone balancing

These labels are often vague and unregulated, which makes it easy for brands to overstate their products' benefits. Unfortunately, this deceptive practice creates a "false sense of health" that may contribute to overconsumption of products that aren't genuinely nutritious.[4] When brands use these terms, it's often an example of *health washing*—the practice of making misleading health claims to sell products.[5]

A silver lining to this trend is that consumers are increasingly learning to see through these tactics. For instance, a study from Austria found that people who were first exposed to misleading claims on food labels were more likely to make healthier decisions after being educated about the strategies used by companies.[6]

BEYOND THE BUZZ: KEY FACTORS ON FOOD LABELS

When navigating food labels and advertisements, it's essential to look past the flashy health claims on the packaging. Instead, focus on these four crucial factors:

1. **Ingredients List** – Ingredients are listed in descending order by weight.[7] If a product highlights a key ingredient, such as almonds in a trail mix, but that ingredient is near the end of the list, it's a red flag. Look for whole and minimally processed foods as often as you can.

2. **Serving Size** – Food labels often present nutrients per serving but serving sizes can be misleading. People frequently consume more than the stated portion, leading to a higher intake of calories, sugar, fat, and other nutrients.

3. **Daily Values** – The percentage of daily values (DVs) listed on food labels is based on a general population guideline, so it's essential to adjust based on individual dietary needs, but seeing these targets can give you a better sense of whether or not the food offers a high or low amount of a certain nutrient. For example, those who are deficient in certain micronutrients should pay closer attention to the DV percentages of those nutrients of concern.

4. **Added Sugars, Saturated Fat, Fiber, and Protein** – Pay particular attention to added sugars and saturated fats. Since 2020, food labels have been required to list added sugars, making it easier to identify hidden sugars.[8] Opt for foods with higher fiber and protein content, as these nutrients contribute to long-term satiety and overall health.

THE MYTH OF SUPERFOODS AND INFERIOR FOODS

The term "superfood" has become a marketing sensation, but it's often misused and misunderstood. It's a term often used for foods that aren't as common to a specific region. So, for many Americans, when they are introduced to foods like goji berries, açaí, quinoa, and anything with an exotic-sounding name, they immediately fall for its magical potential. Marketers capitalize on this by selling the idea that these novelty items from distant, "mysterious" places hold unparalleled health benefits that local foods can't match. The higher price tag only reinforces the illusion that if it costs more, it must be healthier.

In reality, while most whole foods do provide nutritional benefits, none alone can supply everything necessary for optimal health. Labeling any food as "super" implies it vastly outperforms others in nutritional value, which oversimplifies the complex nature of nutrition. Take the sweet potato, for instance, which has gained "superfood" status, while the white potato is often deemed fattening or unhealthy. This perception is problematic, especially since both vegetables offer valuable nutrients. For example, sweet potatoes may be richer in vitamin A, but white potatoes provide more potassium.

Neither is better than the other, but the white potato often falls victim to the *horn effect*, or the opposite of the halo effect. This cognitive bias leads people to make snap judgments based on a single negative trait. With white potatoes, their association with French fries and chips, as well as their lack of vibrant color, fuels their negative reputation. However, a sweet potato fry isn't any healthier than a regular French fry, as both are quite similar when processed.

Ultimately, research shows that both sweet and white potatoes, when consumed in minimally processed forms, offer comparable health benefits.[9,10]

ADDED SUGAR IS ADDED SUGAR

One of the most common marketing strategies in "healthified" recipes is substituting white sugar with alternatives like coconut sugar. However, from a nutritional perspective, these alternatives offer little advantage. Here's why:

• **White Sugar** – Composed of sucrose, a disaccharide made up of 50% glucose and 50% fructose.

• **Coconut Sugar** – Essentially 99% sugar from equal parts glucose and fructose. 1% is leftover moisture and trace micronutrients.

Both types of sugar affect the body in a similar way. This is because your GI tract is not swayed by false advertisements that claim one added sugar is healthier than another. And while coconut sugar is often marketed as a healthy option due to its trace micronutrients, consuming the required amount to gain any notable benefit would involve eating an unrealistic amount of sugar. In essence, your body metabolizes all forms of simple sugars the same way. The key is moderation.

I suspect that those who find there was a benefit to switching to coconut sugar are not accounting for *healthy user bias*. This occurs when the positive outcomes associated with a specific behavior or product are actually due to the overall healthier lifestyle choices of the people making that swap rather than the product itself. People who use alternative sugars are more likely to make better choices in general, so of course, we associate this sugar with better health. Making this swap might also be the first time you didn't fear the inclusion of sugar and the result was a guilt-free enjoyment, even though these sugars are the same.

GUT-FRIENDLY DRINKS

Another recent trend in food marketing is using trendy "gut-friendly" language to sell products. Poppi Prebiotic Soda recently faced allegations for overstating its health benefits within this domain, however.[11] This is really not surprising. Many brands in the functional food and beverage industry tend to exaggerate their claims. The lawsuit cited research showing that consuming 7.5 grams of agave inulin daily for three weeks didn't provide any significant health benefits.[12]

To achieve the effective prebiotic dosage through the soda alone, the amount of sugar consumed would likely be greater than any potential benefits of the inulin, which raises a broader concern in the industry. Many brands make exaggerated claims, but as consumers learn more about nutrition, these companies may face more scrutiny and legal challenges.

Ultimately, relying on prebiotic sodas to boost fiber intake is far less beneficial than consuming fiber-rich foods, which offer a range of other vital nutrients. While these drinks can be healthier alternatives to traditional sodas, they shouldn't replace fiber-rich foods in your diet. Though less visually appealing than colorful sodas, a diet rich in whole plant foods will provide far better digestive health.

BRANDING

Brand power has such a powerful psychological influence on our purchasing decisions. Take when you're shopping for clothes for example; have you ever found that a T-shirt or sunglasses priced at $15 is somehow less appealing than a branded version for $50? Why is that? It's because we're conditioned to believe that wearing luxury brands or consuming expensive foods will raise our social standing. We also tend to associate higher prices with superior quality and reliability, especially when a product is endorsed by a well-known company or celebrity.

Brands often emphasize their commitment to hard work, authenticity, and excellence, persuading us to buy their products, even when cheaper alternatives exist. I remember when I was at Whole Foods and saw a jar of almond butter priced at $20, though similar products could be found elsewhere for $6–8. After comparing labels, I couldn't find a difference between the products; they were both simply ground almonds. The only distinction was the upscale branding and Whole Foods' reputation, which seemingly justified the higher price.

We often pay more for the perceived security and familiarity that popular brands offer. These companies don't just sell us food; they sell us a sense of status, pride, and reassurance. Be careful though. This branding power often leads to poorer financial choices, as we're inclined to spend more than necessary.

TARGETED MARKETING

Food companies frequently engage in "targeted marketing" to promote their least healthy products to children, teens, and communities of color—a practice that has well-documented harmful effects.[13]

A 2019 review revealed that marketing through TV, movies, and packaging significantly influenced children's food preferences.[14] Children were more likely to favor foods wrapped in packaging adorned with promotional characters, illustrating the powerful allure of branding.

One study found that children exposed to food commercials consumed an average of 48 more calories compared to those who watched toy commercials, highlighting how advertising shapes eating habits.[14]

A cross-national study of youth aged 10–17 throughout six countries also found that fast food marketing strongly influenced brand preferences and increased fast-food consumption. Notably, ethnic minorities reported higher fast-food consumption than ethnic majorities, while women consumed less than men, likely exacerbated by targeted marketing.[15]

In the U.S., a 2021 study linked sugar-sweetened beverage ads to higher consumption rates, particularly among low-income households, suggesting that this type of marketing may make existing racial and economic health disparities even worse over time.[16]

Some companies will also host cheap, engaging internet-based games on their websites, where children can play as mascots and earn "health points," a strategy designed to build brand loyalty early on.[17] This engagement is strengthened by interactive content on social media, setting young consumers on a path that could lead to long-term health issues.

FAST FOOD CULTURE

Fast food advertisements work hard to glamorize their products, but the reality often falls flat, quite literally. Ads promise a visually appealing, mouthwatering meal, but what you often get is a lukewarm, squashed burger. The taste isn't necessarily bad; fast food is engineered to stimulate the brain's reward centers, much like other indulgences. However, the disconnect between the glossy ads and the actual experience can be frustrating.

Adding to the irony, fast food companies often feature celebrities in their ads, creating the illusion that these stars regularly enjoy fast food. In reality, many of these famous people have private chefs preparing healthy, gourmet meals while we line up at the drive-thru based on their endorsements.

Fast food culture has also profoundly shaped the American lifestyle, often in problematic ways. The average American spends just 63 minutes a day eating and drinking, which is far less than people in countries like France, Italy, and Greece, where mealtimes seem to be a more cherished ritual.[18] It's not just about time; Americans' cooking and nutrition habits also lag behind those of many other nations.

The U.S. pioneered fast food with the first White Castle in 1921, and over the years, these chains have spread, particularly in urban areas and food deserts.[19] As a result, eating fast food has become a near necessity for many, mostly because of its convenience and accessibility.

While ads might depict families happily gathering around a kitchen table for a perfectly presented fast food meal, that's rarely the reality. For many, fast food is a lifeline, a quick solution when there's little time, energy, or money to prepare meals at home. It also represents an element of hustle culture, where leisurely home-cooked meals are often considered a luxury.

Fast food's role in American culture is complex. It might pose health risks, but it has also provided convenience and fond memories that shouldn't be entirely dismissed. But with research that continues to suggest that banning fast food advertisements could reduce childhood obesity rates by 18% and adolescent obesity rates by 14%, it's hard to consider it a net positive.[20] While doing something as radical as eliminating fast food entirely isn't a necessity, we should focus on resisting the marketing influence these companies continue to push on us. At the same time, we can support broader cultural and socioeconomic changes that could reduce people's reliance on fast food as a whole.

SOCIAL MEDIA

Social media has become a dominant force in how Americans consume news. Nearly 62% of adults now rely on platforms like Facebook, X, and TikTok to learn what's going on in the world, a figure that's steadily increasing.[21] This rapid shift means many, including myself, turn to social media to keep up with trends and stories. After all, it helps in appreciating the range of perspectives and unfiltered ideas it offers. Yet, while it can be a treasure trove of diverse opinions and grassroots insights, finding truly credible nutrition information on these platforms is a different story.

The prevalence of misinformation is especially concerning when it comes to health and wellness. Numerous studies have demonstrated that much of the health content on social media is inaccurate and of alarmingly low quality, often putting users at risk.[22,23]

A study reviewing mental health advice on TikTok found that a staggering 83.7% of the 500 videos analyzed contained misleading information. Shockingly, only 9% of the creators behind these videos held relevant qualifications.[21]

In another investigation of 221 health-related videos with over 300 million views, non-medical influencers were found to frequently post content with low educational value and poor harm/benefit scores. Perhaps most alarming, only 46.7% of these videos from non-professionals were factually accurate.[24]

This issue isn't just frustrating for healthcare professionals; it's a widespread societal problem. In a survey of university students, over three-quarters admitted they struggled to determine the accuracy of nutrition information they encountered online.[25] This is particularly concerning considering that 87% of millennials and Gen Z are turning to TikTok for health advice, with 31% reporting negative effects from following dubious trends they found on these platforms.[26]

Social media's ability to quickly spread content is a blessing and a curse. The low barrier to entry means anyone can share health information, but it isn't always such a great thing. It also allows misinformation to spread as easily as reliable content. Not only that, but social media algorithms often prioritize engagement over accuracy, making it difficult to distinguish sensible advice from sensationalized claims. This issue is unlikely to be resolved soon, especially as platforms continue to reward attention-grabbing content over truth.

BUMMER

Jaron Lanier, a renowned American computer scientist, is one of the loudest critics of social media's darker side. In his book "*10 Arguments for Deleting Your Social Media Accounts Right Now*," he argues that platforms have become dangerous forces, undermining truth in pursuit of profit.[27] One of Lanier's key points is that social media algorithms manipulate users, keeping them trapped in their own echo chambers. He dubs these algorithms the "BUMMER machine," short for "Behaviors of Users Modified and Made into Empires for Rent." This machine constantly analyzes users' behaviors to feed them more of what they already believe, reinforcing their existing viewpoints.

Lanier explains that social media platforms are not designed to serve our best interests. They manipulate our behavior for profit. Essentially, users become the product, and every click, like, or share further fuels the BUMMER machine. Over time, this process creates a feedback loop that reinforces confirmation bias. This makes it harder to encounter content that challenges your beliefs.

Let's say you show even a slight curiosity about a conspiracy theory by clicking on a related post, and then the algorithm will quickly begin to flood your feed with similar content, subtly steering you toward believing it. The same pattern occurs with fad diets. People often feel they've discovered the perfect solution, not because it's backed by evidence, but because they keep engaging with content that resonates with them. The algorithm then inundates them with more of the same, reinforcing their beliefs. This creates a bubble where opposing viewpoints are completely shut out.

While social media may appear to offer endless opportunities for learning and exploration, as Jaron Lanier cautions, if you don't use it wisely, it's more likely to trap you in a cycle of misinformation, reinforcing dangerous ideas and making you susceptible to falsehoods.

JUST GOOGLE IT?

Just like with social media, the way you search for information online can significantly shape your beliefs.

Search engines like Google learn from your search history and personalize results to match your interests. While this is definitely helpful for finding products you enjoy, it can also dangerously shrink your perspective on more critical topics, such as health and nutrition.

What many people don't realize is that the *phrasing* of a search query can dramatically influence the type of information you receive. I recently conducted an experiment using eggs, a food often debated in terms of health. When I searched "Are eggs healthy?", on Google, the top results were overwhelmingly positive, with articles like "6 Reasons Eggs Are the Healthiest Food on the Planet" and "10 Amazing Health Benefits of Eating Eggs."[28,29] I then slightly altered the query to "Are eggs unhealthy?" and the results took a much different tone. I was now given titles such as "Why We Should Not Eat Eggs" and "Health Concerns with Eggs."[30,31]

This change in results highlights an important point: the information you get from a search engine is heavily influenced by how you *frame* your question and your prior search history. Most users trust the top results they see, often without realizing they may be reinforcing their existing beliefs rather than offering a well-rounded view.

The bias in search results works similarly to confirmation bias on social media, guiding content toward what already aligns with existing beliefs. Just like social media algorithms, search engines create an echo chamber that can distort the understanding of important issues.

In the past, traditional ads on TV or billboards presented information uniformly to all viewers without tailoring it to individual preferences. But today, online ads and search results are highly personalized, reflecting back at you based on who you are and what you've previously searched for. While this personalization may seem convenient, it can also dangerously narrow your worldview.

It's particularly concerning that 36.4% of people rely on Google for health and wellness information.[32] If search queries are influenced by strong biases or ambiguity, they can lead to misleading results that shape poor decisions.

To truly benefit from search engines, it's vital to remain aware of these biases and strive for a more objective, critical approach. Otherwise, the risk relying on inaccurate information becomes greater, and this can lead to making unhealthy choices without even realizing it.

INFLUENCERS

We're all familiar with social media influencers—people with an enviously large, engaged number of followers who have the power to sway opinions and shape behaviors. In the realm of nutrition, influencers range from chefs and doctors, to bodybuilders and wellness gurus, each eager to share tips and advice with their audience. However, regardless of their background, many influencers, though often well-intentioned, end up spreading inaccurate or misleading information, primarily to meet marketing goals. Their tactics tend to follow a predictable and well-worn pattern.

THE PLAYBOOK

Whether it's food marketing or social media promotion, influencers typically don't sell ideas grounded in solid, rational information; instead, they sell what's trendy because that's what grabs attention. Today, they might villainize dairy, gluten, sweeteners, or oils, blaming them for a variety of health problems. But soon enough, they'll move on to the next fad, like a child discarding an old toy for something shinier and new. The most problematic influencers, who constantly chase after what's trending, tend to follow the same playbook:

Step 1: The Background – Influencers start by sharing personal struggles with severe health issues, which may or may not be genuine, or by emphasizing their medical or academic credentials, which lends them credibility. This introduction establishes them as trustworthy guides who can lead you on a journey toward better health.

Step 2: The Awakening – Next, they claim to have uncovered a hidden truth, a revelation that supposedly changes everything they and their followers once knew about nutrition. This so called "awakening" is framed as a moment of clarity, positioning the influencer as someone who has broken free from mainstream myths to offer the real truth.

Step 3: The "Ah-ha" Moment – After their dramatic awakening, influencers will identify one single culprit responsible for all health issues, often zeroing in on toxins, sugar, salt, meat, or another easily targeted food group. They then present a specific diet or supplement as the ultimate solution to these problems. Sometimes, they target broader issues like cancer or other incurable diseases, claiming that their approach is the cure-all.

Step 4: Cherry-Picking Evidence – To make their claims more convincing, influencers selectively present so-called "scientific" data that supports their narrative. They often use simple charts or bold, out-of-context statistics to suggest their solutions are foolproof. This approach adds an air of believability to their argument, even if the evidence they cite is far from conclusive.

Step 5: The Urgent Sell – At this stage, influencers create a sense of urgency around their solutions, whether it's a detox plan, a specific diet, or a miracle supplement. By instilling a fear of missing out or by suggesting that time is running out to act, they pressure followers into purchasing their product immediately, leaving little time for thoughtful consideration.

Step 6: Self-Righteousness – Influencers often position themselves as one of the first, or among a select few, to uncover a "big secret" that the rest of the world has yet to see. They promise to guide their followers toward this newfound health truth if only they are trusted and followed. Throughout the process, they frequently remind you of the problem while subtly or overtly promoting their products, often using legal disclaimers to cover themselves. Criticism is dismissed as noise from "haters," without ever needing to engage in a logical rebuttal from others. Over time, this approach develops into what's known as the "big lie technique," where repeated falsehoods or half-truths become accepted as fact.

Step 7: Overpromise, Underdeliver – Once influencers have captured your attention and made their sales, delivering actual results becomes less important. They've already achieved their goal: gaining views, followers, and profits. This leaves their followers with unmet expectations and empty promises. Much like modern movie trailers that generate excitement only for the film to disappoint, influencers often fail to deliver on the hype they create.

This cycle of excitement and disappointment is central to the way many influencers operate, prioritizing profit and popularity over factual, responsible health advice.

BAD BLOGS AND PROBLEMATIC PROFILES

When navigating the blogs, websites, and social media profiles of health influencers, approach their content with a critical eye. While some influencers genuinely aim to help, many are primarily focused on selling products or services.

Here are four classic tactics health influencers use that you should be cautious of:

Testimonials – Testimonials can be persuasive, but they often lack transparency. How can you know if the stories shared are real, unbiased, or even relevant to the claims being made? An influencer may boast about helping "hundreds" of people, but without context, those success stories could easily be cherry-picked from a larger, less successful group of clients.

Before and After Pictures – These images are frequently manipulated using lighting, angles, or editing tools, making them unreliable as evidence of real transformation.[33] Although they may seem impressive, they're often nothing more than outdated and sleazy marketing tactics. True health is measured in far more meaningful ways than just how someone looks in a staged photo.

A Quote from Hippocrates – Nutrition sites love to drop famous quotes like, "Let food be thy medicine" or "All disease begins in the gut." While food undeniably plays a critical role in health, not all diseases stem from poor gut health, and some conditions are purely genetic. For example, those with Huntington's disease, muscular dystrophy, or sickle cell anemia aren't suffering as a result of poor gut health. Moreover, equating food with medicine is misleading. While food supports health, it's not a cure-all. This tongue-in-cheek observation highlights the strong correlation between using old, misguided quotes and promoting fraudulent nutrition advice.

Unnecessary or Pricey Services – It's fair for professionals to charge for their expertise but be wary of services that include unproven tests or generic, one-size-fits-all recommendations. Often, these pricey packages are marketed as "investments" in your health but can lead to unnecessary worry and financial strain. As the saying goes, 'Watch what they say, and then watch what they sell."

CATCHY CONTENT

One common problem with social media is the race to outdo others with clever, provocative posts. The goal often isn't to provide genuine help but to grab attention. A classic example is what I call the "Obvious Health List," which goes something like this:

HEALTH IS EASY. ALL YOU NEED TO DO IS:

- EAT CLEAN

- LIFT WEIGHTS

- MEDITATE

- COLD PLUNGE

- READ MORE

- TALK LESS

- FIND THE FOUNTAIN OF YOUTH

- WORK HARD

- LAUGH OUT LOUD

- FIND PURPOSE

AND YOU'LL BE UNRECOGNIZABLE IN 3 MONTHS. IT'S THAT SIMPLE.

The comments on posts like these will consist of people cheering, saying things like, "Yes, there would be no more sickness if we just did these!" or "I've been saying this for years, it's so simple." While the message is in fact very simple, achieving these goals clearly isn't *easy*. These kinds of posts amuse the masses and make the influencer posting feel insightful, yet they rarely offer any new or useful information. If staying healthy were as easy as following this list, why isn't everyone thriving?

That's because the actual *application* of them is the hard part. To be a valuable health expert, one must have both knowledge and the ability to help others apply it. Simply pointing out that sugary Starbucks drinks are unhealthy (something most people already know) isn't helpful unless practical solutions follow. What alternatives can people choose? Should they try alternative sweeteners, set boundaries on how often they indulge or focus on adding more protein and fiber to meals to curb cravings?

Look for influencers who provide actionable solutions, not just those who criticize. It's easy to point out problems, but it's much harder to offer realistic solutions. The world needs more problem-solvers, not more empty critics who offer zero solutions.

WHAT I EAT IN A DAY

A popular type of content is the "What I Eat in a Day" videos, where influencers post clips of their meals throughout the day. While entertaining, these posts have both pros and cons:

Pros:

- Social media thrives on the sharing of ideas. Seeing what someone's having for lunch or dinner could inspire you to try new recipes or discover new food brands.

- These posts also highlight our differences, showing that everyone has unique preferences. Even if the meals don't appeal to you, they still offer a glimpse into the creator's personality, making them feel more relatable.

Cons:

- Rarely do you see this content from someone who is struggling with obesity, lacks muscle definition, or is unhappy with their body. This creates several problems. First, we tend to compare ourselves to the idealized versions of others on social media, leading to disappointment and potential mental health issues.

- Those posting these videos also feel pressured to maintain a perfect image, curating meals they likely don't eat regularly and using lighting and angles that misrepresent reality. When we don't receive realistic content, we feel inadequate when our own attempts fall short.

- We love to copy the behavior of celebrities and influencers, but simply mirroring their diet won't make you like them. You're more likely to lose sight of your own needs and preferences. It's essential to find your identity in your own personalized eating habits. While you can certainly adopt some useful ideas from influencers, copying them entirely pulls you further from your best self.

BODY IMAGE

Social media's pervasive influence among teens and young adults has been linked to increased body dissatisfaction and a heightened drive for thinness, which puts these groups at greater risk for eating disorders.[34] This troubling trend underscores the need to incorporate social media awareness into general prevention programs and personalized treatment plans. One study even found that reducing social media use improved body image perception among teens and young adults most vulnerable to eating disorders.[35]

Advertising also plays a harmful role in perpetuating negative body image, often objectifying women and girls, which only makes body dissatisfaction, low self-esteem, and eating disorders worse. These issues are widespread across all ethnic groups, and weight-related stigma is closely tied to depression, low self-esteem, and even suicidal thoughts.[36]

STEROIDS AND PERFECT LIGHTING

In today's social media-driven world, portraying a fit, healthy lifestyle is often considered more important than actually living one. And this quest for the "perfect" image has pushed influencers to extreme measures. James Ellis, a personal trainer and bodybuilder, is a cautionary example. Initially committed to a basic fitness and diet routine, Ellis found that to rise to the top, he needed more—so he started using performance-enhancing drugs. His moral compass began to waver as his following grew, and the allure of social media clout outweighed concerns about side effects like high cholesterol, blood pressure, and liver damage. As Ellis put it, "The more entrenched you get in your industry, the more your appearance counts. You start getting accolades, more followers and those moral decisions just go out the window."[37] Unfortunately, his story is far from unique.

Trainer Tobias Holt, an openly steroid-using coach, claims that nearly all top bodybuilding influencers use performance-enhancing drugs (PEDs). According to Holt, "Anyone that tells you they're not is a f-cking liar."

This deceptive culture fosters unrealistic expectations among followers who believe they can achieve similar physiques through diet and exercise alone.

Another notorious example of social media warping our collective sense of healthy living is Brian Johnson, aka Liver King. He built his entire $100 million fitness empire promoting a "primal" lifestyle that was aimed at representing the potential for a remarkably fit body by eating a very restrictive diet of raw liver and only a few other animal products. But what he failed to mention (until he was exposed by another social media influencer) is that he was relying on massive steroid use to fuel his ridiculous physique.[38] While many suspected his body was enhanced, the time leading up to this reveal ultimately misled countless followers, especially the more impressionable ones.

This is not an isolated example either, as many influencers conceal their steroid use. Beyond steroids, many others will manipulate their images through clever lighting and camera angles, fasting, flexing, Photoshop, and now AI, which can make themselves appear more physically impressive than they truly are. This dishonesty can lead even the most dedicated gym-goers to experience body dysmorphia, eating disorders, and other mental health challenges as they strive to measure up to these unattainable, manufactured ideals.

10 INFLUENCER RED FLAGS

So, now that you know more about the potentially misleading nature of many well-known influencers, here are 10 signs that can help you determine if a social media star is prioritizing views and profit over helping others:

1. Over-Selling Products – Endorsing supplements isn't inherently bad but beware of claims like "Everyone needs this product!" Nutritional needs vary, and no single product is universally necessary. A responsible recommendation considers individual diet and lifestyle factors.

2. Universal Quantifiers – Phrases like "always" or "never" oversimplify complex nutritional concepts. Instead of saying we should "never" eat butter or sugar, it's more accurate to suggest a healthy balance, like the 80/20 rule.

3. Grocery Store Puppets – Some influencers spend way too much recording videos in grocery stores, oversimplifying foods as "healthy" or "unhealthy". While this can be helpful in some cases, many are simply parroting trendy terms like "clean" or "inflammatory" without providing proper perspective or evidence for these claims. In most instances they're likely just repeating what they've seen in other popular posts as they lack the ability to explain why certain foods are harmful at a fundamental level.

4. Trend Hoppers – Constantly shifting from one diet trend to another is a red flag. Take Paul Saladino, aka the Carnivore MD, who has swung from raw vegan to paleo to carnivore and beyond.[39,40,41,42,43,44] While a credible expert's views may evolve, drastic shifts suggest a lack of foundational nutrition knowledge.

5. Body-Based Content – Influencers like Lee Tilghman learned the hard way that "my body was my business card."[45] Relying solely on appearance to gain followers can lead to extreme behaviors and mental health issues. Trusting advice based solely on someone's physique overlooks the broader aspects of health, like mental well-being and sound nutritional principles.

6. Personal Experience Only – Personal experience is valuable, but it shouldn't be the sole basis for recommendations. What works for one person may not work for another. Look for influencers who support their advice with scientific research, not just their own story.

7. Claims Lacking Evidence – If an influencer makes bold claims, like "90% of users have lost weight with my supplement!", they should be able to back them up with credible sources. If they can't, it's likely a ploy for clicks.

8. Messiah Complex – Beware of influencers who act like they have all the answers and never admit they're wrong. This "influencer messiah complex" leads to the refusal to update views, even when new evidence is presented, which is the opposite of critical thinking.[46]

9. One-Size-Fits-All – Advice that applies a single rule to everyone is another red flag. For instance, some people may actually need to avoid dairy, while others can incorporate it healthily. Nutrition advice should be tailored to individual needs.

10. Beyond Reason – Diets with extreme promises, like losing 30 lbs. in a month, are likely unsustainable and unrealistic. Good health takes time. If something sounds too good to be true, it probably is, so don't waste your time.

MORE MEDIA MADNESS

We're living in an era where headlines must be sensational to grab attention. With so much information available at our fingertips, only the most dramatic content stands out. These headlines are crafted to evoke strong emotional responses, feeding our dopamine-driven impulses. The marketing strategy is clear: create a bond between the consumer and the product through emotional manipulation, even if that trust is built on shaky ground.

To capture attention, marketers often rely on extreme claims, such as unveiling a "secret food that's killing us" or promoting a new diet as the ultimate cure for all ailments. This tactic, known as "clickbait," isn't about offering genuine value; it's about driving traffic and boosting engagement.[47] The problem is that these exaggerated claims are rarely supported by solid evidence, leaving consumers misinformed and susceptible to manipulation.

CLICKBAIT

The rise of mass media brought with it the evolution of attention-grabbing headlines. In the late 19th century, newspapers began using bold, sensationalist headlines to outshine their competitors.[48] Today, whether it's on magazine covers, news websites, or blogs, headlines are engineered with one goal in mind: to seize attention. And nothing captures attention better than chaos.

In the world of nutrition, chaos is often created by contradictory advice. One day, eggs are deemed to be bad for you, and the next, they're considered a superfood. The truth, however, lies somewhere in the middle. Eggs, for instance, are nutritious, but their benefits depend on how many you consume and your unique health profile.

Unfortunately, nuance doesn't sell. People are drawn to extremes, which is why much of the content from influencers and media outlets is hyperbolic and oversimplified.

The real issue isn't just with the content creators, but it's also with us, the consumers. We fuel the demand for more outlandish ideas, pushing those offering advice to ramp up the insanity. Though it's far from ethical, this cycle persists because it works.

BAD TITLES

While some headlines are sensationalized, others are just downright inaccurate. Take this ridiculous headline as an example:

"Major Study Claims to Identify the Root Cause of Obesity: Fructose."[49,50]

If this were true, it would be groundbreaking. However, after investigating the "study," I found that it wasn't even a study at all. Instead, it was a poorly executed review paper summarizing various obesity hypotheses, not conducting any new research. The conclusion? "More research is required," especially since most studies on fructose's effects were conducted on animals, not humans. This headline is a prime example of misrepresentation. Most people who see this type of headline won't dig any deeper or even know how to tell if it's accurate or not. They'll simply remember the anxiety and confusion it caused. Because of this, some might avoid fructose altogether, even in healthy foods like fruits. As a result, these absurdist headlines leave many of us stressed, misinformed, and none the wiser.

DR. OZ

Dr. Oz is one of the most infamous figures in the health and wellness industry. Once a trusted voice, his show gradually morphed into a platform for dubious health advice and questionable weight-loss products. His egregious promotion of "magic weight-loss cures" and "miracles in a bottle" exemplify how marketing can overpower ethics and truth.

In 2012, for example, Dr. Oz famously touted green coffee bean extract as a miracle weight-loss supplement, claiming it could help users lose 20 pounds in four weeks and reduce body fat by 16 percent in just three months.[51] Sales of the product skyrocketed, but the Federal Trade Commission later sued the company for false advertising behind the supplement.[52] Despite the controversy, Dr. Oz defended himself, arguing that he was simply providing information his audience wanted and needed.[53] However, a meta-analysis of his show found that fewer than half of the recommendations made were backed by solid evidence.[54] This highlights a troubling pattern: sensational claims backed by little to no scientific support, all for the sake of fame and profit.

SHARK TANK SCAMS

Even the popular TV show *Shark Tank*, where entrepreneurs pitch their ideas to potential investors, has had its share of health scams. A notable example from 2019 involved *Minus Cal*, a product that claimed to block fat absorption and aid in weight loss. The investing "sharks" quickly saw through the dubious claims, and the conversation heated up:[55]

Entrepreneur: "Neither one of us claimed that if you take this product, you'll lose weight."

Mark Cuban: "Look at your shirt."

Entrepreneur: "It says 'fewer calories.'"

Mark Cuban: "Right, and how do you lose weight?"

Entrepreneur: "We're not claiming that you're going to lose weight; we're saying we'll take some fat out of your body and help you with your weight."

Robert Herjavec: "Now you're pissing me off... You just said you're not losing weight. What does it say right here?" (points to the product sign, which says *LOSE WEIGHT*).

Investors: "I think we're done here."

The pitch quickly fell apart under scrutiny.

While it's satisfying to see a scam exposed, it's just one example in a sea of fraudulent health products. Sadly, many other scams succeed in the marketplace, misleading consumers desperate for quick fixes. This leads not only to wasted money but also to disappointment and confusion when people realize they've been duped yet again by false nutrition marketing.

Ultimately, all of this confusion and disappointment stems from a media landscape that is incentivized to manipulate and exploit consumer fear. Rationally, many of us know just how misleading media and marketing efforts can be, but our overly emotional investment in some of the most prominent health ideologies continues to diminish our ability to apply critical thinking skills and so we keep falling for nutrition nonsense.

WHERE DID THIS NONSENSE COME FROM?

There are a few biases in nutrition marketing that contribute to a majority of the nutrition nonsense we see every day.

LOW-RISK, HIGH-REWARD

Let's start with the enormous financial motivation behind misinformation. In 2023, the global weight-loss supplement market was valued at an astounding $29.96 billion.[56]

Literally every food, product, and advertisement in the nutrition space includes some form of weight loss promise these days. For businesses, ethical considerations are often overshadowed by the promise of financial gain. Companies knowingly slap buzzwords like "natural," "fat-burning," or "miracle cure" onto products without solid evidence to back these claims, all in the pursuit of profit. Influencers, celebrities, and marketers capitalize on these weight loss and health trends too, realizing that hyping overblown products can boost their social media presence. Algorithms reward sensational content, and influencers who toss around grandiose claims can become Insta-famous overnight.

The lure of this deceptive marketing is strong because there are few real repercussions. Freedom of speech, a fundamental necessity, is vital for protecting the exchange of ideas. Unfortunately, it can be misused by allowing misleading information to spread online with limited regulation or accountability.

Without regulation, there are essentially zero barriers to entry in the realm of social media nutrition advice. After all, anyone can set up a blog, create a social media account, or market themselves as a health expert without any formal qualifications or accountability, which is wonderful for promoting free expression and innovation, but, unfortunately, it can be abused by people knowing fully well they're spreading false information without the risk of facing any consequences. Because of this, the internet has democratized information sharing, but it has also flooded the market with dubious advice. This has made it difficult for consumers to distinguish between reliable and unreliable sources. Influencers and marketers are free to peddle ridiculous products and ideas, leaving consumers to bear the consequences of ineffective, overpriced, or even harmful trends.

SOCIAL CONFORMITY

Social psychologist Solomon Asch's famous conformity experiments, conducted in 1951, revealed a deep truth about human behavior: we often conform to social norms even when we know they're wrong.[57] In these classic experiments, participants were placed with a group of confederates who deliberately gave incorrect answers to simple questions. Despite knowing the right answer, about 75% of participants still conformed to the group at least once.[58]

This tendency to follow the crowd, even when it contradicts our own better judgment, is particularly relevant in nutrition. It's common for people to accept popular beliefs, no matter how unfounded, simply because everyone else seems to be doing it. This bandwagon fallacy drives people to embrace social media-driven diets, new superfood products, or the disordered eating habits of an influencer simply because these ideas have gained popularity and are being promoted online. Social media and marketing teams manufacture these majority beliefs, creating an illusion of consensus and pressuring individuals to conform to bad advice.

SECRETS CAN BE FUN

Pretending that there is some top-secret plan that only a few select people know about optimal health is a powerful marketing tool. The promise of insider knowledge creates a sense of exclusivity and trust. Once consumers buy into the program or product, they're often gaslighted if it doesn't work, and often, the influencer blames the user for not following the instructions correctly. This tactic shifts responsibility away from the product or service and keeps the customer hooked on ineffective solutions. Consumers, therefore, continue chasing results, convinced that the key to success is just one secret away.

FREQUENCY ILLUSION

The *"frequency illusion,"* also known as the *Baader-Meinhof phenomenon*, occurs when something you've recently encountered starts popping up everywhere, creating the false impression that it's more common or important than it actually is. In the world of food marketing and social media nutrition, this illusion often occurs when a new diet or trendy ingredient goes viral. For instance, after hearing about the supposed benefits of celery juice from a colleague, I decided to look into it. Almost instantly, it felt like celery juice was everywhere. My social media feeds were flooded with articles, influencer posts, and ads promoting celery juice detoxes. At first, I thought it must be a huge health trend that everyone was trying out. But the more I saw, the more I realized something odd. The science behind it seemed flimsy, yet the content kept coming. The algorithms picked up on my curiosity, feeding me more and more posts, and suddenly it felt like celery juice was the answer to everything. It made me question how much of what I was seeing was really reliable or just an illusion created by the algorithms.

Similarly, food companies take advantage of the frequency illusion by flooding the market with products labeled as "superfood" and "clean." For example, after seeing a new line of snacks advertised as containing chia seeds, a widely marketed superfood, you might start seeing chia seeds on every food label. This constant exposure almost makes it seem as though chia seeds are an essential part of a healthy diet. The truth is; however, their benefits are only part of a balanced nutritional approach.

The frequency illusion leads consumers to overestimate the importance of certain foods or trends, skewing their health decisions based on what appears to be popular, not what's scientifically proven.

PLAYING ON EMOTION

Marketers frequently exploit emotional triggers to manipulate consumer behavior, especially in regard to nutrition and health products. Fear, hope, and guilt are powerful motivators that companies and influencers use to push their products. These are the exact emotions I felt when I was misled by the almond butter villain at the store and when I had placed too much hope in a smoothie to overcome a complex disease like cancer.

Have you ever been searching the internet only to come across a pop-up ad saying "This One Ingredient in Your Pantry is Slowly Killing You!" Such emotionally charged statements tap into our fear, pushing consumers to purchase certain products that claim to be free of harmful chemicals or toxins, even if the claims lack scientific backing. For instance, gluten-free products exploded in popularity after fear-based marketing convinced many consumers that gluten was harmful to everyone, not just those with celiac disease.

On social media, influencers often use guilt to promote weight-loss products or fitness programs. Posts might feature a perfectly toned influencer with a caption like, "What's your excuse?" or "If I can do it, so can you!" This subtly shames viewers into feeling inadequate about their bodies, pushing them to buy whatever product the influencer is endorsing, whether it's a supplement, workout routine, or detox plan. The emotional manipulation is clear: these posts play on the viewers' insecurities, making them feel like they're not doing enough to achieve the influencer's version of success.

THE VON RESTORFF EFFECT

The *Von Restorff effect*, also known as the *"isolation effect,"* suggests that items that stand out are more likely to be noticed and remembered. In the context of food marketing and social media, brands and influencers take advantage of this psychological principle by using vibrant colors, striking designs, and eye-catching packaging to draw attention to their products.

Brightly colored packaging on the shelves of grocery stores immediately draws the consumer's eye. A product like *Flamin' Hot Cheetos* uses bright reds and oranges, invoking a sense of excitement and spiciness. It's not just the taste that sells the product. It's the vibrant, attention-grabbing visuals that make consumers notice it, creating an emotional link before they even try the snack.

In a more health-focused context, products often use green packaging and earthy tones, tapping into associations with health, nature, and purity. Consumers are more likely to remember and trust products that visually align with their expectations of what healthy looks like.

On social media, the Von Restorff effect is used extensively by influencers as well. You'll often see posts featuring a colorful smoothie bowl with bright pink dragon fruit or vibrant green matcha framed by a well-lit, aesthetically pleasing background. These vivid, attractive visuals stand out in an Instagram feed filled with less colorful content, making users more likely to stop scrolling and engage with the post. Bright, visually striking content garners more likes, shares, and saves, which boosts the influencer's visibility due to the algorithm's preference for highly engaged content. Products that are brightly colored or packaged, like a particular brand of protein powder or vitamin supplements, are more likely to be remembered and purchased by viewers simply because they look good on screen.

These marketing strategies play a role in our natural tendency to notice and trust what stands out. By isolating their product visually through color or aesthetic design, companies and influencers can make their products more memorable and appealing, even if the product itself isn't objectively better than its competitors.

OVERCOMING MARKETING MISINFORMATION

1. **Turn Down the Noise** – Instead of trying to sort through thousands of confusing messages thrown at you every day, limit your exposure in general. Set limits on your phone and computer for the amount of time you use on social media. Unfollow accounts that promote questionable products or rely on sensational claims. By streamlining your media consumption, you not only reduce stress but also create space for healthier, more informed decision-making. This simple shift can improve both your mental well-being and your ability to make sound nutritional choices.

2. **Choose Quality Media** – Media can be a valuable tool if approached with intentionality. Without a strategy, we risk becoming passive consumers, vulnerable to marketing tactics designed to sell rather than inform. Be mindful of where you get your information - prioritize media outlets, podcasts, or experts that base their content on sound research, not style. Before consuming or sharing a post, ask yourself who stands to benefit from this message: is it genuinely helpful for you, or is it aimed at driving sales?

3. **Reject Sensationalized Marketing Tactics** – Sensationalism in marketing preys on our emotions and misplaced desires, often using fear, urgency, or exaggerated claims to manipulate our decisions. It's important to reject these tactics by recognizing them for what they are—attempts to sell us products and ideas, not provide useful information. Be wary of buzzwords, which are often used to make products seem more essential than they are. When you are looking for food products, it may help to rely on shopping lists you created earlier as this keeps you from being distracted by thousands of different marketing techniques used to sell items in the store.

4. **Trust Your Own Needs** – Don't underestimate the importance of trusting your own needs. You are your best advocate when it comes to your health. And remember, what works for someone else might not be the best for you. Pay attention to how your body responds to different foods and health practices; don't feel pressured to follow a trend just because it's popular. Rather than overhauling your lifestyle based on one influencer or article, balance external advice with your own preferences and experience.

5.   **Stay Focused on Specific Goals** – Marketing works by creating distractions and making you believe you need something that, chances are, you probably don't. The key to overcoming this is staying laser-focused on your personal health goals and not getting swept up in hype or sensational headlines. Reflect on what truly aligns with your life and well-being, and resist being led astray by fads or trends that promise quick fixes. Clarity in your goals will prevent others from determining them for you.

Even when you learn to see through marketing's deceptive tactics, the challenge of finding trustworthy nutrition expertise remains—next, we'll explore why it's so difficult to identify credible guidance and how to navigate a world full of conflicting advice.

CHAPTER 4: EXPERTISE

"The whole problem with the world is that fools and fanatics are always so certain of themselves and wiser people so full of doubts."
— **Bertrand Russell**

Becoming an expert in nutrition while navigating through our busy lives and pursuing diverse interests is not something most of us can realistically achieve. Yet, we all understand how crucial food is to our health, and that's why we seek out trusted voices for guidance. Unfortunately, in a world where subjective opinions often overshadow objective facts, finding reliable information on nutrition has become increasingly difficult.

While healthy debates can contribute to our collective knowledge, the lack of clear standards leaves many of us confused about who to believe. In fact, a survey revealed that nearly half of adults' struggle to find trustworthy information on healthy diets, with both experts and media playing a big part in this confusion.[1]

In "*The Death of Expertise*" Tom Nichols argues that shifts in our culture and the rise of the internet have harmed our ability to rely on true experts. Whether it's due to profit-driven education systems, personal biases, or the sensationalist nature of modern media, expert knowledge is now in a precarious position.[2]

In this chapter, we'll dive into why many so-called authorities in nutrition can be misleading, and how you can identify the ones who truly know what they're talking about. We'll also cover essential critical thinking skills that will help you stay skeptical in a healthy way and find the kind of advice that can actually benefit your health.

WHAT SHOULD EXPERTISE LOOK LIKE?

True expertise isn't just about possessing a title or making big claims. Expertise is a trait that's earned through deep learning, hands-on experience, and practical application in a specific field. Whether it's healthcare, education, business, or technology, we count on experts to solve complex problems, guide our decisions, and expand our understanding of the world.

Unfortunately, in the field of nutrition, recognizing real expertise has become harder than ever now because there are far more voices competing for attention. We're bombarded with advice from best-selling books, social media influencers, TV doctors, and even well-meaning relatives. It's easy to get lost in all this noise, but more information doesn't always mean better information. In fact, the overwhelming volume can dilute the quality and clarity of the advice we truly need.

We seem to be at an all-time high of those labeling themselves as "nutrition experts" on social media, even if they lack qualifications or evidence to back up their legitimacy. Now more than ever, it's critical to seek out and recognize genuine experts—those who are not only qualified but have a proven track record of helping people navigate the often-confusing world of nutrition.

SOURCES OF AUTHORITY

When looking for advice on nutrition, there's a variety of sources you can turn to that claim to guide you toward better health. One common source people turn to is popular nutrition books, which have become more widespread as more people focus on healthy living. But the question is, are these books really reliable sources of information? Let's take a look.

BOOKS

After reading over 100 popular nutrition books myself, I can say with confidence that a vast majority of them are full of misinformation. But how does so much bad information make it into best-sellers? A big reason is that many of these books are written by people who don't have the necessary expertise in nutrition. Just take a look at the next graphic on authorship to see who is publishing the most purchased nutrition books.

Author Occupation

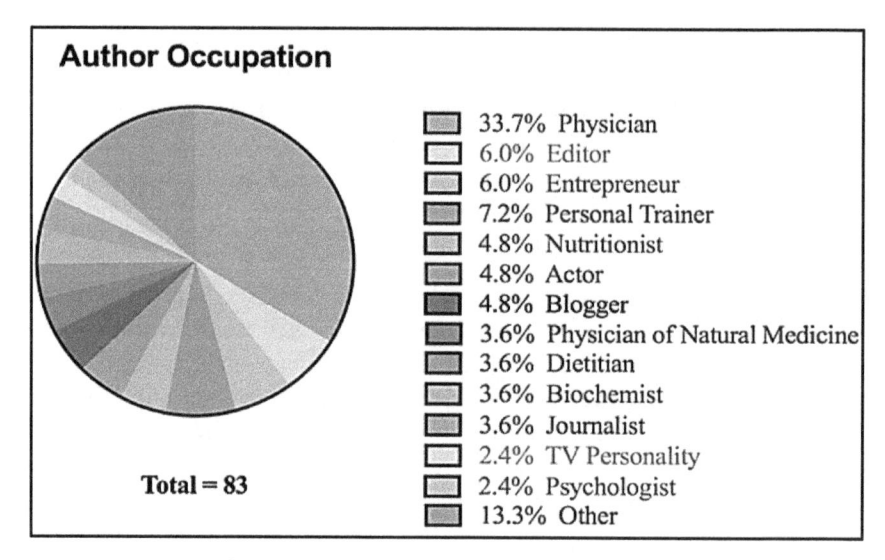

- 33.7% Physician
- 6.0% Editor
- 6.0% Entrepreneur
- 7.2% Personal Trainer
- 4.8% Nutritionist
- 4.8% Actor
- 4.8% Blogger
- 3.6% Physician of Natural Medicine
- 3.6% Dietitian
- 3.6% Biochemist
- 3.6% Journalist
- 2.4% TV Personality
- 2.4% Psychologist
- 13.3% Other

Total = 83

As you can see, it highlights that a significant number of these authors are medical doctors who, despite their credentials, receive fewer than 20 hours of nutrition education during their four years of medical school.[3,4] Certainly, their medical training might give them authority on other health topics, but their limited education in nutrition makes them ill-equipped to provide high-quality, accurate information in this area. We'll explore how certain biases shape the content of these books later on.

A closer look reveals that 31 of the top 100 best-selling nutrition books from 2008-2015 claim to cure or prevent diseases like diabetes, heart disease, cancer, and dementia.[5] While these bold promises may inspire hope, they're often misleading. Especially considering that many of these books actually *contradict* each other. One book may claim that a carnivore diet is the only way to achieve optimal health, while another insists that veganism is the only path forward.

The truth is that many of these authors are simply promoting what worked for them, framing it as a universal solution, complete with flashy promises and rigid meal plans that leave little room for alternatives.[6] While these approaches may sell books, they rarely lead to lasting health improvements.

Another major issue with popular nutrition books is the questionable quality of their references. Many of the citations are either irrelevant, weak or even contradict the points the authors are trying to make. Most readers don't have the time or expertise to fact-check these references, so they often go unchallenged. This gives authors free rein to make nearly any claim they want. In my own experience fact-checking these books, I've found the accuracy of the references to be alarmingly low. Some books don't even bother to include references at all (which is a big red flag).

One study found that only 65 out of 100 U.S. diet and health books had references, a shocking number when you think about how important it is for health-related books to be thoroughly backed by evidence.[7] Another study focusing on Canadian nutrition books found that many authors used their publications to promote their own products and services, revealing how these books are often more about making money than actually helping people get healthier.[8]

Back in 1982, a book called *"The Sense and Nonsense of Best-Selling Diet Books"* called out the same issues we see today in the world of diet literature. Despite being written over 40 years ago, its criticisms remain surprisingly relevant. The author had hoped that the more people became educated about the importance of good nutrition and regular exercise, the more diet books would eventually move away from gimmicks and focus more on promoting lifelong healthy eating habits.[9] Unfortunately, the trend of popular diet books overpromising and underdelivering is still going strong, proving that little has changed in the world of nutrition literature or our collective susceptibility to nutrition nonsense.

DOCUMENTARIES

Documentaries have a unique power to stir up emotions. They often lead viewers to make dramatic lifestyle changes after just a couple of hours of screen time. While some documentaries can be effective tools for social change, many that cover nutrition are heavily skewed toward a particular dietary ideology. Instead of presenting a well-rounded view of health, they tend to cherry-pick data that supports their message, often leaving viewers with a distorted understanding of nutrition. A standout example of this is the 2018 documentary *"The Game Changers."*

"The Game Changers" follows James Wilks, an elite Special Forces trainer and *"The Ultimate Fighter"* winner, as he travels the globe to discover the best diet for human performance.[10] The documentary tells a compelling story, which certainly had me believing every word when I first watched it. But it does so by selectively presenting evidence to support its pro-plant-based argument. For instance, it highlights the 2016 UFC fight between Conor McGregor, who followed a meat-heavy diet, and Nate Diaz, a plant-based athlete.[11] When Diaz won the fight, the documentary implies that his plant-based diet played a crucial role in his victory, conveniently ignoring that McGregor won their rematch later that same year.

By leaving out this detail, the documentary pushes a narrative that diet was the key factor when, really, both fighters' success had much more to do with their individual skills and training regimens than with what they ate. Yes, athletes can excel on a plant-based diet, but they can also perform at peak levels on a diet that includes animal products.

The documentary doesn't stop there. It even manipulates nutrition perspectives to fit its narrative. For instance, the documentary points out that plants have 64 times more antioxidants than animal products and that iceberg lettuce contains more antioxidants than salmon or eggs.[12] While this is definitely true, it's not the whole story when it comes to nutrition. Salmon and eggs, for instance, are packed with essential nutrients like protein, omega-3 fatty acids, and vitamins that are crucial for overall health. Iceberg lettuce, on the other hand, does not offer many of those benefits, so it's really not a beneficial comparison. A more honest approach would have been to discuss the pros and cons of both plant and animal foods, acknowledging that each has unique benefits and limitations.

Lastly, "The Game Changers" critiques industry-funded research, particularly studies funded by the meat and dairy industries, as biased and unreliable. However, it fails to mention that many of the studies it relies on for its pro-plant-based stance were funded by plant-based organizations, like the Hass Avocado Board.[13] This one-sided attack undermines the film's credibility and highlights a common problem with health documentaries in general: instead of offering viewers a balanced array of information so they can make informed choices, these films often push a particular agenda. The result is a distorted view of nutrition that doesn't account for the complexity of diet and health.

Although nutrition documentaries are well-intentioned in trying to point out peak nutritional standards, they never seem to recognize the achievements of other legendary athletes who followed less-than-perfect diets that can still provide plenty of fuel for competition. For example, during his intense training for the 2008 Beijing Olympics, Michael Phelps famously consumed a staggering amount of food, which included fried egg sandwiches, pancakes, and pizza.[14]

Similarly, Usain Bolt was known for eating around 100 chicken nuggets per day during those same Olympics, which was the year he set the record for the fastest 100-meter dash time ever recorded.[15] While these diets might not be ideal in the long run, it's misleading for documentaries to suggest that anything below a perfect diet will completely derail our health or that one specific diet is ideal for humans as we have plenty of examples of athletes who thrive on more varied diets.

PODCASTS

Many listeners tune in to podcasts hoping for trustworthy health advice, only to end up making decisions based on exaggerated or inaccurate statements. Even experts can get caught up in this, presenting oversimplified or misleading information to make their content more engaging.

One podcast that I was always intrigued by that consistently ranks at the top of the science, education, and health charts is hosted by a neuroscientist and professor at a prestigious university.[16] While he's made significant contributions to the fields of brain development and neuroplasticity, he occasionally ventures into topics outside his expertise, such as nutrition. Though he often invites guests to speak on these topics, some of them, including a popular author who has written several nutrition books, are known for presenting low quality information.

In a 2023 episode, this popular author referenced a study on sugar-sweetened beverages but got many of the details wrong. He claimed that participants in the study who were asked to consume full-sugar soda gained 22 pounds, while also claiming that the diet soda group gained 4.4 pounds, and that the water group lost 4.4 pounds.[17] In reality, none of the groups experienced significant weight changes after consuming one liter of soda per day for six months. The actual study found only a small increase in fat mass in the full-sugar soda group and a slight reduction in abdominal fat in the diet soda group.[18] The guest exaggerated the results to make his anti-sugar argument more compelling, glossing over the actual findings in favor of a more sensational narrative.

This kind of misinformation highlights a broader issue in health podcasts: the tendency to distort or oversimplify complex information to fit a particular viewpoint. In this case, the host also failed to challenge the guest's claims, allowing the misinformation to pass unchecked. It's for this reason listeners might walk away with an exaggerated fear of sugar and sugar substitutes despite scientific evidence showing that moderate consumption is not to be feared, but is just something to be mindful of.

It is important to note that sugar-sweetened beverages are indeed linked to higher body weight and an increased risk of cardiometabolic diseases like type 2 diabetes. However, exaggerating these risks, as the guest did, can lead to unnecessary fear and extreme diet beliefs that steer us away from sustainable habits.[19,20]

In another interview, the same podcast host was asked about his habit of promoting supplements even when they have limited evidence to support using them. His response was revealing: "People have different thresholds for what they consider worth trying... For some, it's 20 years of randomized controlled trials. For others, it's a mouse study. For some, it's the guy at the gym."[21] While it's true that people have varying standards for what counts as reliable evidence, a responsible science communicator should aim to raise those standards and not pander to the lowest common denominator.

Podcasts have the potential to educate and inspire, but they also run the risk of spreading misinformation when hosts and guests prioritize engagement over accuracy. For listeners, this means approaching podcasts with a critical mindset and seeking out content that is rooted in solid, evidence-based research rather than falling for persuasive yet unsubstantiated claims.

CELEBRITIES

Celebrities hold a unique place in our lives, often influencing everything from what we wear to how we eat. This influence is rooted in a combination of constant exposure and our innate desire for status. When we see familiar faces endorsing certain health practices or diets, it's easy to trust them, even if they aren't qualified to give that advice. After all, we want to believe that if we mimic their behavior, we might somehow achieve their looks or success.[22]

One particular celebrity who has gained a massive following in the wellness community is Gwenyth Paltrow. Despite her acting success, her health advice is often questionable. In a recent interview, she revealed that she frequently uses IV therapy, claiming, "I love an IV... it's really important to support my detox."[23,24] The problem? Detoxes and routine IV therapy are not supported by credible science. She also mentioned trying to follow a paleo diet, but without having to do much research, none of our ancestors were using IV treatments. If she just consumed more nutrient-rich foods on a regular schedule, she likely wouldn't feel the need for such ridiculous interventions.

Her extreme routines have sparked backlash, with some fans accusing her of promoting disordered eating. She's even earned the title of "almond mom," a term used to describe women who are overly fixated on diet culture and thinness, often at the expense of real health.

Unfortunately, this actress isn't the only celebrity promoting questionable health advice. Another well-known actress recently stirred controversy by claiming that "You really only need about 600 calories per day."[25] Later, she clarified that this extreme restriction was only part of detox—which is still not helpful.

Such statements are dangerously misleading. Every adult needs far more than 600 calories a day to function properly, and promoting such extreme caloric limits is harmful. It's a stark reminder that fame doesn't equal expertise, and many celebrities are far from qualified to offer health and nutrition advice.

FAMILY AND FRIENDS

When it comes to conversations about nutrition, family and friends can be both a blessing and a curse. I've had many productive, meaningful discussions with people in my life, but I've also had my fair share of frustrating ones. I remember one friend who was completely sold on the keto diet. He lost a significant amount of weight, and soon everyone around him was convinced that keto was the magic solution. But a year later, he admitted to me that "I regained all the weight and more" and he just felt like a failure. He ultimately blamed himself, thinking he just didn't have the willpower to stick with it. But the truth is, the *diet* was the problem, not him.

Another friend of mine dove headfirst into the vegan craze a few years ago when acai bowls and goji berries were all the rage. Like my keto friend, he lost weight and felt great at first. But what he didn't realize was that the key to his weight loss wasn't just the plant-based diet. He had also cut out a lot of unhealthy, calorie-dense foods like soda, desserts, and fast food—which he replaced with more nutritious home-cooked meals. The real magic wasn't in the plants alone; it was in the overall improvement in the quality of his diet. So, if he had gone another dietary route—swapping fries for lean meats instead of vegetables, the result would have been similar due to the lower calorie intake and better food choices.

Family members, too, can have a powerful influence on our eating habits, often more than we realize. Growing up, I constantly heard the phrase, "Finish everything on your plate." This kind of well-meaning advice, passed down from one generation to the next, can set the stage for unhealthy eating patterns. Parents often try to give us the tools for a successful life, but if they don't have a solid understanding of nutrition themselves, they can unintentionally pass down bad habits. Children naturally absorb the behaviors of those around them, and this can lead to lifelong struggles with food. While family members usually have the best intentions, their nutrition advice isn't always based on sound science.

SOCIAL MEDIA STRATEGY

Spend any amount of time on social media, and you'll quickly notice a pattern: to attract followers, you need to find your niche. In the world of nutrition, that might mean focusing on gluten-free recipes, keto-friendly meal plans, or vegan eating. A well-defined niche helps influencers stand out in a crowded space, drawing in an audience with specific interests.

One of the strengths of social media is its ability to cater to niche topics, offering targeted advice to people with unique dietary needs. However, the danger lies in how these niches can create blind spots. For instance, following an account like "Keto King" or "Vegan Nutrition Coach" can narrow your perspective. These accounts are often highly focused on promoting a specific dietary ideology, and because their identity is so closely tied to it, they are likely to defend it, even when faced with conflicting evidence.

Many of these accounts start off innocently enough, providing helpful tips and recipes. But as they grow in popularity, some influencers become more concerned with promoting *their* diet as the best option, rather than offering a balanced view. Once an influencer has built their brand around a specific dietary philosophy, there's a lot of pressure to stick with it. The fear of losing followers can make it difficult for them to adjust their message, even if new evidence suggests their approach isn't as effective as they once thought.

Followers of these niche accounts are often just as biased as the influencers they follow. When someone commits to a particular diet, they're more likely to experience positive results, whether due to the diet itself or because of their belief in it. This creates a cycle of confirmation bias, where they only see evidence that supports their existing views, regardless of the diet's actual effectiveness.

Another major issue with social media is the lack of regulation or oversight. If you've spent any time online, you've probably noticed that literally anyone can claim to be a nutrition expert. And in a space where popularity often trumps qualifications, it can be hard to tell the difference between sound advice and snake oil. Some of the top Instagram accounts offering nutrition advice aren't run by registered dietitians or professional nutritionists but by individuals with different backgrounds and qualifications, such as:

- Entrepreneur
- Chiropractor
- Pharmacist
- Neuroscientist
- Biochemist
- Psychiatrist
- Physician
- Personal Trainer

While these influencers might be highly knowledgeable in their respective fields, most of them lack the specialized training necessary to provide high-quality nutritional guidance. Even doctors, scientists, and fitness experts may not have received the in-depth nutrition education required to offer sound dietary advice. And yet, their massive follower counts often lend them an air of credibility that isn't always deserved.

Ideally, social media would be a place for diverse, evidence-based perspectives, but all too often, it becomes an echo chamber of niche ideologies, where personal preferences and unverified beliefs are shared as facts. This is why it's so important to approach social media with caution, seeking out information from qualified professionals and always questioning the claims being made, especially when they come from someone with a strong, niche-driven agenda.

CAN YOU TRUST A DOCTOR IF THEY AREN'T FIT?

In the world of social media, we're often drawn to people who look the part—those with great physiques and polished appearances. It's natural to assume that someone who appears fit might know more about health and wellness. But does physical fitness actually determine how trustworthy their advice is? If you visited a doctor or healthcare professional who wasn't in peak shape, should it impact how much you trust their guidance? While it's easy to think that a fit person is automatically more credible, the truth is far more nuanced and requires considerations like:

Expertise vs. Personal Habits – A person can offer excellent advice without necessarily following it themselves. Circumstances like work stress, genetic conditions, or mental health issues might prevent them from practicing what they preach.

Perception of Trust – I don't expect my mechanic to drive a perfect car themselves to trust their ability to fix mine. Judging their abilities based on personal habits might sometimes line up, but it isn't an accurate way of assessing their ability and expertise. Similarly, a doctor's fitness might not reflect their professional abilities.

Comfort and Bias – Our comfort level and biases play a huge role in whom we trust. Some people feel more inclined to listen to someone who "looks the part," while others might prefer a doctor who doesn't come across as the epitome of fitness. This preference is often rooted in our personal experiences. For example, if you've struggled with weight or fitness yourself, you might feel more connected to a healthcare provider who shares those challenges. Alternatively, if you're seeking a role model or inspiration, you might gravitate toward someone who appears physically fit. Neither preference is wrong, but it's essential to recognize that our biases don't always correlate with someone's actual knowledge or ability to help us.

At the end of the day, expertise, experience, and context should carry more weight than physical appearance. Consider these examples:

- Would you trust an oncologist who has successfully treated countless cancer patients or a cancer survivor with no medical training but a compelling personal story?

- Would you value advice more from Bill Belichick, a Super Bowl-winning coach, or from a high school football star who looks more fit but lacks the same experience and insight?

The point is that while physical fitness can be impressive, it isn't a reliable measure of someone's professional ability. What truly matters is their knowledge, skill, and ability to offer sound, evidence-based advice. Just because someone isn't the picture of fitness doesn't mean they can't guide you toward better health.

REGULATED TITLES

In the U.S., several nutrition and healthcare titles are regulated by strict education and experience standards, but many people don't know what these titles really represent. Understanding the differences can help you figure out if a professional is truly qualified to give the nutrition advice you need. While fancy titles and letters after someone's name don't guarantee a great experience or even outstanding competence, they serve as a good indicator of their education and training background.

REGISTERED DIETITIANS

The term "Registered Dietitian" (RD) can sound outdated and unappealing, often conjuring up the image of the "food police" rather than someone offering practical, everyday advice. It's no wonder that many RDs now prefer to use the title "Registered Dietitian Nutritionist" (RDN) because *nutritionist* sounds more relatable to the average person. Regardless of the title, RDs undergo rigorous training that spans clinical settings, food service, and community education.

Here's a look at the comprehensive training every RD must complete:

- **Educational Requirements** – RDs must hold at least a bachelor's degree in nutrition or a related field, and they are required to complete a 7–12 month accredited dietetic internship. As of 2024, a master's degree will also be mandatory.

- **Licensing Exam** – They must pass a national exam administered by the Commission on Dietetic Registration (CDR), which has a pass rate of just 65%.[26]

- **Continuing Education** – RDs are required to complete 75 hours of continuing education every five years to keep their license active.

- **Scope of Practice** – RDs are trained to assess, diagnose, and treat nutritional issues, providing evidence-based dietary recommendations. Their expertise covers medical nutrition therapy (MNT), calculating tube feedings, creating nutrition policies, ensuring food safety, and counseling individuals on specific dietary needs.[27]

Despite their extensive training, RDs sometimes fall short in addressing the everyday challenges people face. Many individuals seek guidance on navigating social media trends and processed foods or learning practical skills like meal prepping, areas where traditional RD training can be lacking. While RDs are equipped with a strong foundation in nutrition science and clinical skills, the ability to creatively apply that knowledge to real-world problems is often what helps people connect and engage.

It's also important to recognize that RDs, like any professionals, have specializations. Not every RD is equipped to handle every health issue such as eating disorders, sports nutrition, or rare diseases. While RDs offer the best chance at staying in-line with the most ideal nutrition advice, I have seen many of them fall into the trap of promoting non-evidence-based practices like juice cleanses or excessive supplements despite their rigorous training.

That said, RDs remain the gold standard for nutrition professionals, given the stringent education and training they undergo. However, when seeking out their help, it's important to look at their background, specializations, and how well their approach aligns with your personal goals. If you are looking for one to provide professional nutrition advice you may need to try out more than one as sometimes it may not be a good relational match.

Fun fact: The word "dietitian" is one of the most commonly misspelled words in healthcare. Since 1954, when *Time Magazine* listed it as one of the 20 most misspelled words, many people have spelled it "dietician" with a C instead of "dietitian" with a T.[28]

DIETITIANS AND BIG FOOD

The dietitian profession is poised for significant growth, but like many responsible careers, it is also facing challenges. While many dietitians uphold the highest standards, some may not realize how their work is being influenced by large food corporations, often referred to as "Big Food."

In today's food landscape, dietitians are sometimes caught between delivering unbiased advice and facing industry pressure. Because of this, it's not uncommon for biased information to be spread, a growing concern both in the U.S. and internationally. That said, not all ties to the food industry are inherently bad. For many families, especially those facing food insecurity, processed foods can fill a necessary gap, offering affordable and accessible nutrition.

Dietitians can help the general public figure out which processed foods are genuinely beneficial and how to strike a balance between modern food products and whole foods, which can be tricky to figure out. Because of this, navigating the balance between corporate influence and practical nutrition advice is essential. Dietitians must remain objective, avoiding industry bias, while still providing realistic, applicable guidance that includes both whole and processed foods in a responsible way. From my experience, this balance is achievable, but is something RDs need to be mindful of as it can be easy to get pulled into either extreme direction—over promoting processed foods or fear mongering all of them.

Nevertheless, we should continue to hold dietitians to high standards, expecting them to deliver unbiased, effective advice that meets the modern-day challenges of nutrition. Personally, I choose not to accept money or gifts from food companies in exchange for endorsements as I want to stay vigilant to the concerns of industry influence. However, positive and transparent relationships between dietitians and the food industry can still have beneficial outcomes, provided they are rooted in integrity and clear communication.

STAYING WITHIN YOUR SCOPE

As an RD myself, I also realize the limits of my scope of practice. I know fully well I'm not qualified to diagnose medical conditions, crack backs, or provide mental health counseling. While I can appreciate their importance and promote basic guidelines from other areas of health. I also know when to refer patients and clients to those with knowledge that I simply do not have, as it would be irresponsible for me to overstep into areas where I am untrained. While holistic care is valuable, sticking to your professional scope is also very important. Ethics should never be compromised for the sake of ego or attention, yet too often, they are. This goes the other way too—other healthcare professionals have a tendency to offer nutrition advice to patients and clients when it really is not appropriate.

CERTIFIED NUTRITION SPECIALIST (CNS)

The title Certified Nutrition Specialist (CNS) is relatively new but is also a regulated designation that signifies a higher level of competency in providing nutritional care, depending on where they practice. The requirements for becoming a CNS include:

- **Educational Background** – A master's or doctoral degree in nutrition or a related healthcare field from an accredited institution.

- **Coursework** – Completion of courses in nutrition, biochemistry, physiology or anatomy/physiology, and other sciences such as biology, microbiology, and organic chemistry.

- **Supervised Experience** – A minimum of 1,000 hours of supervised practice.

- **Licensing Exam** – Passing a national exam with a current pass rate of 70.5%.[29]

CNS professionals are trained to provide evidence-based dietary recommendations, personalized nutrition plans, and counseling to address various health concerns.[30]

While I've personally encountered very few CNS professionals before, it appears that the training they receive is extensive enough, and it's likely we'll be seeing more of them in the future. However, it's essential that we hold them to the same high standards that apply to other nutrition professionals.

NUTRITION PhDs

Possessing a PhD in nutrition from an accredited university represents one of the highest levels of expertise a person in the field can achieve. Individuals with this degree often have advanced knowledge in research and education, and they excel in critical thinking and analyzing complex nutritional data. Although their focus is more on research and academia than on direct patient care, they offer a deep and thorough understanding of nutrition science.

In my experience, PhDs in nutrition can offer incredibly valuable insights, especially when it comes to interpreting research. However, their effectiveness in working directly with patients or clients may vary, depending on their background and practical skills. Like any professional, a PhDs ability to apply their knowledge in real-world situations is what sets them apart.

SO, WHAT IS A NUTRITIONIST THEN?

The term "nutritionist" is perhaps the most misleading in the nutrition field. Unlike "dietitian," the term isn't regulated in the U.S., so anyone can call themselves a nutritionist regardless of education or qualifications. My toddler could literally call himself a nutritionist and no one would bat an eye. This lack of regulation is unfortunate because the term nutritionist carries weight in the *public's* eyes, which seems like credible expertise that may or may actually exist.

The Cleveland Clinic offers a great analogy for understanding the difference between a "nutritionist" and a regulated professional. It's like choosing between getting a haircut from a friend with a pair of clippers or going to a licensed barber. Both might cut your hair, but you're more likely to trust the barber's skills.[31] While some nutritionists do have legitimate expertise, the title alone doesn't guarantee it.

Personally, I don't mind if people refer to me as a nutritionist because they trust my expertise, but it's critical to remember that without formal education and training, the term lacks credibility.

CERTIFICATION CONFUSION

The world of health, nutrition, and life coaching is crowded with minimal barriers to entry. While some coaches excel, many lack the depth of knowledge needed to provide credible advice.

When I first started my path of nutrition exploration, I completed a 12-month online nutrition certification. While it gave me a basic foundation of nutrition principles, most online certifications today are much shorter, some as brief as 4 to 6 weeks, and lack the depth required for real expertise. It's like comparing basic math to advanced calculus; you can't expect the same level of understanding from a short program as you would from years of formal education.

Virginia Aronson, a journalist, dietitian, and textbook author, explored these types of online nutrition certifications to find out just how they operated. She went undercover and purposely provided wrong answers in a nutrition certification course, yet received high grades and even a diploma with honors.[32] This experience revealed just how low-quality some certification programs can be:

"When I took the first test, I deliberately gave some answers that contradicted information in the school's lesson. My exam was returned to me with a surprisingly high grade. On the second exam, I again gave some answers that contradicted information in the lesson. To my surprise, I received a grade of 100 percent and an accompanying note congratulating me on the 'excellent manner in which you have completed the Nutrition course.' I then sent $10 for the 'Nutritionist' certificate to hang on my office wall. Although the certificate includes an attractive gold seal and indicates that I graduated 'Cum Laude,' my colleagues in the Harvard Nutrition Department seem unimpressed by it."[32]

Many of these certifications are essentially "diploma mills" designed to churn out graduates quickly and profitably. They require minimal educational effort and offer content that can be easily acquired after 10 minutes on the internet.

While alternative certifications can be valuable starting points, they often fail to provide the rigorous education needed for true expertise. This isn't to say that more traditional degrees are perfect; they, too, deserve scrutiny. But if we applied consistent, fair criticism to all those claiming expertise, many unqualified coaches and nutritionists would likely fade from the public eye.

Having gone through both alternative certification programs and an RD program, the difference in expertise is as clear as night and day. During my RD rotations, I was pushed by doctors and professionals who questioned every health decision and made me apply the most rigorous science. On the other hand, my certification program often focused more on personal diet preferences than on solid scientific principles. While affordable and accessible nutrition certifications with high standards are important, most certifications available today don't provide the level of expertise needed—so watch out.

MISPLACED TRUST IN OTHER TITLES

Whether it's a psychologist, scientist, movie star, self-proclaimed biohacker, or even the Pope, holding a title outside the field of nutrition doesn't equate to expertise in it. Just because someone eats food and has an impressive title next to their name doesn't mean they're qualified to discuss nutritional biochemistry or provide dietary counseling. Even individuals with some background in nutrition may not possess the depth of knowledge required for truly effective guidance.

If you're seeking solid, in-depth nutrition advice, it's crucial to choose someone with the right education, training, and experience to deliver meaningful results. On the other hand, if all you need is someone to tell you that fruits and vegetables are healthy or to confirm your own biases, nearly anyone can do that. Don't be swayed by impressive titles that lend false credibility to superficial advice.

HOW TO SPOT TRUE EXPERTISE

Although sorting through the various titles and educational backgrounds of those claiming nutrition expertise can be challenging, there are reliable ways to assess someone's true competence. My goal isn't just to tell you which titles to trust but to help you identify the qualities of genuinely knowledgeable professionals. Ultimately, what matters most are results—effective, practical advice that improves nutrition habits. To help you distinguish between nutrition scams and legitimate experts, here are 12 key green and red flags to look for:

THE 12 GREEN AND RED FLAGS OF AN EXPERT

Green Flags	Red Flags
1. Embraces Criticism: Uses feedback as an opportunity to educate or learn and shows humility towards other sources of authority.	**1. Dismisses Criticism:** Rejects feedback without valid reasons, labeling critics as "haters" and feeling threatened by intelligent people.
2. Contextual Advice: Offers general advice but acknowledges the need for context and admits to gray areas when necessary.	**2. Rigid Thinking:** Makes absolute statements and applies a one-size-fits-all approach, ignoring nuance.
3. Open-Mindedness: Willing to change their mind when presented with a better argument, recognizing errors and striving to learn.	**3. Stubborn Beliefs:** Clings to beliefs despite overwhelming evidence to the contrary, often responding with hostility.
4. Continual Learning: Actively learns from resources like textbooks, rescarch, and mentors, rather than just focusing on teaching.	**4. Neglects Learning:** Spends more time "teaching" others than continuing their own education.
5. Skeptical of Trends: Approaches new ideas with skepticism and requires substantial proof before adopting them.	**5. Trend Follower:** Embraces new trends without questioning the evidence behind them.
6. Clear Explanations: Can explain complex subjects in simple terms, demonstrating a deep understanding of the topic.	**6. Complicated Jargon:** Uses overly complex jargon and scientific-sounding terms without clear understanding.

7. Consistency in Principles: Applies the same principles consistently across different scenarios.	**7. Cognitive Dissonance:** Displays contradictory behavior, such as promoting non-toxic cleaners but using Botox injections.
8. Trusted Experience: Has applicable experience in their field, with a career that reflects their knowledge and expertise.	**8. Lacks Relevant Experience:** Oversteps their expertise, claiming to have all the answers without legitimate experience or recognition.
9. Focus on Solutions: Prioritizes idea-driven, lasting solutions over quick fixes.	**9. Focus on Quick Fixes:** Prioritizes fast, easy solutions and seeks external validation.
10. High Standards and Character: Upholds strong ethical standards and quality in their work.	**10. High Charisma, Low Integrity:** Charismatic but lacks concern for the quality of information or the well-being of others.
11. Balanced Knowledge: Can state both obvious and new facts, showing a strong grasp of foundational knowledge.	**11. Repeats Statements:** Repeats obvious facts like "added sugar is bad" without offering new insights or understanding deeper concepts.
12. Confident, yet Cautious: Speaks with confidence but uses language that acknowledges uncertainty when appropriate.	**12. Overconfidence:** Displays excessive confidence and certainty, ignoring the complexity and nuance of nutrition.

CRITICAL THINKING HABITS

If you're still unsure which experts to trust, it might be time to step back from the noise and focus on building a foundation of critical thinking. True nutrition experts tend to agree on key principles, while the contradictions you often hear come from less qualified voices, such as media outlets or self-proclaimed health gurus without proper education.

Developing critical thinking skills can help you evaluate true expertise more effectively. It's not about being negative; it's about being objective, open-minded, and inquisitive. Critical thinking involves analyzing information based on evidence, not personal opinions or biases. This approach leads to deeper understanding and better decision-making.

CHAPTER 4: EXPERTISE

WHERE DID THIS NONSENSE COME FROM?

True expertise is not just about titles or popularity. It's about providing a depth of practical knowledge that can stand the test of time and bear the weight of criticism. Having a high level of authority shows trust that was gained over time, but it doesn't necessarily mean every idea or action is trustworthy. Here are some of the reasons we fall for bad advice from those claiming expertise.

DUNNING-KRUGER EFFECT

The Dunning-Kruger Effect is a cognitive bias where people with limited knowledge in a field overestimate their abilities. When I first started learning about nutrition, my confidence was sky-high, even though my actual understanding was shallow. As I pursued more education, my confidence dipped and has never returned to that early peak, thankfully, because it's allowed me to keep learning and growing. Recognizing this bias is crucial because it takes humility to admit when you're wrong and to continue improving. The more you learn, the more you realize how much you don't know, which can be both humbling and liberating.

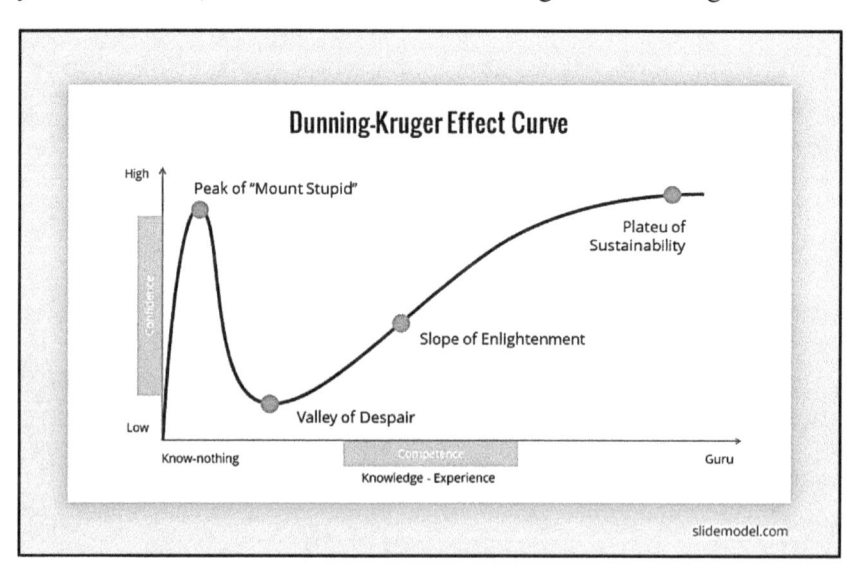

NOBEL PRIZE SYNDROME

Perhaps the opposite extreme of the Dunning-Kruger effect is the *Nobel Prize Syndrome*. Nobel Prize Syndrome refers to the phenomenon where Nobel laureates, after winning their prize, mistakenly believe their expertise extends to other fields.[33] This can lead them to make bold, unfounded claims outside their domain of expertise.[34] A prime example is Linus Pauling, who made groundbreaking discoveries in chemistry (winning the Nobel prize in 1954) but later became obsessed with vitamin C, claiming it could cure the common cold and even cancer, which is unsupported by evidence.[35,36]

Other examples include:

Brian Josephson (Physics Nobel Prize - 1973) – Promoted beliefs in telepathy and cold fusion.[37]

Nikolaas Tinbergen (Physiology/Medicine Nobel Prize - 1973) – Wrongly claimed that poor parenting causes autism.[38]

Luc Montagnier (Physiology/Medicine Nobel Prize - 2008) – Suggested antibiotics could treat autism.[39]

James Watson (DNA Discovery Nobel Prize - 1953) – Made claims about black people having lower intelligence and that sex drive was related to skin color.[40,41]

Nobel Prize Syndrome reminds us that even brilliant minds can fall prey to misguided ideas. If someone claims to know everything about multiple complex fields, it's a red flag. Expertise in one area doesn't grant authority in all areas.

APPEAL TO AUTHORITY

The "appeal to authority" is a cognitive bias where someone's opinion is trusted solely because of their title or status. This is most recognizable in celebrity worship or blind loyalty. But just because someone is a TV doctor, celebrity, or influential figure doesn't mean their advice is sound. Authority, even when backed by impressive credentials, can be misleading. Because of this, it's important to remain skeptical and evaluate all information critically, even from experts.

So as not to get too easily taken in by a person's status, remember to focus on the quality of their evidence and the logic behind their advice. By doing so, you empower yourself to make informed decisions rather than

EVERYBODY EATS

One of the most common biases in nutrition is the idea that everyone is an expert simply because... wait for it—everyone eats. Food is essential for survival, so naturally, most people have basic knowledge and experience about the subject. But for some, they feel that this makes them competent in the field of nutrition. Because, unlike fields such as physics or engineering, where specialized knowledge is required, food is something we engage with daily, making us feel like we've mastered it. This often leads to overconfidence in understanding complex aspects of nutrition science, research, and health counseling.

FALSE EQUIVALENCE FALLACY

Not all opinions hold equal weight. Just because two sides exist doesn't mean they deserve the same consideration. Teaching that 1+1=2 doesn't mean we should equally value the idea that 1+1=3, just because it's "it's offering another side". Similarly, the views of someone with no formal nutrition training shouldn't be placed on par with those of a professional who has dedicated years to studying and practicing in the field. Just because someone is likable or believable doesn't mean their argument holds water. It can often help to separate someone's advice from our previously held opinions about them.

MOTTE AND BAILEY FALLACY

The Motte and Bailey Fallacy happens when someone mixes a safe, easy-to-defend idea (the "Motte") with a more controversial one (the "Bailey").

A nutrition influencer might say, "Eating more vegetables is crucial for good health" (the Motte), which is a widely accepted and defensible statement. But they might also claim, "Therefore, you should only eat raw, organic vegetables and avoid all cooked foods because cooking destroys nutrients" (the Bailey). The first statement is solid advice, but the second is a much more extreme and controversial position that's not supported by evidence. The sensible advice to eat vegetables is essentially weaponized to give undeserved support to the more extreme claim. Just because someone offers good advice in one area doesn't mean their more controversial opinions are valid. Even a broken clock is right twice a day, so don't be swayed by selective truths.

HOW TO SEPARATE EXPERTS FROM CHARLATANS

1. **Question Experts and Those Claiming Expertise** – Remember, even highly respected experts can be wrong (and often they are). Stay critical and open-minded; understand that no one is immune to mistakes, regardless of their credentials. I've been critical of popular health influencers like Peter Attia before, but I also respect his willingness to admit when he was wrong, such as in past posts that overly promoted intermittent fasting and unnecessary biohacking.[42] When an expert changes their stance after being challenged with better evidence, it's a good indicator of credibility.

2. **Notice the Details** – Pay attention to the solid evidence behind the claims you encounter. There's a big difference between advice grounded in solid research and opinions based on personal experience alone. A resource like Red Pen Reviews, which fact-checks nutrition books, can help you separate credible information from unsupported assertions.[43]

3. **Be Skeptical but Productive** – Use skepticism not just to criticize but to deepen your understanding. If something doesn't add up, don't simply dismiss it. Seek out better solutions. Skepticism should lead to better answers, not just negativity.

4. **Activate Your BS Meter More Often** – Even sources you trust should be regularly questioned. Don't let familiarity or popularity cloud your judgment. Evaluate every claim with the same critical eye, no matter where it comes from.

5. **Demand Clear Explanations from Those Giving Advice** – A true expert should be able to break down complex concepts in a simple, understandable way or at least be honest about what they don't know. Be cautious of those who overcomplicate, deflect, or avoid giving straight answers.

Even when you learn to separate experts from charlatans, the complexity of nutrition science itself can still feel overwhelming—next, we'll dive into why the science of nutrition is often so confusing and how to navigate its many uncertainties with confidence.

CHAPTER 5: SCIENCE

"True scientists look for evidence to disprove their hypotheses, but pseudoscience looks for evidence to support it"

— **Karl Popper**

These days, science is pretty divisive. People react to it strongly, either positively or negatively. The chaos of COVID-19 and how the government responded have contributed to a decline in Americans' trust in scientists and science itself.[1] While a lot of this skepticism is understandable, it's crucial to refocus our understanding of science on the scientific process and critical thinking, not just the people or institutions we associate with them.

At its core, science is about using doubt and skepticism to refine knowledge. Through the scientific method, we can find answers to some of the most challenging problems. In nutrition science, this approach helps us identify the most relevant health recommendations by looking at a variety of independent sources that come together to form a consensus.

This chapter will explore the history of the field of nutrition and how current research methodologies can improve health span and lifespan. The goal isn't to push belief in any one person or institution but to highlight the value of curiosity and observation in understanding the world. Because of this, this chapter aims to differentiate between good and bad approaches to science to make more informed health and nutrition decisions.

WHAT IS SCIENCE?

A lot of people think science is an elitist discipline with rigid rules dictating our lives, but its fundamental principle is a structured process that helps us make more unbiased observations. As you may remember from school, the scientific method is a step-by-step approach that blends observation with skepticism, helping to limit the biases that can cloud our understanding of the world. Many of the nutrition myths debunked in this book would not have existed in the first place if we all applied a more skeptical perspective using the scientific method. To avoid falling into these traps, let's revisit the seven steps of the scientific method using a practical nutrition example:

STEP 1: Problem and Question

Example: You feel tired and hungry most mornings around 10 a.m., so you often overeat unhealthy snacks to maintain focus until lunchtime.

STEP 2: Observation and Research

You notice that your mornings are typically busy, and your breakfast usually consists of just a piece of toast or plain oatmeal. After researching healthy breakfast options, you find that they tend to include more protein-rich foods.

STEP 3: Hypothesis

You wonder if adding a protein-rich food, like an egg on toast or Greek yogurt to your oatmeal, might improve your mid-morning hunger.

STEP 4: Experiment

Design an experiment over two weeks:

Week 1 – Eat your usual breakfast.

Week 2 – Eat a higher-protein breakfast each day.

Keep other variables, like breakfast timing and portion size, consistent.

STEP 5: Data Collection

Record your hunger levels from breakfast until lunch on a scale of 1 to 10 for both weeks. Note any snacks you consume and how they affect your hunger.

STEP 6: Analysis

Compare hunger levels and snacking frequency between the two weeks. If week two shows lower hunger and fewer snacks, you might conclude that a high-protein breakfast helped. If there's no significant change, other factors may be influencing your hunger, prompting further investigation.

STEP 7: Report

Share your findings with a spouse or friend and keep your data for future reference. You might adjust your breakfast choices based on the results to better manage your hunger. I know I personally need a significant amount of both protein and food volume to keep me full until lunch every day.

CONTINUING THE SCIENTIFIC METHOD

To be a good scientist in your own life, don't settle for the first answer you stumble upon either. Continue applying a critical eye to any nutrition discovery and use skepticism to refine your understanding.

It's easy to stop at the most convenient answer, but true scientific inquiry always goes deeper. In the example above, even if you reduced your snack cravings, you shouldn't assume that protein was the sole factor, or that eggs are a universal solution for every nutrition problem you encounter.

Other factors, such as added fat, calories, or food volume, could have played a role in this scenario. Or perhaps it was this new motivation and belief at play that ultimately influenced your results. To truly understand your own personal nutrition findings, it may help to consult trusted expertise or continue collecting data from your observations.

The goal of the scientific method isn't to confirm what you want to believe, but to find the *most* correct answer. By applying this approach, you can make informed decisions about nutrition choices, like which breakfast habit can mitigate snack cravings throughout the day. This exact same scientific method has been applied to nutrition research efforts over the past 300 years, which has provided all of us with a wealth of fundamental knowledge.

A BRIEF HISTORY OF NUTRITION SCIENCE

Food has always been crucial for survival, but the science behind *how* it nourishes the human body has only recently begun to unfold. Modern nutrition research has made it possible to measure and understand the specific effects of individual food components. Although significant progress has been made, much of what is known about nutrition has only emerged relatively recently.

I personally love exploring the evolution of nutrition science and discovering what history can teach us about what we now know about our health. Let's take a quick look at some of the most intriguing milestones in this field.

CHAPTER 5: SCIENCE

NUTRITION DISCOVERY TIMELINE

1747 – One of the earliest nutrition discoveries occurred in 1747 when Dr. James Lind identified vitamin C as a cure for scurvy, a disease that caused weakness, anemia, gum disease, and poor wound healing, which claimed the lives of thousands of British sailors.[2] Lind conducted what is now considered one of the first randomized controlled trials. He divided twelve sailors with scurvy into six pairs, each receiving a different potential treatment. The two men, who were given citrus fruits like oranges and lemons, recovered within days, allowing them to care for other sick sailors.[3] Although the underlying mechanisms weren't fully understood at the time, we now know that their scurvy was cured by resolving a vitamin C deficiency. This pivotal discovery laid the groundwork for preventing and treating conditions with known nutritional remedies.

1780 – Antoine Lavoisier, the "father of modern chemistry," made a significant contribution to human health by describing metabolism and respiration. He demonstrated these processes by placing a guinea pig in a container connected to an ice-filled chamber.[4] Lavoisier found that animals generate heat by burning energy through respiration.[5] The heat produced by the guinea pig melted the surrounding ice, proving that respiration is a form of slow combustion that allows humans to convert food into energy.[3] This understanding also revealed that most of the energy we lose when burning fat exits the body as carbon dioxide through breathing.[6]

1897 – Dutch physician Christiaan Eijkman discovered that a vitamin B1 (thiamine) deficiency was the cause of beriberi, a disease that led to muscle weakness, speech difficulties, and shortness of breath.[7] While investigating a microbial cause in the Dutch East Indies, Eijkman observed a similar illness in chickens.[8] He noticed that chickens recovered from the illness when fed unpolished rice, which retained the outer layer rich in vitamin B1. This finding showed that restoring vitamin B1 in the diet could reverse beriberi symptoms, marking one of the first discoveries of the essential role of vitamins in human health.[9]

1912 – Researcher Gowland Hopkins found that his lab rats failed to develop properly without milk in their diet, suspecting an essential nutrient was missing.[10] In 1913, Elmer McCollum isolated "factor A" from butter and egg yolk, now known as vitamin A, which led to higher growth and survival rates in rats.[11] This breakthrough revealed the critical role of vitamin A in immunity, growth, reproduction, and vision.[12]

1920 – The discovery of vitamin D, which acts as a crucial hormone in the body, was pivotal in the treatment of rickets, a disease marked by bone weakness. Although the link between vitamin D and rickets had been observed since the 16th century, it wasn't until the 1920s that effective treatments emerged.[13] Cod liver oil, sunlight exposure, and irradiating foods to increase vitamin D levels were all used successfully to prevent rickets. This discovery was part of a broader understanding of vitamins that emerged in the early 20th century.[14]

1960s – Norman Borlaug, who began his work in agriculture in the 1940s, developed dwarf wheat strains resistant to disease and rust. By the 1960s, Borlaug introduced these wheat crops to India and Pakistan, which were facing food shortages due to population growth. The new wheat strains nearly doubled crop yields between 1965 and 1970, helping these countries become agriculturally self-sufficient. Borlaug's work, credited with saving over a billion people from starvation, earned him the title "father of the Green Revolution."[15]

A Glimpse into Nutrition History – This timeline offers only a small taste of some key discoveries that shaped our understanding of nutrition, from identifying essential vitamins to developing methods for combating global food crises. While there are many more milestones in this field, these examples underscore our fundamental nutritional needs and illustrate how the scientific process deepens our understanding of how to meet them.

CURRENT NUTRITION RESEARCH

We often take the discoveries made by previous generations for granted, yet these breakthroughs continue to shape our daily choices, particularly in health and nutrition. The scientific method is more than just a fascinating way to explore the world; it's the foundation of the reliable knowledge we depend on. One of humanity's greatest strengths is our ability to share this knowledge and build upon it. Without this shared understanding, every new generation would be stuck reinventing the wheel.

Think about electricity. Thanks to pioneers like Thomas Edison, we can flip a switch and light up our homes without a second thought. If we had to rediscover electricity from scratch every time, progress would be impossible. The same idea applies to nutrition. Much of what we know about which foods benefit our health has already been discovered, and we have easy access to this information through scientific literature. There's no longer a need to re-discover certain principles, only the need to continue learning more and applying them appropriately.

However, there's still much we don't know about nutrition. That's why it's crucial to build on existing knowledge. Diet fads and unproven theories persist because people often ignore the historical lessons that disprove them. Instead of relying on guesses or trends, we should turn to the best available evidence—data that's been rigorously collected, reviewed, and cataloged over the years.

Today, health and nutrition information is more accessible than ever, but it's also overwhelmed by a flood of misinformation. This makes it all the more important to rely on reliable evidence when making decisions. The way we approach and evaluate information can save us time, effort, and resources. One of the best tools we have for distinguishing between good and bad information is through a hierarchy of evidence.

THE HIERARCHY OF EVIDENCE

The hierarchy of evidence ranks different types of scientific studies based on the strength and reliability of their findings. This system helps researchers, nutrition experts, clinicians, and policymakers evaluate the quality of evidence when making health-related decisions. In short, not all evidence is created equal. By giving priority to higher-quality studies and considering the entire body of research, we can form a more accurate and well-rounded understanding of nutrition.

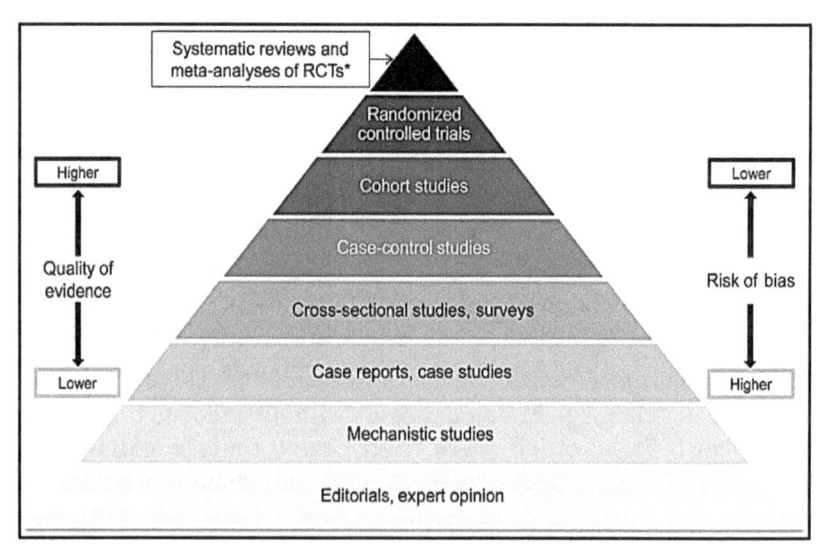

Here's an overview of the hierarchy of evidence:

SYSTEMATIC REVIEW

At the top of the research hierarchy is the systematic review, a comprehensive compilation of all relevant empirical evidence that meets predefined criteria to answer a specific research question.

Its goal is to reduce bias by carefully identifying, evaluating, and combining studies on a specific topic.[16] Think of it as an exhaustive book report on a subject. If you wanted to know if eating apples daily benefits your health, a systematic review would analyze every single study on apple consumption and health.

STRENGTHS

Structured and Transparent – Systematic reviews follow a strict, predefined protocol to ensure a thorough and unbiased assessment of all relevant studies on a particular topic.

Comprehensive Overview – They provide a broad understanding of the current evidence, highlighting gaps in knowledge and helping to guide future research.

LIMITATIONS

Time-Consuming – Conducting a systematic review requires significant time and effort to search, assess, and synthesize all relevant studies, making them labor-intensive.

Limited by Available Data – Systematic reviews rely on existing studies, and if those studies are of poor quality or lack critical data, the review's findings may be limited or inconclusive.

REAL SYSTEMATIC REVIEW:

A systematic review analyzing 30 studies with 3,230 participants found a significant link between reduced salt intake and lower systolic blood pressure, regardless of age, gender, or ethnicity. This suggests that reducing salt intake could significantly lower blood pressure, a key factor in preventing cardiovascular disease.[17]

META-ANALYSIS

A meta-analysis, often part of a systematic review, is a quantitative technique that combines results from multiple studies to produce a more precise estimate of an effect or intervention.[18] This matters in health and nutrition because looking at just one study can give you a skewed perspective. By pooling data from many studies, a meta-analysis can reveal whether a diet or intervention truly works.

STRENGTHS

Comprehensive Data Synthesis – Meta-analyses combine results from multiple studies, providing a more powerful and comprehensive understanding of a particular question or intervention.

Increased Statistical Power – By pooling data from various studies, meta-analyses can detect effects that individual studies may have been too small to identify, offering more robust conclusions.

LIMITATIONS

Quality Dependence – The overall reliability of a meta-analysis depends on the quality of the included studies. If poor-quality studies are incorporated, the findings may be misleading.

Heterogeneity – Variations in study design, populations, or methodologies across the included studies can make it difficult to draw definitive conclusions or generalize results.

REAL META-ANALYSIS:

In a 2020 meta-analysis, researchers combined data from 36 studies involving 616,905 participants to explore the connection between dietary sodium and cardiovascular disease. They found that for every 1g increase in sodium intake, the risk of cardiovascular disease was raised by 6%.[19]

RANDOMIZED CONTROLLED TRIAL

A randomized controlled trial (RCT) is the gold standard of research studies. In an RCT, participants with similar conditions are randomly assigned to different groups, typically one receiving the treatment and another receiving a placebo.[20] Randomization ensures that the groups are similar, reducing bias. This setup allows researchers to see if the treatment has a real effect beyond a placebo.

STRENGTHS

High Internal Validity – By randomly assigning participants to treatment or control groups, RCTs minimize biases, allowing researchers to isolate the effect of the intervention with a high degree of reliability.

Causality – RCTs are one of the few study designs that can establish clear cause-and-effect relationships between an intervention and an outcome.

LIMITATIONS

Costly and Time-Consuming – RCTs require significant resources, both financial and logistical, and can take a long time to complete, especially when studying long-term outcomes.

Ethical Constraints – In some cases, random assignment to treatment or placebo groups may not be ethical, especially when withholding treatment could harm participants.

REAL RANDOMIZED CONTROLLED TRIAL:

In a 2021 RCT in rural India, 502 participants were randomly assigned to use either regular salt or a reduced-sodium, added-potassium substitute.[21] The salt substitute significantly lowered blood pressure in hypertensive patients, demonstrating its potential as a low-cost intervention.

COHORT STUDIES

Cohort studies are longitudinal studies that follow a group of participants over time, often years, to observe how certain factors influence health outcomes.[22] For example, the famous Nurses' Health Study tracks nurses' dietary habits and their impact on health, such as comparing the health of nurses who eat five servings of fruits and vegetables daily versus those who eat only two. By controlling for confounding factors like smoking, researchers can glean valuable insights into long-term health effects.

STRENGTHS

Efficiency – Ideal for studying rare diseases, as it's easier to find cases after they occur.

Cost-Effective – Quicker and cheaper than cohort studies, especially for rare outcomes.

LIMITATIONS

Recall Bias – Relies on accurate recall of past exposures, which may be flawed.

Causality – Cannot establish a clear cause-and-effect or the timing of exposures.

REAL COHORT STUDY:

In a large cohort study in rural China, over 20,000 participants were observed for nearly five years. Those using a salt substitute had lower rates of stroke and cardiovascular events compared to those using regular salt.[23] Despite the many uncontrolled variables, the large sample size and long duration offer valuable insights into the potential long-term effects of sodium intake on cardiovascular health.

CROSS-SECTIONAL STUDIES

Cross-sectional studies are used to quickly assess the prevalence of diseases or conditions within a population.[24] These studies are relatively fast and inexpensive, providing a snapshot of the situation at a single point in time. They are often used as a preliminary step before conducting more in-depth research, like cohort studies. However, because they measure exposure and outcome simultaneously, they cannot establish cause-and-effect relationships.

STRENGTHS

Quick and Efficient – Allows for rapid data collection and analysis.

Prevalence and Associations – Useful for identifying the prevalence of diseases and associations with risk factors.

LIMITATIONS

Causality – Cannot determine cause-and-effect relationships due to simultaneous measurement of all variables.

Temporal Relationships – Cannot establish whether an exposure preceded the development of a condition.

REAL CROSS-SECTIONAL STUDY:

A cross-sectional study in Bagalkot City, India, examined hypertension among 20- to 40-year-olds, identifying stress, tobacco use, BMI, and family history as common risk factors. Factors that can improve blood pressure include abstinence from smoking and a decreased salt diet.[25]

CASE-CONTROL STUDIES

Case-control studies investigate diseases or outcomes by looking back at what might have caused them. Unlike cohort studies that follow people over time, case-control studies start with people who already have a condition and compare them to those who don't. For example, researchers might compare people with lung cancer to those without and look for differences in their past behaviors, like smoking.

STRENGTHS

Efficiency – Ideal for studying rare diseases, as it's easier to find cases after they occur.

Cost-Effective – Quicker and cheaper than cohort studies, especially for rare outcomes.

LIMITATIONS

Recall Bias – Relies on accurate recall of past exposures, which may be flawed.

Causality – Cannot establish a clear cause-and-effect or the timing of exposures.

REAL CASE-CONTROL STUDY:

A 2007 case-control study found that a no-added-salt diet significantly lowered blood pressure in people with high sodium intake.[26] While this suggests an association between salt intake and blood pressure, it does not prove causation.

CASE STUDIES

A case study is a detailed report on an individual patient's treatment, response, or diagnosis, often offering insights into rare conditions or unique treatment outcomes.[27] Case studies can generate new research questions, though their findings are not widely generalizable.[28]

STRENGTHS

Detailed Insight – Offers in-depth information on specific cases, especially for rare conditions.

Hypothesis Generation – Can inspire new research questions and hypotheses.

LIMITATIONS

Generalizability – Findings are limited to the specific case and may not apply broadly.

Bias – Subjective interpretation by authors can influence the results.

REAL CASE STUDY:

In a case study, a patient who adopted a DASH diet after a heart attack saw significant improvements in blood pressure, lipid levels, and overall health.[29] Case studies, like this DASH diet, offer some interesting insight for the person being studied, but is not very useful to everyone else.

MECHANISTIC STUDIES

Mechanistic studies explore the biological processes behind a particular effect, often using animal models or cell cultures. While they help form ideas for future research, their findings don't always apply to humans because of biological differences and can sometimes be poor predictors of actual health outcomes.[30]

STRENGTHS

Biological Insight – Provides detailed understanding of the underlying mechanisms of an effect.

Hypothesis Generation – Lays the groundwork for future research and clinical trials.

LIMITATIONS

Complexity – May oversimplify biological interactions by focusing on isolated components.

Translation to Humans – Findings in animals or cells may not always apply to humans.

REAL MECHANISTIC STUDY;

Mechanistic studies have shown how sodium influences blood pressure by affecting the renin-angiotensin-aldosterone system.[31] For example, one study found increased aldosterone levels in response to low-sodium diets, indicating how sodium can impact blood pressure regulation.[32]

EDITORIALS AND EXPERT OPINIONS

Editorials and expert opinions are articles written by journal editors or invited experts that offer commentary, perspectives, or insights on specific topics, issues, or recent research findings. These pieces are based on the author's professional experience and expertise.

While an article provides valuable insights from an expert, it's important to remember that this is the cardiologist's opinion, not new research. The advice is based on their interpretation of existing studies and their professional experience, but it doesn't offer new evidence. It's a useful perspective, but it should be considered alongside other types of research for a fuller understanding. The purpose of these articles is to provide context and perspective on current issues, trends, and advancements. It also helps interpret and comment on recent research, offering expert insights and recommendations, while stimulating discussion and debate within the scientific community.

STRENGTHS

Expert Insight – Offers valuable perspectives from leading experts, helping to contextualize and interpret complex issues. Provides guidance that can inform clinical practice, research, and policymaking.

Stimulates Discussion – Encourages critical thinking, debate, and further investigation, while highlighting gaps in knowledge and suggesting new hypotheses.

LIMITATIONS

Subjectivity and Bias – Reflects personal viewpoints, which may be influenced by the author's biases and experiences. Lacks empirical data, so conclusions are not directly supported by new evidence.

Variable Quality – The rigor of these articles varies widely, depending on the author's expertise and the journal's standards.

REAL EDITORIAL:

Many people mistakenly use editorials as solid evidence, not realizing they represent opinions rather than well-supported facts. For example, an editorial by Andrea Grillo and colleagues discusses the impact of sodium on blood pressure, summarizing existing research and emphasizing the risks of a high-salt diet.[33] While informative, it's important to recognize that this is not a research study but rather a synthesis of existing evidence, potentially influenced by the authors' perspectives.

CULMINATION OF EVIDENCE

Public health policies and dietary recommendations, like reducing sodium intake to lower the risk of cardiovascular disease (CVD), are based on multiple lines of solid evidence. If only one type of study supported the idea of lowering sodium intake, it wouldn't be convincing enough to spark widespread change. But when different types of studies—from observational research to clinical trials—keep showing the same strong results, it really drives home the point that cutting back on sodium is key to better health. That's why each "real study" example from the different levels of evidence above was focused on the health impact of salt and sodium—it allows you to see that the culmination of different findings can produce the most reliable results.

Organizations like the American Heart Association base their guidelines on this process, pulling together extensive research to offer sound advice. In populations with high rates of CVD and hypertension, especially where salt consumption is excessive, reducing sodium intake is a sensible public health strategy.

While some might argue that these guidelines are simply about making food less enjoyable, they are grounded in rigorous analysis of vast amounts of evidence, providing the best advice available. If you disagree with such recommendations, you will need to produce stronger evidence than the thousands of studies involving millions of participants that currently support them.

It's important to note that public health guidelines are general, and individual needs absolutely vary. This is part of why you should not eliminate salt entirely from your diet. Sodium and chloride, which make up table salt, are essential for bodily functions. But knowing the dosage that you need is important. So instead of focusing on the small amounts of salt you add at home, it's more practical to be mindful of the hidden salt in processed and fast foods, which contribute 75% of our sodium intake.

REAL PEOPLE, REAL EVIDENCE

When applying scientific evidence, nutrition experts must consider how the research translates to each individual, tailoring their advice to ensure it's both relevant and practical. For example:

- Is the patient similar to those studied in the research?
- Does the treatment offer benefits that outweigh any risks for this individual?
- Which specific health outcomes are being targeted?
- Are the patient's personal values and circumstances aligned with the proposed intervention?

The most effective approach is shared decision-making, where healthcare providers engage in open discussions with patients about their views, preferences, and unique health conditions. This collaboration is the foundation of evidence-based practice, ensuring that clinical decisions are informed by both scientific data and the individual's needs.

It's also crucial for experts to question sensational headlines like "Superfood X Prevents Disease Y." Evaluating the level of evidence, understanding the context, and determining whether findings apply to the individual patient are critical steps in ensuring appropriate use of scientific data.

No study is perfect; there will always be some degree of error, bias, or misinterpretation. But when enough well-designed studies are conducted, reliable patterns emerge. Human judgment is essential in applying these patterns in real-world situations. Science lays the groundwork, but it's the human touch that turns data into meaningful, personalized solutions.

WHAT DOES EVIDENCE-BASED MEAN?

Evidence-based science, closely linked to evidence-based medicine, emerged in the mid-19th century as a method of integrating the best available research with practical expertise and individual preferences.[34] It combines rigorous knowledge with hands-on experience to provide the most effective strategies for healthy living.

This balanced approach relies on three key elements:

1. **Validated Scientific Evidence** – Data from well-conducted research.

2. **Practical Expertise** – The skills and insights of professionals in applying the data.

3. **Individual Values** – The unique preferences and circumstances of the person involved.

Focusing too heavily on one element can lead to problems:

- Relying solely on scientific evidence might overlook personal needs or creative solutions.
- Focusing exclusively on practical expertise risks introducing unchecked biases.
- Prioritizing individual preferences limits the exploration of more effective, data-driven options.

By integrating all three elements, health professionals can offer unbiased yet personalized care, making decisions that are both data-informed and tailored to the individual.

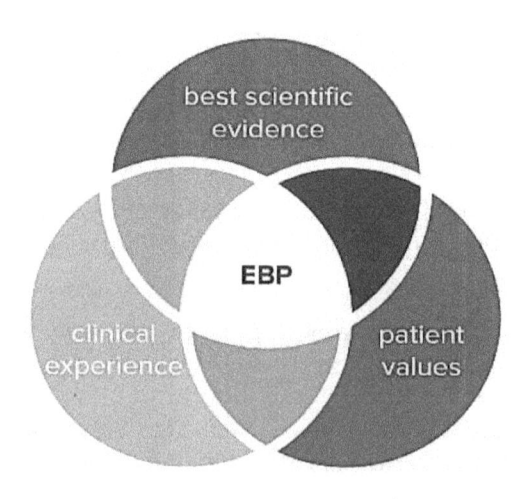

THE POWER AND PITFALL OF ANECDOTES

Humans are naturally drawn to stories over statistics, which is why compelling personal anecdotes, like a friend's dramatic weight loss or a cancer survivor's diet, can easily influence our decisions.[35,36,37] However, anecdotal evidence can mislead us when compared to broader, systematic research. Here's why anecdotes are often unreliable:

Small Sample Size – A single story (N=1) doesn't represent a general truth. What works for one person may not apply to others.

Outliers – The most extreme voices are often the loudest, distorting our perception of what is typical.

Investment Bias – People deeply invested in a particular diet or method may lack objectivity, much like sports fans rooting for their favorite team.

Short-Term Thinking – Anecdotes tend to focus on short-term results and often ignore long-term health outcomes.

Recall Bias – Human memory is unreliable, and people may unintentionally distort their recollection of past experiences.[38,39]

Association Bias – Anecdotes often attribute success to the wrong factor, failing to recognize the true cause.

Relying on anecdotal evidence can lead to poor decisions. Instead, it's important to seek out layered, high-quality evidence from experts who follow the scientific method, steering clear of pseudoscience. Many fall into the traps of pseudoscience because it offers quicker, more gratifying answers. To avoid bad nutrition advice, it's essential to understand the clear differences between scientific thinking and pseudoscience.

SCIENCE VS. PSEUDOSCIENCE

Understanding the difference between science and pseudoscience is essential for making informed nutrition decisions. While science relies on evidence-based research, rigorous testing, and peer-reviewed studies, pseudoscience often presents untested or misleading claims as fact, exploiting common biases and misconceptions. Here are eight key differences between the two:

1. Challenges Assumptions: Actively seeks to identify and question false assumptions.	**1. Confirms Biases:** Seeks evidence that aligns with pre-existing beliefs, ignoring contradictory data.
2. Relies on Peer Review: Weighs findings against a broad spectrum of evidence.	**2. Relies on Anecdotes:** Bases conclusions on personal stories, rejecting broader evidence.
3. Considers Total Evidence: Uses the collective body of research to inform decisions.	**3. Cherry-Picks Studies:** Highlights individual studies that support biases, disregarding conflicting research.
4. Contextualizes Findings: Prioritizes human studies over lab or animal research w	**4. Ignores Applicability:** Gives undue weight to irrelevant or non-human studies.
5. Shoulders Burden of Proof: Demonstrates how something can be true, even when the evidence is difficult to obtain.	**5. Shifts Burden of Proof:** Expects opposing viewpoints to disprove claims.
6. Recognizes Media Bias: Uses media to generate questions, not as definitive proof.	**6. Trusts Biased Sources:** Relies on opinion blogs, videos, and social media aligned with preconceptions.
7. Adapts to New Evidence: Changes conclusions in response to stronger evidence.	**7. Clings to Disproven Ideas:** Adjusts hypotheses to fit outcomes when proven wrong.

| 8. Applies Consistent Skepticism: Evaluates all ideas with the same level of scrutiny. | 8. Selective Skepticism: Questions evidence only when it opposes existing beliefs, accepting favorable ideas uncritically. |

HOW TO "DO YOUR OWN RESEARCH"

In a world full of misleading information, many advocate for "doing your own research." While it's wise to be cautious and informed, effective research requires more than just internet searches. Here's how to approach it:

Understand Research Complexity – High-quality research demands resources and expertise that most individuals lack. Instead of attempting to conduct original research, adopt a journalistic approach: sift through existing research and compare credible sources.

Build Scientific Literacy – To critically assess scientific literature, consider taking a course on science literacy. Without this training, distinguishing between good and bad research can be challenging.

Improve Your Search Skills – Be mindful of algorithms and the types of questions you ask online, as these can lead you down biased paths. Apply critical thinking to evaluate the information you find.

Recognize Limitations – While many aspire to find evidence-based answers, few have the time or inclination to do so thoroughly. This is where reputable experts come in as they can distill complex information and provide balanced insights.

Avoid Superficial Content – Don't rely on short, entertainment-focused videos or social media snippets for research. Genuine insight requires time, effort, and a methodical approach. Consuming content is not the same as gaining knowledge.

By approaching research thoughtfully and relying on trusted experts, you can avoid the pitfalls of pseudoscience and make more informed decisions.

CHAPTER 5: SCIENCE

WHERE DID THIS NONSENSE COME FROM?

Nutrition studies are often misused, intentionally or unintentionally, to fuel food myths and create confusion about health. A range of cognitive biases plays a significant role in spreading this misinformation. Here are a few common ones that lead us astray:

FREE SPEECH FALLACY

Everyone is entitled to their own opinion, but not all opinions are equally valid or informed. It's like someone insisting that a simple blue dot on a canvas has more artistic value and beauty than the ceiling of the Sistine Chapel. One can hold that opinion, but it doesn't make it more credible.

Or let's take another look at how people talk about the dosage of salt in our diet. Despite strong evidence linking high salt consumption to hypertension and heart disease, some people still argue that high-salt diets are harmless or even healthy. Often, this contrarian stance comes from research funded by the food industry, which has a vested interest in promoting salt (looking at you, electrolyte mix companies). The scientific consensus, backed by extensive research, supports reducing salt intake for most people. Yet, the contrarian opinion persists, often due to distrust in health organizations or a desire to push back against mainstream advice, even when it defies logic.[40]

SCIENCE CAN BE BORING

Let's face it: science, especially when it comes to nutrition, can seem dull. Extreme and unvalidated ideas often gain traction because they're more exciting than the tried-and-true scientific consensus. People love novelty, and the thrill of discovering a radical new diet is much more appealing than the steady drumbeat of "balance" and "moderation."

Fad diets like the carnivore diet get attention because they offer a dramatic alternative to conventional wisdom. Eating nothing but meat sounds rebellious and intriguing, even though mountains of evidence show that diets rich in fruits, vegetables, and whole grains are healthier in the long run. The thrill of breaking the norm often overshadows the reliable but less glamorous truth.

POOR SCIENTIFIC COMMUNICATION

One of the biggest challenges in nutrition is the poor communication of scientific findings. While often brilliant, scientists sometimes struggle to convey their discoveries in a way that's accessible to the public. On the flip side, influencers, who may misunderstand or even misrepresent the science, often excel at grabbing attention.

A headline claiming, "Eating too much protein can damage your kidneys" might stem from a rodent study but gets blown out of proportion in media coverage, misleading readers into thinking the same automatically applies to humans. This kind of poor communication allows sensational, yet inaccurate ideas to spread rapidly. It highlights the need for scientists to bridge the gap between complex research and public understanding.

EPISTEMOLOGY AND IDENTITY

Epistemology is the study of knowledge or how we know what we know. It explains why people arrive at different beliefs and how they interpret information. In the context of nutrition, the way people value personal experience over scientific evidence can lead to vastly different conclusions about the same facts.

In scientific epistemology, statements like, "fruits and vegetables are healthy", are based on years of research, logic, and empirical evidence. But for some, personal experiences or anecdotal stories carry more weight than scientific data. This can make nutrition feel more like a belief system than an objective science.

Dietary choices often become entangled with personal identity. People who identify as vegan, paleo, or keto may consider these choices to be extensions of who they are, leading to emotional attachment. When they come across evidence that contradicts their lifestyle, they might take it as a personal attack and reject scientific facts to protect their identity. This can lead to the promotion of shaky science and unfalsifiable ideas, which persist because they're harder to disprove.

COGNITIVE DISSONANCE

Cognitive dissonance occurs when new information conflicts with what we already believe. This discomfort can lead people to cherry-pick data that supports their current views while ignoring evidence that challenges them. It's common for people to embrace science when it confirms their beliefs but reject it when it doesn't align with their desires.

For instance, someone might enthusiastically drive across the country to witness a solar eclipse, relying on precise scientific predictions, but then dismiss solid research showing the benefits of whole grains for health. This selective acceptance of science shows how people only embrace what's convenient or exciting while disregarding evidence that challenges their current thinking.

LEADING THE WITNESS FALLACY

The "*Leading the Witness*" fallacy occurs when someone asks a biased or sarcastic question solely to elicit a specific, predetermined answer. It's a tactic used to manipulate the response rather than seeking genuine insight.

In nutrition debates, this might look like, "So are you saying we should all just live on rabbit food forever?" This kind of question isn't meant to foster discussion—it's designed to provoke a reaction. Instead of addressing the evidence that supports a balanced diet, the conversation is steered toward extremes, making it harder to have a thoughtful exchange about real nutrition science. This fallacy fuels misunderstandings, making it easier to dismiss scientific advice and cling to more emotionally appealing ideas.

NUTRITION RESEARCH PROBLEMS

Finally, conducting nutrition research can be limiting and challenging, leading to natural gaps and issues within some studies that can reduce their impact or credibility.

Here are key issues to be aware of:

Dietary Data – Assessing diet-disease connections relies heavily on dietary data, often obtained through self-reported methods like food records, food frequency questionnaires, and 24-hour recalls. These methods frequently produce errors. Participants may misreport or forget what they ate, and food records require the respondents to take precise measurements of food intake. These flaws can lead to unreliable data and misleading conclusions.[41]

Funding Bias – Research funding can introduce bias, particularly when a study is financed by a company with a vested interest in the results.

However, funding sources must be disclosed in research papers, offering transparency. While biased funding doesn't automatically discredit research, it's crucial to take a closer look at the study's methods and design. You shouldn't just dismiss a study because of who funded it—understanding how the research was done is key to judging how reliable it is.

Research Fraud – Although fraudulent studies do happen—more than 11,000 papers have been retracted—it's important not to dismiss all research because of a number of bad examples. Recognizing the errors in certain studies underscores the need for using multiple sources and understanding raw data. Avoid binary thinking; use critical analysis to sift through flawed and valid studies alike.

Journal Quality – Not all journals are equal. Some, like "Nutrients," are criticized for publishing lower-quality, opinion-driven articles. These journals may give the appearance of legitimacy but often lack rigorous scientific backing. To discern quality research, focus on the raw data and critically evaluate the findings rather than relying on journal reputation alone.

Replication Issues – Non-replicable studies—those that provide results that can't be reproduced—are often cited more than replicable ones, leading to widespread misinformation.[42] Always prioritize research that has been replicated and verified by independent studies.

Missing Data – Many studies overlook minority groups and women, leaving significant gaps in understanding how nutrition affects diverse populations. This lack of representation limits the applicability of research findings and underscores the need for more inclusive studies.

USING NUTRITION SCIENCE PROPERLY

1. Understand How to Read a Study or Find The Right Sources – If you're up for sifting through research yourself, first learn how to do so by using reliable platforms like Coursera's Medical Research course or subscribe to reputable resources such as Sigma Nutrition, which offers classes and content that break down complex nutrition science. If you're like most people, however, resources like Examine.com's guide provide a solid foundation for understanding different types of studies and their implications without needing a scientific background. This knowledge helps you discern the quality and relevance of the research you encounter.

CHAPTER 5: SCIENCE

2. **Apply Bayes Reasoning** – Adopt Bayesian reasoning, which assesses the probability of a hypothesis based on evidence. This approach helps you view truth on a spectrum rather than as absolute, encouraging more nuanced understanding and decision-making.

3. **Balance Intuition with Science** – While scientific data provides a critical foundation, don't completely dismiss your personal experience or intuition, especially when it aligns with established facts. Science can guide broad decisions, but your body also gives you data in the form of how you feel after eating certain foods. Just be cautious of falling into the trap of "Broscience," where personal anecdotes are treated as universal truths.

4. **Maintain Childlike Curiosity** – Adopt the curiosity of a child when approaching nutrition and health. This mindset allows you to explore new ideas without preconceived notions, fostering a willingness to change your perspective when confronted with better evidence. Curiosity encourages ongoing learning and questioning, keeping you engaged with new developments in nutrition science.

5. **Value Science as a Method, not a Belief** – Remember, science is not a belief system; it's a method for uncovering the truth about the world. This means being open to change and questioning even long-held views. Rather than treating science as a set of unchangeable rules, view it as a flexible process of continuous discovery.

Using nutrition science effectively can empower better decisions, but many people struggle with its nuances—next, we'll explore how the tendency to view nutrition in black-and-white terms creates challenges and limits a more accurate understanding of health.

CHAPTER 6: DUALITY

"Things are seldom black and white, even when we wish they were and think they should be, and I like exploring this nuanced terrain."

— **Emily Griffin**

In the complicated world of nutrition, our understanding is often skewed by oversimplified beliefs. These ideas, often rooted in false dilemmas, can limit how we view health's true complexities. This chapter will break down three major false dilemmas that often shape conversations about nutrition and wellness:

1. **The Obesity Conundrum** – Many believe obesity is either society's most urgent health crisis or something entirely irrelevant. This kind of black-and-white thinking fails to capture the nuanced reality of how body weight impacts health. The truth lies somewhere in between. While obesity can negatively affect health, it's not always a catastrophic issue. So, while we cannot disregard the importance of weight issues, we need to be careful not to over fixate on it. Embracing this complexity is key to developing a healthier, more balanced view of weight and well-being.

2. **The Calorie Paradox** – Another widespread misconception is that calories either don't matter at all, or are the only thing worth paying attention to. This false dichotomy ignores the intricate role that other factors play in weight management. Calories are important and still a part of these other factors, but we must consider the bigger picture of health as well.

3. **The Health Data Debate** – We often find ourselves at odds over health measurements, viewing them as either essential to understanding our health or completely pointless. This extreme thinking overlooks both the value and the limits of health metrics. Personalized data can be incredibly useful, but relying on numbers alone can lead to an incomplete understanding of well-being. A balanced perspective recognizes that health metrics provide valuable insights without being the whole story.

By challenging these misconceptions, this chapter will help you take a more balanced, informed approach to nutrition. Finding the middle ground is essential for navigating the complexities of nutrition science and fostering a healthier, more realistic view of wellness.

WHAT IS DUALITY?

Duality means having two opposing forces or ideas within a single concept. This often happens in nutrition, where we often encounter confusing and contradictory beliefs. The presence of duality can lead to false dilemmas, making us feel like we have to choose between two extremes.

In nutrition, dualities shape how we view food and health. We might see food as "good" or "bad," weight as "healthy" or "unhealthy," and calories as either "vital" or "irrelevant." These black-and-white perspectives fail to capture the true complexity of these issues, where there's often truth on both sides.

Understanding duality helps us recognize that health and nutrition aren't about picking one extreme over the other; they involve balancing different forces, acknowledging that both sides contribute to the overall picture. Breaking down these dualities can help us move beyond false dilemmas and develop a more balanced, comprehensive approach to nutrition. The first false dilemma we will look at: obesity.

THE OBESITY CONUNDRUM

False Dichotomy – Obesity is seen as either one of the biggest health problems *OR* it's seen as a completely irrelevant factor that should be ignored.

Realistic Duality – Obesity can have a significant impact on health *AND* obsessing over it can be problematic, doing more harm than good.

MY PASSIVE WEIGHT LOSS

After college, I lost 50 pounds over the span of three years. I remember stepping on the scale during my sophomore year and seeing I weighed 225 pounds. As someone who had always been active in contact sports, it felt like a significant achievement to have gotten to that point, yet I was deeply insecure. I was much heavier in middle school and college, and I constantly indulged in the most calorie-dense foods I could find. Late nights were spent making batch after batch of Eggo waffles and mini corn dogs while watching TV. My friends and I laugh about it now, but the sheer volume of food I could put away was staggering.

CHAPTER 6: DUALITY

Even today, when someone boasts about how much they can eat, I think, "That's nothing. You should have seen what I could put away." My meals used to consist of a half-gallon of ice cream, boxes of waffles slathered in peanut butter, corn dogs, pizza rolls, chips, leftovers, and more ice cream. My eating habits were driven by boredom and a search for comfort, as I was constantly seeking distraction and a reliable hit of dopamine.

While it's normal for weight to fluctuate in your teen and young adult years, maintaining a healthy weight or a significant weight loss over the long term is less common. After losing weight, I joined the National Weight Control Registry, a study that tracks people who have lost at least 30 pounds and kept it off for over a year. I found the common traits among participants fascinating:[1]

Average weight loss: 66 lbs., maintained for 5.5 years

Diet modification: 98% changed their diet to lose weight

Increased physical activity: 94%, mostly through walking

Daily breakfast: 78%

Regular weighing: 75%, at least weekly

Limited TV: 62%, less than 10 hours per week

Daily exercise: 90%, averaging about 1 hour per day

These statistics shed light on what it takes to pursue lasting weight loss but also highlight how weight has become a national obsession. As a dietitian, I guide others on their weight management journeys, yet I know firsthand how challenging it can be to achieve long-term success.

My own weight loss wasn't just about the numbers on the scale. It was about reshaping my relationship with food. Growing up, I didn't think much about how food impacted me. But as I started making healthier choices, influenced by environmental changes, my health improved.

At my heaviest, 225 lbs., with a BMI of 31.4 (classified as obese), I didn't fully understand why I weighed so much. When I dropped to 170 lbs., with a BMI of 23.7 (in the "normal" range), the weight loss felt almost accidental. My summer working as a camp counselor played a significant role: I walked more, slept better, ate structured meals, and thought less about food. The weight came off without much effort on my part. Every choice I made was mine, but the *circumstances* made those choices easier.

Looking back, I recognize that luck contributed to my weight loss. Although it wasn't the sole factor, it was part of the equation. This reminds me that weight management often involves a mix of willpower and external factors, making it more complex than we might think. My experience taught me that addressing obesity isn't just about personal choice; it's about understanding the influences around us and taking meaningful action.

The benefits of weight loss, at least in my case, have been transformative. But I also recognize how personal, sensitive, and difficult this topic can be for many. Weight management is never as simple as "just making a choice," and approaching it with compassion is crucial.

DOES OBESITY DEFINE US?

Obesity is a polarizing topic in health and nutrition. Given its complexity, it's important to approach the subject with an open mind. While obesity certainly can influence health, it's rarely the sole determinant of well-being. More importantly, we must consider the many factors that contribute to obesity.

First, we need to consider all aspects of the problem. Body size influences cultural perceptions of beauty, health, and personality, making it difficult to separate physical appearance from self-identity. With body size playing such a big role in how we see ourselves and how others see us, it's vital to approach this conversation with sensitivity and understanding.

Amidst all this complexity, one truth remains: it's essential to love your body at any weight. The endless pursuit of an "ideal" body, much like the pursuit of wealth, can lead to an unfulfilling cycle of dissatisfaction. It's perfectly fine to want to change your appearance, but it's important to reflect on whether those desires stem from a personal sense of fulfillment or from external pressures.

Embracing your body with love and acceptance doesn't mean ignoring the potential health effects of higher body fat. Loving yourself and striving for health aren't mutually exclusive, as they can and should coexist. By understanding these nuanced realities and confronting the complexities of obesity, we can cultivate a more compassionate and informed approach to health and well-being.

A POTENTIAL RISK FACTOR

Although it's uncomfortable, we can't ignore the fact that obesity carries certain health risks. These risks vary across a spectrum and are often influenced by other factors, but research shows that crossing the obesity threshold increases the likelihood of the following:[2-10]

- High blood pressure and cholesterol
- Strokes
- Certain cancers
- Type 2 diabetes
- Asthma and sleep apnea
- Joint issues such as osteoarthritis
- Gallstones and gallbladder disease
- Depression and anxiety

Beyond health, obesity has financial implications. In 2019, U.S. medical costs related to obesity soared to nearly $173 billion. Additionally, life insurance companies often charge higher premiums for individuals with higher body weight, using weight and BMI as indicators of potential health risks.[11] While these facts may seem to clash with the body positivity movement, they highlight the real-world impact of weight on health and finances.

It's important to remember that obesity exists on a spectrum, and BMI, a debated but widely used metric, plays a major role in how we define it.

BMI: WAY OVERUSED BUT NOT WORTHLESS

Body mass index (BMI) remains the standard tool for determining obesity in healthcare settings.

BMI has its controversies, but it's not inherently flawed; it just needs to be put in the right context. For many, even discussing BMI can lead to bad feelings, but at its core, BMI is just a simple calculation: weight in kilograms divided by height in meters squared.[12] It's a broad indicator of health, most often used in population studies to identify links between body size and disease risk. But this simplicity can lead to misinterpretation.

BMI doesn't account for differences in muscle mass versus fat mass or reflect individual lifestyle habits.[13] For example, a bodybuilder may have a high BMI due to muscle mass, but their actual body fat is quite low. While BMI can offer some helpful insights, especially in large population studies, it shouldn't be relied on as the only measure of individual health. Focusing too much on BMI can overlook other important health factors. It's a quick and useful tool for healthcare professionals and researchers, but it's not the best way to assess personal health habits—which is why most people don't need to pay attention to it.

IS WEIGHT THE BEST METRIC?

Health is about more than just weight. Numerous studies show that physical fitness can reduce the risks associated with obesity, even without significant weight loss. For instance, one study found that physically fit individuals had health outcomes similar to those of normal-weight individuals.[14] Another study revealed that exercise capacity is a more reliable predictor of mortality risk than BMI.[15]

While BMI serves as a useful tool, its relevance shifts across different populations, largely due to genetic factors. More specific measurements, such as body composition analysis, can give us better insights into individual health risks. Achieving balance is critical as being underweight comes with its own set of health issues, which can cause equal potential for concern.

True health is about much more than just weight. Physical fitness, diet, sleep quality, and stress management all contribute significantly to overall well-being. Consider two individuals: one with a BMI of 23 (normal weight) and another with a BMI of 28 (overweight). If the person with the higher BMI eats more fruits and vegetables, sleeps better, and manages stress effectively, they may actually be in far better health than the person with a "normal" BMI. A great example of just how limited BMI can be is Ilona Maher, an Olympic rugby player who recently shared that although her BMI is just shy of being "obese", she is clearly physically fit. In no way should her BMI change how she lives her life as an incredible Olympic athlete and person.

SHAME ON US

For a lot of us without great lifestyle habits, however, carrying excess weight can impact health over time. But using shame as a tool to address the high rates of obesity only makes the problem worse. Fat shaming can lead to emotional eating, increased anxiety, and reduced self-esteem, all of which undermine health goals.[16] I know I personally was never more motivated to lose weight just because I felt shame about my weight. True body positivity should center around healthy habits and movement rather than focusing on weight loss alone. Appearance is a shallow way to measure health, and the emphasis should be on encouraging long-term habits that promote overall well-being.

Discipline is often praised in weight management, but willpower is influenced by psychological and environmental factors. Focusing on holistic health, self-compassion, and behavior change usually works better than shame-based approaches. Rather than shaming ourselves or others, we should consider the factors that affect whether obesity is truly a personal choice.

THE MYTH OF "CHOICE ACTING ALONE"

The idea that obesity is purely a result of personal choice is a misconception. In reality, obesity is influenced by a complex mix of genetics, environment, and individual physiology. It's not simply because of a lack of willpower or motivation; it's shaped by powerful forces that create a "passive choice" environment in which making healthy decisions is incredibly difficult.[17] Those who don't struggle with obesity often underestimate how challenging it can be to make consistently healthy choices, especially when every meal feels like an uphill battle. Over a lifetime, winning that battle at every meal is nearly impossible.

MULTIFACTORIAL

Obesity can't be solely defined by personal choice. While individual decisions do influence body weight and should not be neglected, they are deeply connected with genetic, environmental, and physiological factors. Most people find themselves influenced by a mix of these elements.

CHAPTER 6: DUALITY

Making healthy choices is undoubtedly important, but maintaining a healthy weight requires a lifetime of consistently making good decisions. For some, these choices are made easier by their body's natural responses, access to nutritious foods, and a positive relationship with food. For others, the same decisions are far more difficult.

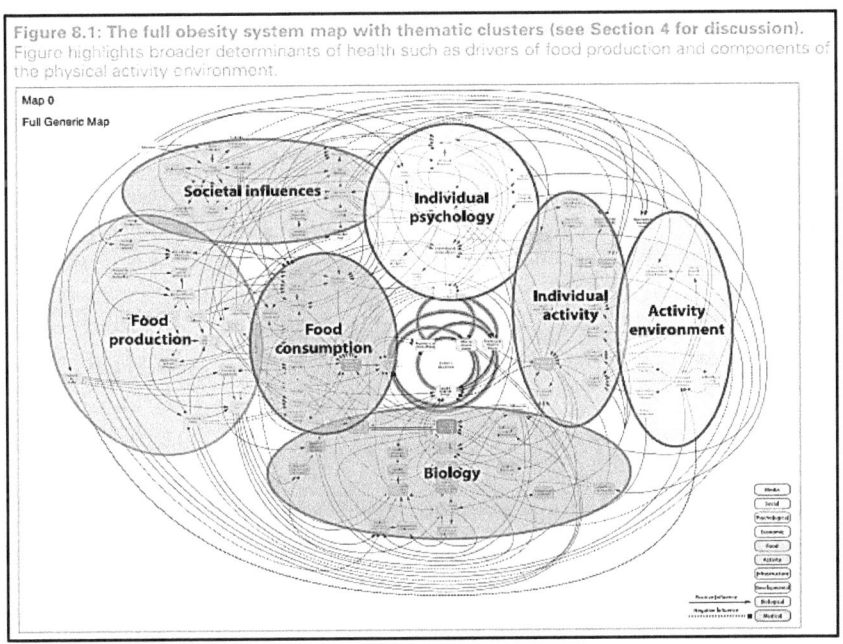

Figure 8.1: The full obesity system map with thematic clusters (see Section 4 for discussion). Figure highlights broader determinants of health such as drivers of food production and components of the physical activity environment.

Here are some of the factors that can make weight management much more difficult:

GENETICS AND PHYSIOLOGY

Studies have revealed that obesity is significantly affected by genetic and physiological factors.[18] For instance, individuals with obesity often exhibit lower levels of peptide YY (PYY), a hormone that reduces appetite, which can lead to increased food intake.[19]

Genetics also plays a substantial role. Studies on twins have shown that identical twins, who share all their genes, tend to have more similar body weights than fraternal twins, suggesting a strong genetic component in weight regulation.[20,21]

NEUROLOGY

Obesity is linked to heightened food reward responses, similar to those seen in substance addiction. Although the *dependence* on food and *addiction* to drugs are very different, both situations share one key factor: most people cannot simply "will" their way out of obesity.[22] The unique neurological responses in some individuals make it much harder for them to regulate their eating behavior.[23]

MODERN CONTEXT OF OBESITY

If genetics and physiological factors play such a significant role in obesity, why were obesity rates lower in the past? The answer lies in the balance between energy intake and expenditure *through the environment*. In the past, our ancestors faced different circumstances than us—they had limited access to calorie-dense foods, and a more active lifestyle kept obesity rates low.

In contrast, today's world bombards us with food choices that are high in energy but low in nutrients. Some people succeed in maintaining a healthy weight due to high motivation and favorable physiology, while others struggle with stronger genetic hunger signals, a more rewarding mental response to food, and economic factors that make it exponentially harder to stay healthy.

The modern environment promotes this idea of "passive obesity," where a combination of sedentary lifestyles and the easy availability of high-calorie, low-cost foods lead to weight gain. Reports show a clear decline in physical activity paired with an increase in the consumption of energy-dense foods, illustrating the multifactorial model of obesity.

TRAUMA

Trauma, particularly in women who have experienced abuse, is another significant factor in obesity. Research indicates that exposure to multiple adverse childhood experiences (ACEs) can increase the likelihood of developing obesity by as much as 46% in adulthood.[24,25] This connection highlights the psychological and emotional layers of the obesity issue, making it very challenging and complex.

STIGMA AND PERCEPTION

Obesity is essentially a chronic condition that may require medical intervention, yet it's frequently framed as a reflection of personal choice alone. This overlooks the intricate interplay of factors involved in weight management. In many cases, medications or other treatments may be necessary for long-term success, given the environment we live in. If our modern world were to shift heavily, this reality may change, but as of now it makes sense to consider the potential of medical insight.

Unfortunately, body weight is also unfairly used as a basis for judging someone's personality or attractiveness, leading to harmful stereotypes and negative perceptions.[26,27] It's crucial to separate body size from personality traits and understand that obesity is multifaceted. People in larger bodies are not lazy or undisciplined, and this assumption is both damaging and inaccurate.

WHAT MATTERS MOST

While body measurements like BMI can offer some insight into health, our collective obsession with weight loss, as seen in the $89.9 billion industry in 2023, is detrimental to overall well-being.[28] If awareness alone could solve obesity, the problem would have been resolved long ago. Nearly half of U.S. adults try to lose weight every year, yet the focus on dieting and body size hasn't led to widespread success.

The difference between body positivity and obesity treatment is subtle, but neither should be used to define someone's worth. Obesity is certainly a health concern in many cases, but being underweight is also a concern, so there's clearly a healthier range in which most people should land in for lower risk. Our culture often overlooks the health consequences of consistently eating too little, yet this is a serious issue that can mirror the effects of obesity on long-term health.

Rather than fixating on weight, we should focus on adopting healthy habits, which often lead to better health outcomes regardless of the scale. Both the food industry and personal responsibility play important roles in the obesity epidemic, and a balanced approach, one that considers healthy habits, individual abilities, and a supportive environment, is essential. Reducing shame and promoting overall well-being should be the main goals, with weight management being a possible side effect, not the primary focus.

Understanding the intricate web of genetic, environmental, physiological, and psychological factors behind obesity is crucial in addressing the epidemic as well. This knowledge can help us support individuals in achieving better health outcomes without resorting to oversimplified or stigmatizing views of obesity.

THE CALORIE PARADOX

False Dichotomy – Calories are viewed as an unreliable metric and should never be tracked *OR* it's often believed that calorie counting is the only way to manage weight effectively.

Realistic Duality – The principle of "calories in, calories out" does ultimately govern every human's weight and adiposity levels *AND* it's a very complex equation with stressful ramifications so relying on calorie counting as your only approach to weight maintenance is not a practical approach for a majority of people.

BEST DIET EVER?

Imagine a diet that promises you can lose 27 pounds in 10 weeks, improve your cholesterol levels, and still satisfy your sweet tooth. Would you try it? Mark Haub, a professor of human nutrition at Kansas State University, tested this concept by going on an all-Twinkie diet in 2010.[29] Despite eating ultra-processed foods like Twinkies, sugary cereals, and Doritos, Haub lost significant weight and saw improvements in his blood lipids as his triglycerides dropped by 39%, LDL cholesterol by 20%, and HDL cholesterol increased by 20%. Although Haub was a perfect example of how calories dictate weight loss, he cautioned against following such a diet. He thought it was better to raise questions about what "healthy" truly means and whether our understanding of health outcomes might be incomplete.

THE MCDONALD'S DIET

Mark Haub's experiment wasn't the only time someone revealed the reality of how calories do dictate overall weight. Tyler Whitman maintained his 215-pound weight loss by eating two bowls of Chipotle and two S'mores-flavored Quest bars daily.[30] Jeff Wilser also lost 11 pounds in a month by eating only junk food and drinking whiskey.[31] Kevin Maginnis, a grandfather from Nashville, somehow lost 58.5 pounds on a 100-day McDonald's diet, and his wife also experienced significant weight loss

CHAPTER 6: DUALITY

from this approach.[32] These stories challenge the traditional narrative around weight loss, illustrating that some people can maintain specific weight outcomes while consuming fast food regularly. This is a good reminder that although food processing is important, it still comes down to the context in which it's consumed and the severity of intake.

METABOLISM AND WEIGHT LOSS

Understanding weight loss and the confusion around calories, first requires a grasp of metabolism. Metabolism is the sum of chemical processes that sustain life, converting energy from food and drink into fuel for the body.[33] This includes catabolism (breaking down molecules) and anabolism (building up molecules), both requiring energy measured in calories.[34] Your own metabolism is measured by a "metabolic rate" which is basically just how many calories you need to carry out different bodily functions each day. Here are five myths about metabolism and our own metabolic rates that may change your previous perception of it:

1. **Big People Have Slower Metabolisms** – Larger bodies need more energy, and muscle mass, which is more metabolically active than fat, plays a significant role in burning calories.

2. **A Fast Metabolism Guarantees Easy Weight Loss** – Weight loss is governed by the balance between calorie intake and expenditure. The difference between individuals with "fast" and "slow" metabolisms is often minimal after adjusting for size and activity.

3. **Your Metabolism Can Be Broken** – Metabolism can't "break" or else you would not be alive. And believe it or not metabolic rates stay relatively stable from ages 20–60. What often changes that lead people to see differences in weight though is a shift in lifestyle, not the metabolism itself.[35]

4. **Skipping Meals Slows Metabolism** – While skipping meals doesn't significantly affect metabolism, *severe* restriction can definitely slow it down, though it doesn't lead to the dramatic "starvation mode" many fear. Skipping meals is not ideal for most of our health goals, but it also won't destroy your metabolism.

5. **You Can Significantly Boost Metabolism** – While certain foods and activities can slightly increase metabolic rate, the impact is minimal. Sustainable weight loss involves long-term habits, not quick fixes. Even building muscle, touted as a metabolism booster, only increases energy expenditure by roughly 13 calories a day for every 1kg of muscle gained.[36]

And while our overall energy expenditure doesn't increase by as much as we think from exercise, it can become significant, as evidenced by extreme populations such as elite athletes.[37]

THE COMPLEXITY OF CALORIES

As already stated, weight management revolves around the balance between calories consumed and calories expended. Calories (while not a tangible part of our food) are just a unit of measurement—which quantifies potential energy. While the principle of "calories in, calories out" is correct in the sense that overall no amount of energy being used or stored in the body is unaccounted for, the effects of different foods on this balance can vary. For example, blending almonds into almond butter changes how much energy your body absorbs and uses to break it down, as well as how full you feel afterward.[38] While calorie counting and exercise are part of the weight management equation, they must be viewed within the larger context of overall health.

Statements like "I didn't lose weight in a deficit" or "I don't gain weight despite eating more" are often inaccurate due to errors in *calculation*, not because the principles of energy balance are flawed. Errors in fitness trackers or food logging often lead to misjudgments. Calorie counting requires more accuracy and sophisticated measurement tools than many people realize. This is why calorie counting may not work for everyone.

So, while most people misjudge their metabolic rate, or the daily speed at which calories are used, it shouldn't be assumed that calorie counting can't be done well or that your metabolism is broken. It just means that it's hard to measure accurately, which is the actual reason that calorie counting seems to doom most people. A shift away from rigid calorie counting toward healthier habits often yields better results. The core issue lies not in the principle itself but in the complexity of physiological math.

WHY YOU MAY BE THROWN OFF

Many people believe that metabolism and calorie balance don't actually account for other physiological factors, but there is no stone unturned when it comes to energy balance. Consider the following factors that impact calorie intake and expenditure:

Calorie Intake Factors:
- Absorption levels/Bioavailability
- Appetite-regulating hormones
- Food environment
- Types of food and how they are eaten (timing, combinations)
- Sleep patterns

Calorie Burn Factors:
- Body size and total muscle mass
- Activity levels
- Hormone utilization
- Incidental movement (non-exercise activity thermogenesis, or NEAT)
- Thermic effect of food

While these factors can complicate energy balance, the good news is that they aren't completely out of our control.

ENERGY BALANCE: THE GATEKEEPER

While energy balance is the gatekeeper of weight outcomes, the factors outlined above are a reminder of just how multifaceted and challenging this balance can be. For instance, those going through menopause or those with PCOS do experience changes that can alter metabolism. But because most of us do not actually have access to a calorimeter in a laboratory setting, the chance of knowing your exact metabolic rate is pretty slim. But instead of giving up entirely, we can all have the appropriate balance of calories in and calories out by focusing on better habits.

As discussed earlier, however, practical changes are not merely about willpower or effort but involve systemic changes to mental health, food access, and environmental factors. Instead of fixating on uncontrollable aspects of metabolic rate or the perfection of calorie tracking, we need to simplify our approach. Many are tired of the "calories in, calories out" mantra because traditional calorie counting has failed them.

Because the average daily energy intake in America is currently around 3,500 calories, and daily activity is less than 20 minutes per day, there is certainly room to improve our daily routines.[39]

CHAPTER 6: DUALITY

It's crucial to understand that this is not an attack on anyone's failed attempts or methods, because it's really not an easy area to master. Luckily, there are many ways to succeed, and most of them do not require strict calorie counting. While the principle of energy balance remains true, focusing on practical, relatable advice is far more beneficial.

DIETS: EATING LESS AND MOVING MORE

The "eat less, move more" motto is also very worn out and offers us little practical advice. This is why many people end up loving diets for a short time–they all ultimately promote weight loss by generating a more exciting version of this calorie deficit, even if we attribute it to some other magical principle. But what each of these popular diets have in common is that they help us eat to eat less overall:

Low Carb/Keto – Reducing carbohydrates limits food choices, making it harder to combine fats and proteins in hyper-palatable ways. These diets often focus on whole, unprocessed foods, which are more filling due to their high protein content.

Plant-Based – Rich in fiber and naturally low in calorie-dense foods, plant-based diets help reduce overall calorie intake. They emphasize whole foods, which tend to be lower in fat and more satisfying.

Intermittent Fasting (IF) and Time-Restricted Eating – By shortening the eating window, these approaches reduce opportunities for snacking and calorie consumption. While bodybuilders eat frequently to boost calorie intake, IF allows for larger, more satisfying meals within a limited time frame.

Carnivore – Eating only meat limits food variety, reducing the likelihood of consuming hyper-palatable, high-calorie combinations. Additionally, protein is extremely satiating, which can naturally lower calorie intake.

Clean Eating, Paleo, Whole Food – By avoiding ultra-processed, hyper-palatable foods, these diets help control calorie intake. They emphasize fiber-rich, protein-packed whole foods, leading to greater satiety, improved digestion, and better energy balance, which can also support increased physical activity.

Instead of opting for these restrictive diets that are not actually sustainable, we need to find more exciting and personally helpful ways to manage our energy intake. For those who continue to struggle, it may be necessary to work with a professional nutrition expert as it can be hard to rely on ourselves, given that people often under report calories by up to 50%.[40]

It's also helpful to get outside help as nearly 75% of Americans believe that they are currently following a healthy diet, despite oppositional evidence.[41]

So, although it would benefit many people to strike a more appropriate balance of calories in their diet, we need to explore more sustainable ways of eating less and moving more. This shift needs to start with nutrition, which is the result of the environment that we (or others) create every day. To put it frankly, we all need to set certain boundaries and goals for eating and moving, but the way we get there will be based on your unique circumstance—and it must be sustainable.

THE HEALTH METRICS DEBATE

False Dichotomy – Health measurements are seen as an essential part of staying healthy *OR* they're cast aside as completely unnecessary, providing no benefit.

Realistic Duality – Health measurements are valuable tools that can help us better understand our health *AND* they can sometimes lead to overly narrow thinking, causing us to lose sight of the bigger picture.

IMPORTANCE OF INDIVIDUAL METRICS

Tracking health metrics can be incredibly useful, providing feedback that helps prevent or manage health conditions and can improve both the quality and length of life. However, it's essential to strike a balance between these metrics and our natural intuition. This is because while subjective feelings are valuable, they can be biased. In the end, we need both *objective data* and *personal insights* for a fuller understanding of our health. Here are some important metrics worth keeping tabs on.

BLOOD PRESSURE

Blood pressure offers crucial insights into cardiovascular health. Consistently high blood pressure (hypertension) can lead to serious conditions like heart disease, stroke, and kidney damage. On the other hand, low blood pressure (hypotension) can cause dizziness and fainting and could indicate underlying health problems. Regularly tracking blood pressure encourages healthier lifestyle choices, such as reducing salt intake, increasing physical activity, and managing stress. If you are not typically going to a healthcare provider and having this checked, home monitors are

CHAPTER 6: DUALITY

relatively inexpensive and can give you a sense of where you stand on this important metric.

STRESS

Stress is the body's natural response to perceived threats or challenges. While short-term stress can be motivating, chronic stress can have significant negative effects on health. Stress can be measured through self-reported assessments, physiological indicators like heart rate or cortisol levels, and behavioral observations. Though more subjective and challenging to track, monitoring stress is essential for maintaining long-term health.

Methods for Tracking Stress:

Self-Reported Assessments – Tools like the Perceived Stress Scale (PSS) and the Stress Appraisal Measure (SAM) can help gauge how stress is affecting your daily life.

Physiological Indicators – Metrics like heart rate, blood pressure, and cortisol levels offer objective data on how stress impacts the body.

Behavioral Observations – Noting changes in sleep patterns, eating habits, or work performance can provide insights into your stress levels and areas needing improvement.

A1C

Understanding A1C levels is crucial for those at risk of diabetes and to know how your body is handling blood sugar. The A1C test measures the percentage of red blood cells coated with sugar. Since red blood cells regenerate every three months, this test reflects your average blood sugar levels over that time.[42] Higher A1C levels mean a higher risk of developing diabetes and related complications.[43] This long-term view gives a better understanding than short-term glucose monitors, guiding more informed choices. High A1C can indicate a lack of physical activity, excess weight, or diets high in saturated fats and sugars, showing the need for lifestyle changes to reduce the risk of diabetes.[44]

CHOLESTEROL

Cholesterol, a fatty substance in the blood, is essential for building cells and producing hormones. It's transported through the bloodstream by lipoproteins, primarily Low-Density Lipoprotein (LDL), High-Density Lipoprotein (HDL), and Triglycerides. Cholesterol levels are usually assessed through a blood test that breaks down these types.[45]

While LDL cholesterol is associated with an increased risk of heart disease, the role of HDL ("good" cholesterol) is more complex than previously thought, especially in diverse populations.[46] Recent studies show that HDL's protective effects aren't as straightforward as once believed. As one study's author noted, "It could mean that in the future, we don't get a pat on the back from our doctors for having higher HDL cholesterol levels."[47]

Newer markers like ApoB and Lp(a) offer more detailed insights into cholesterol's role in health. Apolipoprotein B (ApoB), which can penetrate arterial walls and cause plaque buildup, is a key indicator of heart disease risk, while Lp(a) is heavily influenced by genetics.[48] Reducing LDL, which carries over 90% of ApoB, remains the best approach for most people, achievable through fiber intake, lowering saturated fats, and regular exercise.

The importance of routine cholesterol testing can't be understated because high cholesterol often presents no symptoms until it causes serious problems. Remember, though, it's important not to fixate solely on cholesterol numbers. Other factors like exercise, nutrition, and smoking cessation are equally crucial for cardiovascular health.

THE DANGER OF OVER-FOCUSING ON HEALTH METRICS

It's easy to become overly focused on a single health metric and lose sight of the bigger picture. Health decisions should be based on a broad range of factors, not just one metric. Here are a few ways of measuring health that may not help as much as you think.

PURSUIT OF ABS

Aesthetics, like visible abs, are often seen as indicators of health, but pursuing this look can be unhealthy, especially for women who require higher body fat to maintain hormonal and reproductive health. Striving for visible abs at all costs can lead to health issues such as amenorrhea, osteoporosis, cardiovascular disease, and infertility.[49] Health should never be compromised for aesthetics.

HYPERFOCUS ON SUGAR

Sugar often gets blamed for many health problems, but cutting it out entirely doesn't guarantee better health. Diets with both high and low sugar can lead to similar body compositions if overall calorie intake is controlled.[50] Focusing too narrowly on sugar ignores the importance of a balanced diet. Foods like pasta and bread, often labeled simply as "carbs," contain fiber, protein, and other nutrients. Similarly, sugary foods like ice cream and pastries often also contain high levels of fat. Avoiding sugar alone won't necessarily solve overeating or other health issues.

Many people obsess over details, like the size of an apple, and lose sight of the bigger picture. For example, some health experts have fixated on the sugar content of fruits, neglecting the other beneficial nutrients they offer.[51] This kind of narrow focus overlooks the fact that many people choose candy over fruit, which, despite both containing sugar, have vastly different impacts on health. Similarly, concerns over bananas "ruining" smoothies due to their glycemic index are trivial compared to the overall nutritional value of the whole food. Such misleading claims can discourage people from making healthy choices like homemade smoothies, potentially leading them to consume more ultra-processed foods instead.

REALITY OF INFLAMMATION

Chronic inflammation is indeed a serious health issue, but many people try to reduce it without knowing if they even have a problem with inflammation. Inflammation can be measured through many tests, two of which measure ESR (erythrocyte sedimentation rate) and CRP (C-reactive protein), which are useful for monitoring conditions like rheumatoid arthritis.[52,53] However, outside of a specific condition, tests like CRP and ESR are nonspecific markers that may indicate elevated inflammation without identifying the root cause.

Routine testing isn't always necessary unless specific symptoms or risk factors are present, so this excessive use of tests can lead to unnecessary stress or interventions. Following influencer advice on reducing inflammation without evidence for needing it is typically not harmless, but also just nonsensical. Instead, adopting habits like eating more fruits and vegetables, exercising, and cutting back on ultra-processed foods that are crowding out healthier options, will naturally help with chronic inflammation.

STEP COUNTS

The popular goal of 10,000 steps a day is not a magical number.[54] Research shows that significant health benefits can still be achieved with 6,000 to 8,000 steps daily.[55] The overall *quality* and *consistency* of physical activity matters more than hitting an arbitrary number, so setting a sustainable step goal that suits your lifestyle can be more beneficial. That said, if counting steps is useful for you, by all means keep tracking. But be aware of the obsession that can lead to discouragement if you don't always hit that "perfect" number.

METABOLIC AGE

Metabolic age, often used in fitness assessments, is not scientifically validated and oversimplifies metabolism. It can be misleading, as it relies on generalized equations that don't account for individual differences in health or metabolism.

EXPANDING VIEW OF HEALTH

Narrowing your focus to one health aspect can mislead you, and feeling good in the short term doesn't always equate to long-term health. Serious conditions like atherosclerosis or cancer can develop silently without immediate symptoms showing. As Dr. Idz, a prominent debunker of nutrition myths, rightly says, "You can't feel your arteries clogging or cancer cells replicating."[56] The focus should be on long-term health outcomes, not just immediate feelings or short-term metrics. Achieving lasting well-being requires patience and a broad, balanced approach.

WE EAT FOOD, NOT NUTRIENTS

Nutrition is tricky because we consume foods, not isolated nutrients. In the same way that calling bread or pasta "carbs" overlooks the fiber, protein, and other nutrients they contain. And when people aim to increase protein intake, they often forget that foods providing protein also contain other compounds, such as fat or carbohydrates. Focusing on one nutrient without considering the entire food can make nutrition goals confusing. Remember, foods are made up of hundreds of different compounds, each working together. A balanced diet is one that takes these complexities into account rather than focusing narrowly on one nutrient's potential impact.

NO, SERIOUSLY, ARE EGGS HEALTHY?

The question of whether eggs are healthy depends on various factors, and determining their place in your diet requires considering several criteria.

Dosage – Eating 40 eggs a day or completely avoiding them are both unnecessary extremes. Eggs offer a range of nutritional benefits, so most people who don't get enough of the nutrients found in eggs will improve their diet quality. But if you happen to eat a lot of them and it pushes out other healthy foods, you might reconsider the amount.

Size – This one is simple: if you are larger, you will likely need more of every food, which might include eggs. Eat the amount that is right for you, not someone else.

Genetic Predisposition – Saturated fat and cholesterol from eggs is not usually a cause for concern, but it can affect people at a much more extreme level who have certain genetic predispositions. Genetic testing may help you know if you are at risk.

Taste – If you don't like eggs, don't force yourself to eat them. Conversely, avoid falling prey to fear mongering about them.

Allergies – If you're allergic, don't eat them.

Overall Diet – Are eggs filling a nutritional gap, like providing extra protein, or are they just adding empty calories?

Substitution Effect – What foods are eggs replacing in your diet? Are they pushing out something more or less nutritious?

Ultimately, eggs are neither a superfood nor a villain. Most foods have trade-offs, and your decision to eat eggs should depend on your individual health, nutritional needs, and personal preferences. Eggs are just one of the classic foods that get demonized and then praised back and forth, so they are worth examining. But all food choices should go through a quick run-through using the ideas above. This will help you understand how to implement foods in a more individually suitable way.

WHERE DID THIS NONSENSE COME FROM?

When it comes to nutrition certain heuristics can actually oversimplify ideas that require complexity. To avoid extreme ideologies let's look at which shortcuts and biases may sabotage our eating habits.

EITHER-OR FALLACY

Throughout this chapter, we've explored how nutrition is often viewed in black-and-white terms, when in reality, it's much more nuanced. This kind of either-or thinking can obscure the complexity of health and nutrition, leaving out meaningful solutions. In health and fitness circles, many people falsely believe that you either need to be on a strict diet or you might as well give up and eat whatever you want. But plenty of people fall somewhere in between. In fact, it's often the people who avoid these extreme ends of the spectrum that end up with much better health outcomes.

PLAIN TRUTH FALLACY

An example of the *Plain Truth Fallacy* in nutrition is the claim that "calories in, calories out" is outdated or no longer works. Statements like, "It's obvious that just cutting calories won't help you lose weight anymore," imply that it's self-evident that "calories in, calories out" is ineffective simply because it didn't work for someone in a specific context.

In reality, while the principle of energy balance, calories in versus calories out, remains true, accurately measuring and controlling these variables can be difficult. Factors like genetics and lifestyle make the equation more difficult. By completely dismissing the reality of calorie importance, this argument oversimplifies a complex issue when it is actually a nuanced and complex topic.

THIRD-PERSON EFFECT

The *Third-Person Effect* in nutrition misinformation occurs when people believe others are more susceptible to false claims while they see themselves as immune. For example, someone might view a fad diet, like a "juice cleanse to heal inflammation," as something only naive individuals fall for. They assume they are too informed to be influenced by the marketing of such trends yet may still be subtly swayed by similar claims over time.

This bias can prevent people from critically engaging with nutrition information, as they believe they are *above* being misled. At the same time, they worry about others being influenced by misinformation. This effect perpetuates the spread of dubious health advice while downplaying its potential influence on personal decision-making. So instead of preaching the sermon to someone else, preach it to yourself first.

HASTY GENERALIZATION

Hasty generalizations arise when broad conclusions are drawn from limited evidence, leading to oversimplified views, especially in nutrition, where individual variability is significant.

Hasty Generalization Example – "All carbs are bad because some high-carb foods are unhealthy."

Reality – Carbohydrates come in many forms, and whole grains and fruits, which are high in fiber and nutrients, are part of a healthy diet. Labeling all carbs as harmful ignores this variety.

SINGLE-CAUSE THINKING

Single-cause thinking, or *reductive reasoning*, occurs when a complex issue is attributed to one factor, ignoring the multiple contributors to a problem. This leads to oversimplified solutions and misunderstandings in nutrition.

Single Cause thoughts about health outcomes – "Obesity is solely due to overeating."

Reality – Obesity is influenced by a combination of genetics, environment, mental health, and socioeconomic factors. Addressing it requires a holistic approach, not just focusing on diet alone.

Health and nutrition are complex topics that should be viewed through a broad lens, considering the interplay of multiple factors, including diet, lifestyle, genetics, and environment. Simplistic and generalized ideas often fail to address the root causes of health issues. A more nuanced approach that takes into account these various influences is essential for achieving long-term well-being.

HOW TO APPROACH COMPLEX NUTRITION TOPICS

1. **Diversify Your Health Metrics** – Evaluate your health using a variety of metrics, such as waist circumference, body fat percentage, fitness levels, blood pressure, cholesterol, and blood sugar. This multi-faceted approach provides a more complete understanding of your overall health beyond just weight or BMI.

2. **Prioritize Mental and Emotional Well-being** – Prioritize your mental health by practicing self-compassion and mindfulness and seeking professional support when needed. Shifting the focus away from calories or weight (if these become obsessions) can reduce stress and improve body image, fostering a healthier relationship with both food and your body. This holistic approach helps prevent the anxiety and depression often associated with weight fixation, promoting long-term emotional well-being.

3. **Integrate Your Health Goals** – Set goals that address multiple areas of health - physical fitness, mental wellness, social connections, and healthy lifestyle habits. This ensures that progress in one area, like improving physical fitness, doesn't come at the expense of mental or social well-being. The key is a balanced, sustainable approach that nurtures all aspects of health without sacrificing one for another.

4. **Educate Yourself on True Holistic Health** – Understand the limitations of relying on a single health measurement, like BMI, and advocate for a more comprehensive view of health. This awareness prevents overemphasis on numbers and encourages a broader approach that values overall quality of life. Recognizing that health is multifaceted helps reduce the pressure to hit specific numerical targets, making space for a more compassionate and individualized understanding of well-being.

5. **Think Directionally on a Spectrum** – View health and diet choices as part of a spectrum rather than a set of binaries, "all-or-nothing" decisions. Strive for balance by making healthier choices most of the time while allowing yourself the flexibility to enjoy indulgences without guilt.

For example, occasional treats can fit into a nutritious diet as long as they are balanced with wholesome foods. This mindset reduces stress and promotes a positive relationship with food, understanding that health is about progress, not perfection. Whether you're on a more positive or negative end of the health spectrum, it's your ongoing direction that matters most, and there's always room for improvement and growth.

Understanding nutrition as a complex, multifaceted topic helps us embrace balance and long-term well-being, but even the best intentions can falter when the way we communicate about nutrition fails. Next, we'll uncover why nutrition communication often misses the mark and how to foster clearer, more effective dialogue.

CHAPTER 7: CONVERSATION

"Conversation isn't about proving a point; true conversation is about going on a journey with the people you are speaking with."

— Ricky Maye

Effective communication is key when it comes to sharing nutrition information. After all, it affects how we apply that knowledge to our health and well-being. Unfortunately, today's nutrition discussions are often filled with divisive rhetoric and rigid beliefs, with many people sticking to dietary "tribes" that reinforce their existing views. This isn't just a social phenomenon; it's a major roadblock to progress in the nutrition space. In fact, research shows that 60% of people are more likely to favor information that is comparable to their pre-existing beliefs, no matter how inaccurate it is.[1,2] This polarization creates echo chambers where misinformation reigns, making it harder for science-based nutrition advice to reach a broader audience.

In this chapter, we'll explore the vital role that clear, accurate communication plays in the world of nutrition and the challenges posed by groupthink and tribalism. We'll also take a closer look at how we communicate our own nutrition beliefs, both to ourselves and to others, offering fresh perspectives on food and health.

WHAT IMPACTS OUR NUTRITION CONVERSATIONS?

Healthy communication is essential for progress. Open dialogue has always been a key driver of human advancement, but it can also damage relationships, affect mental health, and lead to poor decisions when mishandled. Conversations about different eating approaches can be constructive if approached with curiosity and respect. But all too often, they end up doing more harm than good.

To encourage healthier conversations around nutrition, we need to focus on three key areas:

1. **Conversation Shaping**: Are we aware of the underlying beliefs that drive our discussions? Do we acknowledge our biases, and are we willing to challenge them?

2. **Talking at Each Other**: How we engage with others is crucial. Are we actively listening to understand or just waiting for our turn to dismiss opposing views?

3. **Internal Dialogue**: How we reflect on these discussions matters, too. Do we critically evaluate our stance or simply double down on our initial beliefs?

By addressing these core areas, we can start to shift the narrative from one of divisiveness to one of understanding and progress. In the sections that follow, we'll take a deeper dive into each of these three elements to lay the groundwork for more productive nutrition conversations.

CONVERSATION SHAPING

IDENTITY

Our food beliefs, and the subsequent conversations we have around nutrition, are intimately tied to our identities. In many ways, this is a positive connection as food can reflect our culture, upbringing, and traditions, creating a deep sense of belonging and personal meaning. Whether it's a family recipe passed down through generations or pride in maintaining a local or ethical diet, these rituals contribute to our sense of self. Nutrition identities often extend beyond personal preferences, however, and can negatively evolve into rigid worldviews that shape not only how we eat but also how we perceive health and wellness. Many people are drawn into dietary "tribes" or communities formed around shared beliefs about food that offer validation and a sense of safety. This sense of belonging is natural; humans are inherently social creatures, and we are wired to seek acceptance from like-minded groups. While we naturally feel good getting together with those who share our beliefs, it can also backfire.

Take movements like "clean eating," for example. This promotes the purity of food and avoidance of anything deemed harmful or unnatural. While this seems like a reasonable goal, it can quickly spiral into extremism if taken too far. The language and rituals within these groups, terms like "toxins," or "detoxes," and strict definitions of what's acceptable, create a strong in-group mentality. Members adopt these practices not necessarily because they are the healthiest but because they align with the group's values. In this environment, food choices often reinforce a nutrition identity rather than support growth or genuine health.

We naturally protect our sense of self, so we tend to accept information that supports our existing beliefs and push away anything that threatens them. As a result, even when presented with healthier options or new evidence, people may reject these ideas if they feel they undermine their belonging to a dietary tribe.

This dynamic can negatively impact both physical and mental health. People who adopt rigid nutrition ideologies often feel guilt, anxiety, or fear when faced with food that falls outside their chosen framework. The line between mindful eating and obsessive restriction becomes blurred, leading to behaviors that can damage well-being. For instance, someone who strongly identifies with the clean eating lifestyle may avoid food that could benefit them, such as a non-caloric sweetener or a nutrient-dense food that doesn't align with their group's philosophy. Even when a choice might improve their health, they may resist for fear of betraying their identity.

Dr. Sarah Ballantyne is a great example of this problem when it comes to forming rigid nutrition identities. Initially gaining success as a vocal advocate for the Paleo and AIP diets, she grew a large following online as she practiced what she preached. She would later realize that her health improvements were actually more about eliminating bad habits than strictly following her Paleo or AIP framework.

When she began promoting foods like legumes, which are excluded from the Paleo diet, she faced significant backlash from her community and questioned whether or not it was worth giving up her social status to speak up about the truth of her discoveries.[3] She continues to be ostracized from certain groups, just because she updated her thinking when better evidence was presented to her. Different nutrition circles will view her and many others poorly for questioning the legitimacy of their original ideas. Her story underscores how deeply people will cling to their nutrition identities, even when those identities no longer serve them well.

When our identities are wrapped up in nutrition ideologies, we often struggle to evolve our thinking. The desire to belong, to be part of a group, can become more important than pursuing real health benefits. Conversations about food have become less about what works best for us as individuals and more about defending our way of life. This rigidity stifles progress and fosters divisive rhetoric in broader nutrition discussions.

CHAPTER 7: CONVERSATION

REALLY, POLITICS?

Did you know that liberals are more likely to adopt vegetarian or vegan diets than conservatives?[4,5] Or how about the fact that conservative voters, on average, are less likely to try unfamiliar foods when compared to liberals?[6,7] Honestly these might both seem to make sense based on our perspective of these groups, but why does it seem to be in-line with our expectations?

For conservatives, eating familiar foods may stem from their values of upholding tradition—and trying to adopt a vegetarian diet would be way harder if no one else in your social circle is doing it.[8] For liberals, the higher rate of vegan diets may be a result of their values around animal or environmental welfare—and perhaps the basic value of progressivism pushes them toward new foods. Although these original statistics are true, the reasoning behind them is more speculative, but it does bring up an interesting point: It's probably pretty easy to predict someone's nutrition behaviors and beliefs based on the social groups that they come from and the values they prioritize. None of this is inherently a problem, but it can become one if we aren't careful.

I once had a client who was closely connected to a group of people who were tried and true low-fat vegans. While everyone else in the group may have been doing fine, my client's health was clearly suffering. Despite this they hesitated to explore food options that didn't fit their social club's nutrition identity. This person's fear of being ostracized and losing social ties kept them tethered to dietary practices that no longer serve their best interests. When trying to help them see other options, it appeared that there was always a way to see benefits of the diet while downplaying the chosen diet's weaknesses. This is so common among all extreme diet circles—overhype the positive attributes of their diet and resist acknowledging any downsides to it. But in order to have more productive conversations and find the best answers possible, we need to be honest about our nutrition choices and where they come from. Even if it's hard to do.

Rather than viewing nutrition as a battlefield of competing enemies, we must embrace the idea that our food choices, like our identities, can evolve.

Health is not static, and our beliefs about what nourishes us should be adaptable and open to change. By allowing room for growth, we can create a healthier, more productive conversation about food. One that prioritizes individual health outcomes over the need to conform to a group identity.

In the end, it's not about rejecting identity or the social support that comes from belonging to a group; it's about ensuring that these identities don't become *barriers* to better health. We should all adopt more flexible nutrition identities that allow for personal growth and inclusion of better ideas when they come along.

ARE YOU IN A NUTRITION CULT?

Health and nutrition circles can sometimes mirror the behaviors of cults, where rigid adherence to certain diets or ideas overshadows rational thought and open dialogue. Here are some cult-like behaviors to watch out for:

Leader Dependency – When prominent figures within a nutrition community become central to its identity, followers may develop a dependence on their guidance, resisting new ideas and stifling independent thought. If a single person is viewed as the ultimate authority on your diet, it's worth questioning how much that shapes your thinking.

Proportionality Bias – A tendency to oversimplify complex health issues, such as attributing the obesity crisis to one cause, like sugar, can lead to misguided beliefs. In reality, most health problems are the result of many small, interconnected factors.

Biased Questioning – Asking questions with an agenda can block genuine exploration. True inquiry involves approaching topics with curiosity, not just seeking to confirm pre-existing beliefs.

Exaggeration of Benefits – Certain diets or health practices are often overhyped, with proponents amplifying benefits and downplaying risks. This can lead to unrealistic expectations and disappointment when results don't match the claims.

Condescension and Dogmatism – Condescending attitudes toward those with different views, paired with dogmatic statements, can shut down conversations and prevent growth. An inability to confront contradictory evidence signals a narrow mindset and leaves no room for new information.

Ridiculing Divergent Ideas – Mocking or dismissing new or unconventional ideas can push individuals away and limit productive discussion. Adults, like children, need spaces where they can explore new concepts without fear of ridicule.

HEALTHIER HABITS IN NUTRITION CONVERSATION

To move beyond cult-like behaviors, we can foster healthier dialogue around nutrition. Here are some open-minded habits that can transform conversations and lead to better outcomes:

Encourage Resilience – Create environments where people feel safe exploring new ideas without fear of mockery or ostracism. This fosters resilience and a willingness to consider alternative viewpoints.

Foster Open Inquiry – Support genuine questioning that seeks to understand rather than confirm existing biases. Welcoming diverse perspectives can enrich collective knowledge and foster mutual respect.

Challenge Extremes by Addressing Stress – Recognize the role of stress in fueling extreme ideas and conspiracy thinking. It's often a previous bad experience that leads people to adopt more unbelievable beliefs. Unpacking the roots of extreme thinking is often necessary to see where our beliefs come from.

Provide Evidence-Based Information – Counter misinformation by sharing well-researched, reliable data. Recognizing the complexity of health issues helps dismantle overly simplistic narratives.

Embrace Nuance – Move away from black-and-white thinking by acknowledging that health and nutrition are multifaceted. Encourage conversations that reflect this complexity and remain open to change as new evidence emerges.

EMBRACING OPEN-MINDEDNESS

A crucial element of healthy discourse is the ability to *separate one's identity from one's ideas*. When nutrition beliefs are challenged, it's easy to feel defensive, as if questioning our food choices can feel like a personal attack on our character. However, in order to learn, we must embrace curiosity and prioritize growth over the comfort of familiar ideas.

Embracing open-mindedness means recognizing that our current understanding is not absolute. In nutrition, where personal identity is often tightly tied to dietary choices, fostering respectful dialogue and an evidence-based perspective is essential for personal growth and better health outcomes. By understanding how our beliefs, values, and identity shape our thinking, we can reduce bias and promote a more thoughtful, balanced approach to nutrition.

TALKING AT EACH OTHER

When it comes to discussing nutrition, it's important to recognize that conversations in public settings, like social media or podcasts, often differ significantly from private, more personalized discussions. In public forums, people feel freer to share opinions, even if those ideas are not fully formed or scientifically accurate. While these platforms can spark curiosity and bring awareness to new topics, they also open the door to misinformation, especially when important context is left out.

GENERAL VS. SPECIFIC INFORMATION

One key challenge in nutrition discussions is understanding the difference between *general* guidelines and *specific* advice. General guidelines, like those from health organizations, provide a broad framework intended to benefit the *average* person. For instance, recommendations to limit sugar intake or eat more vegetables are helpful starting points for the general public. However, they may not be suitable for everyone's unique health needs or circumstances.

In contrast, specific advice is tailored to the individual. For example, while public health guidelines suggest reducing sugar intake, the recommendations for someone managing diabetes would be much more nuanced, perhaps focusing on precise carbohydrate counting or monitoring blood sugar levels throughout the day.

CONTEXT IS KEY

Public health guidelines play a vital role in spreading general advice to the masses to give us some ideas of where to start. However, they often don't address the cultural, environmental, or individual nuances that can significantly affect how that advice is applied.

Take the general guidelines around coconut oil as an example. Public health guidelines typically caution against consuming too much saturated fat, which is the majority component of coconut oil. In Western diets, where saturated fat intake is already high, adding more could pose health risks. However, in certain traditional Pacific Island cultures where coconut oil has been a dietary staple for centuries, they may not experience the same negative health impacts.

While limitations are likely still necessary, these limits may be different depending on what other foods are included in the diet. The difference in potential outcomes highlights how specific contexts—like cultural, dietary, and lifestyle factors—matters when applying general nutrition advice.

Dietary trade-offs are another important piece of context when discussing nutrition outcomes. These trade-offs were overlooked by companies and the general public when the American dietary guidelines were introduced in the 1980s. These guidelines aimed to reduce heart disease risk by cutting fat intake, but Americans and food production companies misunderstood the assignment as they ended up replacing fats with refined carbohydrates and sugars instead. The result? It did not address the energy intake problem, so we saw a continued increase in obesity and type 2 diabetes.[9] It's crucial to understand that while general advice is a helpful starting point, it can sometimes be problematic when we don't consider the context of the rest of our diet, food trade-offs, or differences in genetics and culture.

ONLINE CHALLENGES

In the digital age, social media and online platforms have become primary arenas for discussing nutrition. However, they often exacerbate the spread of misinformation. Let's explore the key challenges of online nutrition discourse and strategies for encouraging more productive conversations.

Myths Travel Faster Now – Social media, while sometimes offering independence from corporate food narratives, has also become a breeding ground for health myths. Sensational headlines and charismatic influencers often overshadow well-researched dietary advice, leading to widespread confusion.

For instance, viral posts may promote extreme diets like carnivorism, boasting miraculous benefits while ignoring potential health risks. These simplified and emotionally charged narratives are designed to capture attention quickly, which explains why misinformation often travels faster than factual content.[10] Since sensationalized content draws more engagement, social media algorithms tend to favor it, pushing more myths and misleading information our way.

Echo Chambers and Confirmation Bias – Social media's structure reinforces existing beliefs through echo chambers, making it difficult to encounter opposing viewpoints. Algorithms tailor content to individual preferences, ensuring that users mostly interact with those who share similar views.[11]

A 2021 study found that users were three times more likely to follow bots whose partisanship matched their own, regardless of the bot's strength of identification.[12] Another study revealed that even small influences, such as "unfriending," can rapidly lead to the formation of segregated, homogenous communities.[13]

For example, a user who follows mostly vegan influencers may rarely see content that challenges the health claims within that community. This can create a distorted understanding of nutrition, where balanced perspectives are overlooked, and critical thinking is stifled. To break free from this cycle, it's important to actively seek diverse viewpoints and engage with information that challenges your beliefs.

The Nature of Conversing Through Technology – The nature of online interactions—short, impersonal, and often anonymous—poses significant challenges to meaningful discourse. Unlike in-person conversations, where accountability and ongoing dialogue are expected, online exchanges often end abruptly or descend into unproductive arguments.

- **Commentary Pitfalls** – Online comment sections are full of flawed thinking, personal attacks, and attention-seeking one-liners. A user might dismiss a well-researched post on the benefits of a balanced diet with, "That's not my experience!" without engaging further.

- **Soundbite Culture** – Social media platforms like X encourage short, catchy statements that lack context. While these sound bites may spark initial interest, they don't encourage a deeper understanding of complex nutrition issues; the focus on novelty and controversy often overshadows truth and thoughtful analysis.

- **Behind the Keyboard** – Online anonymity makes it easy to spread misinformation without accountability. Someone can claim that "vegetables are unhealthy" without facing real-time counter arguments or having to support the claim with evidence. In-person conversations, however, require us to think critically and engage in constructive dialogue, where baseless statements are more easily challenged.

IMPROVING CONVERSATION ONLINE

Improving the quality of online nutrition discussions requires a conscious effort to move beyond these common pitfalls and embrace more constructive communication strategies.

Active Listening – Instead of rushing to respond, take time to think and listen. Try to fully understand opposing viewpoints and the evidence behind them. This approach, often used in evidence-based practices and motivational interviewing, leads to more effective communication.

Critical Evaluation – When confronted with bold nutrition claims, ask follow-up questions such as, "How does this process work?" or "What evidence supports this?" These questions can help uncover the depth of understanding and distinguish credible advice from sensationalism.

Situational Awareness – Conversations online differ greatly from those held in-person because we lack many of the contextual clues that are present during face-to-face interactions, such as tone, body language, and personal background. Online, we often have very little knowledge about the people sharing ideas or their level of expertise. This requires us to adjust our approach and be more mindful of the situations at play. It's important to recognize that while general advice may be shared online, it's not tailored to individual needs, and we should engage with these conversations accordingly, avoiding assumptions about others' experiences or expertise.

CAN WE COMPARE THE USA TO OTHER COUNTRIES?

Many people believe that countries outside the U.S. have more favorable food environments and healthier populations. Nations like Japan or Spain, where traditional diets and lifestyles are seen to promote better health, are often held up as examples. However, attributing all of America's health issues solely to these generalized dietary guidelines is an oversimplification.

While it's true that factors like the influence of large food corporations and a culture of convenience have lowered the quality of food and health in the U.S. by some margin, the claim that healthy food options don't exist at all is very misleading. The issue isn't that every food is unhealthy; rather, it's more of a cultural and behavioral challenge. Some believe that U.S. dietary guidelines are inferior or even harmful, but this view ignores the fact that our guidelines are *fundamentally the same* to those in countries with far better health outcomes.

THE FOOD PYRAMID AND AMERICAN GUIDELINES

The food pyramid was introduced in the 1990s, and even at the time, it was terrible in several ways, like failing to clearly distinguish between types of fats, refined versus whole grains, and appropriate portion sizes.[14] Industry pressures also played a role in shaping these guidelines, which contributed to public confusion and inconsistent adherence.[15]

Despite these shortcomings, the core message, encouraging a balanced diet of fruits, vegetables, lean proteins, and whole grains, aligns with global standards. The real issue is not the guidelines themselves, but our failure to follow them. For example, less than 10% of Americans actually adhere to these recommendations, making it difficult to assess their true effectiveness.[16] With 90% of Americans not meeting fruit and vegetable intake goals, the majority of us are, in fact, eating contrary to the guidelines.[17]

In 2011, the USDA replaced the food pyramid with MyPlate, a more straightforward visual guide that breaks down healthy eating into meal components.[18] Although MyPlate is easier to understand, the issue of adherence, not reliable information, persists. Problematic cultural habits are deeply ingrained in the modern American mealtime, which means no set of guidelines would change these behaviors.

COMPARING GLOBAL GUIDELINES

When comparing food guidelines globally, most nations with solid nutrition programs, such as Spain and Japan, promote a healthy eating pattern remarkably similar to the U.S. guidelines.[19] In fact, as you can see in the following images, Japan's guidelines are essentially an upside-down version of our old guidelines, and Spain's guidelines look nearly identical to ours as well. The difference lies in how closely people in these countries follow the advice. They may not consciously try to adhere to the guidelines, but their traditional diets and lifestyles naturally align with the recommendations. In Japan, for example, there is a strong cultural emphasis on portion control and mindful eating, habits less common in the U.S.

CHAPTER 7: CONVERSATION

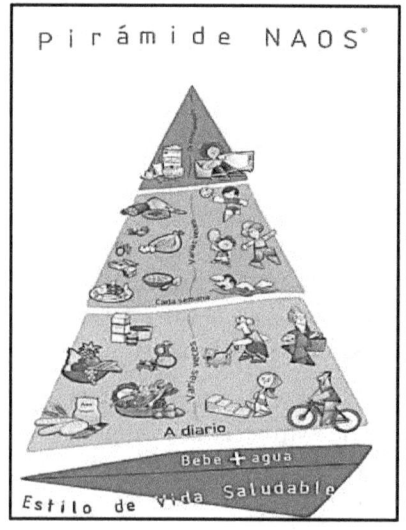

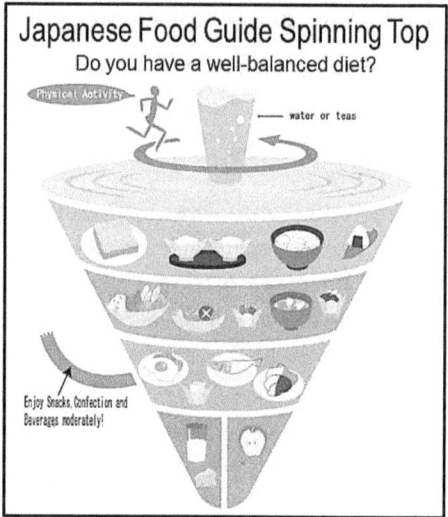

Meanwhile, many popular influencers in the U.S. advocate for eating in direct opposition to these guidelines, suggesting diets that would reduce fruit, vegetable, and whole grains intake. Such approaches not only conflict with established nutrition science but also risk promoting unbalanced and unhealthy eating habits.

But many people who think the guidelines are to blame don't realize that other countries with healthy populations have the same ideals. They also tend to miss the more important conversations around environmental differences that exist between countries. Factors like better urban planning, which encourages walking and physical activity, are one big difference in health outcomes.

It's also worth noting that countries with universal healthcare systems have an economic incentive to promote effective public health measures, including dietary guidelines. If these nations had discovered a superior nutritional approach, it would be in their best interest to implement it widely to reduce healthcare costs. But it turns out they have come up with the same nutrition recommendations that we have in the U.S.

THE REAL ISSUE: ADHERENCE AND CULTURE

The takeaway is that America's dietary issues are not rooted in flawed guidelines but in our lack of following them. Cultural, economic, and behavioral factors play a significant role in why many Americans struggle to follow dietary recommendations. The fast pace of our modern schedule and the reduction of importance on families and family mealtimes often set us up for poorer health choices, both now and over the course of our lives.

To improve public health, we need to shift the focus from simply critiquing the guidelines to addressing the underlying challenges in behavior and culture. This means creating an environment where healthier choices are more accessible, affordable, and integrated into daily life. Beyond guidelines, broader strategies, like education, policy changes, and community support, are essential to encourage healthier living.

While it may be tempting to blame America's health problems on the dietary guidelines themselves, the truth is that similar guidelines are offered in other countries with less deleterious results. The real challenge, then, is fostering a cultural shift toward better adherence to healthy dietary patterns and making these healthy choices easier for everyone to adopt.

THE JUNK FOOD NARRATIVE

The term "junk food" is often used as a catch-all for ultra-processed and fast food, offering an easy way to identify foods we should limit in our diets. While this shorthand can be helpful when we talk to each other about nutrition, it also oversimplifies the foods we're discussing and can lead to misunderstandings. Not all foods labeled as "junk" are inherently bad. Take protein bars, for example: while some are basically candy bars in disguise, others can support workout recovery, aid in weight management, or help increase protein intake. So, not all protein bars deserve the "junk food" label.

The language we use to describe food really can matter. Calling something "junk" will not only stigmatize the food itself but the people who rely on it. For those with limited financial resources, fast food may be one of the few affordable options, but calling it "junk" can imply that their food choices make them "junk people." While this term can motivate some of us to make healthier choices, for others, it can create unnecessary stress and contribute to disordered eating. It's crucial to be mindful of the impact our words have when discussing food, recognizing the nuances behind why people make the choices they do.

For example, pointing out that Cheetos are unhealthy is often redundant and serves very little purpose—most people already know this. The real challenge is understanding how to actually replace these foods on a consistent basis. While using "junk food" as a heuristic can help us quickly categorize foods to limit, terms like "indulgent food" might be more effective. This language signals that these foods can still be enjoyed occasionally, without attaching moral judgment to the choice.

A pivotal moment for me occurred when I was still in high school. I was on a day trip with friends to San Francisco when I saw a large group of people, who were likely homeless, eating at a Burger King. For whatever reason, my attention was pulled toward them while they were ordering food and I had a profound realization. For them fast food may not just be a place to eat; it was a place of comfort and survival. It offered affordable calories, even if it wasn't considered "optimal nutrition." This observation made me rethink the term "junk food." Labeling food in this way ignores the complex realities of why people eat what they do and implies that those who rely on these foods are somehow lesser. Even foods that are dismissed as having "no nutritional value" usually still provide some level of essential nutrients.

My former boss is another great example of why all foods can fit, depending on the level of intake. He ate fast food regularly, albeit in a portioned controlled manner, and maintained shockingly good health. While I don't have access to his lab results, his case shows that moderation, even with so-called "junk food," can be part of a healthy lifestyle. The idea that all fast food is harmful oversimplifies the issue, and dosage really does matter. Language, context, and dosage are all important factors to consider when we talk about our food choices.

WHY EXACTLY ARE SOME FOODS LESS HEALTHY THOUGH?

No single food causes disease, and no single food can cure it. Nevertheless, some foods consistently push our diets in an unhealthy direction. For example, a single bagel isn't "bad," but a diet of low-nutrient, high-sugar, high-fat, or high-salt foods can lead to long-term health problems. While there are foods that may not be nutritionally ideal, they might offer joy or comfort, both of which are important for overall well-being.

You may hear from some wellness circles that there are secretive ingredients and toxins at the root cause of less healthy foods; but in reality, we know which components make the biggest difference. So, here's why fast food and ultra-processed foods are lower quality on average:

1. High Sugar, Fat, and Salt – Fast food tends to be loaded with sugar, fat, and salt, which can encourage overeating and increase calorie intake. Over time, this can lead to excess weight and related health problems.

    2. Lack of Essential Nutrients – Many fast foods are low in essential nutrients like fiber, protein, and micronutrients. This lack of nutrition can put the body at higher risk for disease and compromise overall health.

    3. Reduction of Non-Nutrient Components – Ultra-processed foods tend to lose beneficial compounds like antioxidants, polyphenols, and phytochemicals, which aren't required for short-term survival but significantly promote long-term health.[20]

These factors highlight how fast food differs from whole foods or homemade meals, which generally offer more health benefits.

THE SUBSTITUTION EFFECT

One of the biggest issues with fast food is its impact on overall diet quality through the substitution effect. When fast food becomes a staple, it displaces healthier options. Studies show that increased fast food consumption is associated with lower intake of fruits, vegetables, and whole grains, leading to a decline in diet quality and an increased risk of obesity and related diseases.

On the other hand, prioritizing healthier foods can create a positive substitution effect. Swapping soda for water or choosing fruit over sugary snacks can greatly improve overall diet quality and allow indulgent foods to remain occasional treats rather than mainstays of the diet.[21]

Understanding why fast food can be unhealthy requires basic knowledge of specific nutritional factors, not reliance on arbitrary rules or conspiracy theories. By addressing the real issues, like a lack of nutrients, and instilling a positive use of the substitution effect, we can make smarter food choices that promote overall health.

Based on the current health metrics, many Americans could benefit from cutting back on the frequency of indulgent foods in our daily diets, while others might benefit more from easing the fear and guilt that we attach to them. While we should engage in conversations that push for cultural shifts toward healthier eating, we should also avoid extreme stances on "junk" food. Rather than labeling these foods as "cheat meals" or "guilty pleasures," which carry a sense of moral failure, we can call them indulgences. Recognizing that occasional treats, like Oreos, can fit into a balanced diet is important as long as we prioritize health-promoting meals first and understand the ratio needed for each person.

INTERNAL DIALOGUE

While conversations with others shape our views on nutrition, the internal "conversations" we have with ourselves can be just as impactful. Self-talk and the beliefs we internalize from what we read, hear, or experience often shape our relationship with food, sometimes in problematic ways.

THE ALL-OR-NOTHING DIET

One common form of negative self-talk is the "all-or-nothing" mindset, where you might think, "I have to stick to my diet perfectly, or I've failed." This rigid mentality sets an impossibly high standard, making any deviation from the plan feel like a total failure.

When perfectionism takes over, a minor slip, like eating a slice of pizza or skipping a workout, can cause intense feelings of guilt and frustration. This often spirals into abandoning the diet altogether, followed by regret and more negative self-talk. For instance, eating something sweet might prompt thoughts like, "I'm being bad," or "I shouldn't eat this." This type of thinking frames food choices as moral decisions, linking indulgence with failure. The all-or-nothing mindset can set off a cascade of unhealthy behaviors:

Impact on Behavior – The all-or-nothing mindset can set off a cascade of unhealthy behaviors:

Yo-Yo Dieting – A strict adherence to a diet is often followed by overeating or binging once the diet is "broken." This back-and-forth makes weight management difficult and contributes to a negative relationship with food.

Binge-Restrict Cycle – Guilt-driven self-talk leads to cycles of restriction followed by binge eating. This unhealthy cycle can create feelings of loss of control and reinforce negative self-perception.

Emotional Eating – When dietary slip-ups cause stress and disappointment, food can become a coping mechanism, complicating efforts to maintain a healthy diet.

Reframing the Conversation: Flexibility and Progress – healthier internal dialogue focuses on progress, not perfection. A flexible approach to eating allows for the occasional slip-up, seeing it as a normal and recoverable event rather than a failure. Instead of punishing self-talk, try phrases like, "One slip-up doesn't define my success; I'll get back on track with my next meal." This mindset fosters resilience and keeps you focused on long-term goals.

FOOD EXPECTATIONS: THE MILKSHAKE STUDY

Expectations can have a massive influence on health outcomes. A great example this comes from a 2011 study, where participants were given the same milkshake on two different occasions but were told two different stories about it each time.[22] Here's how it worked:

• **Study Design** – Participants were told that one version of the milkshake was indulgent and high-calorie, while the other was marketed as sensible and low-calorie. Despite both drinks being *perfectly identical* in terms of ingredients and calories, the participants' physiological responses differed based on their expectations.

• **Key Findings** – Even though the milkshake was identical both times, the way participants felt afterward changed based on what they *thought* they were drinking. A lot of this change came from a difference in ghrelin, the hormone that signals hunger. Participants who believed they were drinking the indulgent milkshake experienced a more significant drop in ghrelin levels, meaning they felt more satisfied. Meanwhile, those who thought they were drinking a low-calorie shake had a smaller drop in ghrelin, leaving them less satisfied.

• **Implications** – What we believe about the food we eat can affect how satisfied we feel, regardless of the food's actual nutritional content. Both the placebo and nocebo effect are alive and well in our relationship with food, so shifting away from such negative beliefs of individual ingredients might change our dietary experiences. Food expectations might just matter as much as the food itself.

IBS PERSPECTIVE

Mindset and food expectations also play a significant role in managing conditions like irritable bowel syndrome (IBS). Patients who believe certain foods will trigger their symptoms often experience worse reactions, even if the food itself isn't problematic.[23]

Psychological Stress and IBS – Stress and anxiety are well-known triggers for IBS symptoms. Worrying about food choices can exacerbate these symptoms, creating a feedback loop of stress and digestive discomfort.[24,25]

Cognitive-behavioral therapy (CBT) and mindfulness-based stress reduction (MBSR) techniques can improve IBS symptoms by helping patients change negative thought patterns about food and reduce food-related anxiety.[26,27] These techniques can help patients manage their condition more effectively, but should not be seen as a cure-all, as food-based interventions are almost always part of the equation as well.

Gut-Brain Axis – The gut-brain connection is an important part of IBS. Anxiety can alter gut motility and physiology, which worsens IBS symptoms. Studies also show that changes in mindset can improve gut function, further highlighting the power of mental attitudes in managing physical health.[28]

GLUTEN

In general, gluten is often unfairly blamed for many health issues. While it's a serious concern for those with celiac disease (affecting 0.3% to 1.2% of the population), most people who avoid gluten don't actually have a true sensitivity to it.[29] In fact, studies have shown that gluten doesn't trigger inflammation in the intestines of people without celiac disease.[30] Research even indicates that consuming between 20 and 70 grams of gluten doesn't increase problematic symptoms or risk of chronic diseases like gastric cancer.[31,32,33]

Understanding the difference between true gluten sensitivity and other factors, such as FODMAPs or negative expectations, is essential for making informed dietary choices:

FODMAPs – A review involving 1,312 adults found that only 16% of those who responded positively to a gluten-free diet actually had gluten sensitivity.[34] Many participants experienced worse symptoms after consuming a bar containing fructans but showed no difference in symptoms after eating a gluten-containing bar.[35] Fructans, a type of FODMAP (fermentable short-chain carbohydrates), can cause gastrointestinal symptoms and are often found in foods that also contain gluten. This overlap makes it challenging to identify the true cause of symptoms.

Nocebo, Expectations, or Lifestyle Effects – Other factors such as stress, hormones (e.g., menstrual cycle, ovulation), and eating habits (e.g., eating too quickly or going too long between meals) can also contribute to bloating and discomfort. Often, the real issue is the difficulty in moderating consumption of ultra-processed gluten-containing foods like bread and pasta. In controlled environments, very few people actually experience issues with gluten itself, suggesting that the problem lies elsewhere.

To understand the nocebo effect and the power of psychosomatic experience, another study looked at ways to physiologically change results after patients had altered negative perceptions. In this study, patients were given a harmless saline solution but were told that it would increase their pain following surgery. Remarkably, these patients did report higher levels of pain. Researchers believed it could have been because of an increase in cholecystokinin (a hormone associated with pain, particularly abdominal pain), as well as anxiety. To explore this further, they administered a cholecystokinin antagonist alongside the saline solution to a separate group of patients. Interestingly, the nocebo effect, along with the heightened pain, disappeared. This goes to show that such beliefs can physically trigger hormones linked to anxiety and pain, potentially contributing to symptoms of IBS and gluten sensitivity.[36]

OTHER FACTORS TO CONSIDER

Beyond FODMAPs and the nocebo effect, stress, hormones, and even eating habits (like eating too quickly) can contribute to digestive issues. Now, there are still people who have checked off the boxes above and are still searching for answers. For those that do have another autoimmune condition, it's possible you might have undiagnosed celiac disease or a rare gluten-related issue like Non-Celiac Gluten Sensitivity (NCGS).

A recent study led by Daniel DiGiacomo of the Celiac Disease Center at Columbia University estimated that the national prevalence of NCGS is just over 0.5%, about half the prevalence of celiac disease.[37] Remember, though, it's essential to recognize that gluten-free diets can sometimes lead to lower nutritional quality if processed gluten-free products replace nutrient-dense whole foods.[38,39,40]

While NCGS is real, at least 80% of people who believe they have it do not actually have a gluten sensitivity. This can be tricky to sort out, but working with a nutrition professional can clarify the potential culprits. Just as we discussed the need to not oversimplify, it would be egregious to assume that every case of IBS or gluten issues stems simply from psychosomatic results. But it's worth noting that most people with nutrition problems would benefit from exploring this idea.

WHERE DID THIS NONSENSE COME FROM?

Miscommunication in nutrition often stems from biases distorting how we process information, leading to poor online and in-person dialogue. These biases can reinforce false beliefs, hinder open discussion, and perpetuate myths.

THE BACKFIRE EFFECT

The *backfire effect* is evident when people hold even more tightly to their beliefs after being presented with opposing evidence. A common example in nutrition is the belief that "organic food is always healthier" than non-organic options.

While research shows that the nutritional differences between organic and conventional foods are often minimal, those committed to the superiority of organic products may reject this evidence. They might argue that organic food is inherently better despite studies indicating that factors like overall diet quality and variety have a greater impact on health than whether the food is organic. Instead of reconsidering their stance, they double down, insisting on the health benefits of organic food while dismissing scientific findings to the contrary.

SOCIAL PRIORITIES

Group identity plays a powerful role in shaping dietary beliefs. People often adopt nutritional views that align with the norms of their social circles, regardless of scientific support. Emotional attachment to these group beliefs often outweighs logic, making extreme or fear-based nutrition ideologies easier to spread.

This also ties into the concept of *social proof*, where people follow the actions of others, assuming they reflect the "right" choice. In nutrition, this could manifest as a group of friends adopting a juice cleanse simply because it's trendy, not because there's any credible scientific backing. The herd mentality strengthens these trends, making it harder for individuals to question them critically.

COGNITIVE DISSONANCE

Cognitive dissonance arises when someone holds two conflicting beliefs, causing discomfort that they attempt to resolve by dismissing one of the conflicting ideas. In the realm of nutrition, this might look like someone who champions getting all nutrients from whole foods but also spends large amounts on dietary supplements. To reconcile this conflict, they might justify the supplements as a necessary "backup," even though this undermines their belief in the sufficiency of whole foods.

A similar contradiction is seen in those who avoid "toxins" in the food supply while regularly consuming alcohol, an undeniable toxin. The internal conflict between these beliefs often goes unexamined, leading to inconsistency in discussing and practicing nutrition. This dissonance can distort conversations around diet, as people may cling to one side of the argument while acting in ways that contradict it.

AD HOMINEM ATTACKS

When nutrition discussions turn heated, personal insults or *ad hominem* attacks often replace constructive dialogue. Instead of engaging with the evidence, one side might dismiss their opponent as "ignorant" or "unhealthy," avoiding the actual argument altogether. For instance, a proponent of a strict vegan diet might ignore a scientific critique and instead label the critic as "uneducated" or "biased by the meat industry." This shuts down meaningful discussion and shifts the focus away from the facts. Personal attacks not only damage the quality of the conversation, but also polarize the discussion, making it more difficult to find common ground.

DIFFERENT GOALS

Miscommunication in nutrition discussions often happens because participants have differing goals that aren't clearly expressed. Before engaging in a conversation about diet or health, it's important to clarify your intentions. Are you aiming to exchange information, persuade someone, or share a personal experience? For example, if one person is sharing emotional stories about their struggles with food, and the other is focused on presenting hard data about nutrition, the conversation can quickly become unproductive. Clearly establishing the purpose of the discussion helps keep it focused and constructive, preventing it from veering off into conflicting directions.

ILLUSORY TRUTH EFFECT

The illusory truth effect explains why nutrition myths persist: when people hear a statement repeated frequently, they are more likely to believe it's true, even if it's false. A famous example outside of nutrition is the myth that "we only use 10 percent of our brains," a statement debunked by science yet still widely believed.[41]

Similarly, in the nutrition world, the idea that "eating after 8 PM causes weight gain" lingers despite research showing that weight gain is more about total daily calorie intake than meal timing. Repetition of these false ideas, whether in casual conversation or online, solidifies their perceived truth, making it harder to debunk them.

HOW TO APPROACH NUTRITION DISCOURSE

1. **Be a Bridge Builder** – Focus on fostering understanding and connection rather than trying to win an argument. Effective communication involves listening and absorbing diverse perspectives, not just sharing your own. Prioritize constructive dialogue that builds relationships and common ground, acknowledging when others have valid points and collaborating toward mutual understanding.

2. **Have Thick Skin and Stay Professional** – Not everyone will agree with you, and that's okay. Learn to accept criticism without taking it personally and use feedback as an opportunity for growth. Respond professionally, treating criticism objectively and avoiding emotional responses. Part of maintaining professionalism is applying symmetrical logic, ensuring consistency in your arguments and avoiding the influence of cognitive dissonance. This strengthens your ability to stay open to valid points without compromising your integrity.

3. **Embrace Flexibility and Collaboration** – Avoid strict, rigid rules when discussing nutrition. Instead, embrace guidelines that allow for flexibility and nuance. Acknowledge when you're wrong and be open to adjusting your views based on merit and evidence. Collaboration and a willingness to budge on positions foster progress in discussions and lead to better outcomes.

4. **Be a Learner** – Prioritize being informed and continuously learning, recognizing that meaningful exchanges are only possible when both sides are well-versed in the topic. Encourage thoughtful, well-researched discussions that rely on critical thinking. By approaching conversations with curiosity and a desire to understand, you not only contribute to civil discourse but also deepen your knowledge and avoid the pitfalls of misinformed debates.

5. **Avoid Misinformation and Toxic Influences** – Steer clear of individuals or groups who spread misinformation or engage in discourse solely to reinforce their own beliefs. Seek out those committed to authenticity, growth, and truth. Recognize that some people will cling to unfounded beliefs, and sometimes, it's best to disengage rather than waste energy on unproductive debates. And remember, not all lightbulbs can be turned on.

Approaching nutrition discourse with empathy, professionalism, and a willingness to learn can improve conversations, but mass communication often overlooks the unique needs of individuals—next, we'll explore how to recognize and address the diverse nutritional requirements that make each person's health journey different.

CHAPTER 8: UNIQUE

"Remember always that you not only have the right to be an individual, you have an obligation to be one."

— **Eleanor Roosevelt**

All of us have unique nutritional needs, which are shaped by factors like biology, lifestyle, and personal goals. Nutrition isn't one-size-fits-all; our bodies respond differently due to individual variations in genetics, activity levels, and health conditions. Yet, much of the nutrition advice we encounter is too generalized and often overlooks these critical differences.

Without contemplating where we come from or where we're headed, cookie-cutter nutrition plans are bound to fall short. That's why a personalized approach is essential for achieving and maintaining optimal health. In fact, studies show that personalized nutrition can be up to 1.6 times more effective in improving health outcomes compared to standard guidelines.[1]

However, embracing our uniqueness doesn't mean falling for fad diets that masquerade as "personalized plans." While our individual needs vary, we all share the basic requirement for balanced nutrition—an adequate intake of macronutrients like carbohydrates, proteins, and fats, along with essential vitamins and minerals.

The goal is to craft a personalized eating plan that fits within the framework of proven nutritional guidelines. By respecting our bodies' unique needs while adhering to sound, well-rounded principles, we can develop a sustainable and fulfilling approach to health.

WHAT DOES IT MEAN TO BE UNIQUE?

We all know we're different from one another, but we may not fully grasp how these differences shape our nutritional needs. While I often see a worthwhile focus on differences based on gender or micronutrient needs, I think we tend to miss a myriad of other factors that potentially play bigger roles. To truly support holistic health needs, here are some underrepresented traits that will be the focus of this chapter on unique nutrition needs:

Childhood and Culture – Our upbringing and cultural traditions often shape food preferences, which play a large role in developing a sustainable diet.

Health Conditions – Chronic illnesses, allergies, and intolerances demand specific dietary adjustments to support overall health and manage symptoms.

Genetic Makeup – Our genes influence how we metabolize foods, affecting everything from digestion to food reward experiences, which is why new treatments like GLP-1s work well for some.

Body Size and Composition – Height, weight, and muscle mass influence our nutrient and energy needs.

Habits and Schedule – Meal timing and daily routines impact how our bodies process and use nutrients. Our needs can change over time, such as during pregnancy or seasonal shifts.

Goals – Whether it's weight loss, muscle gain, or managing a condition, personal goals shape nutritional strategies, and they can extend beyond health, like supporting local farms or eating for pure pleasure.

Food Environment and Access – What's available to us, from fresh produce to social influences, can shape what we eat.

Mental Health – Stress, anxiety, and other mental health factors can shift appetite and nutritional needs.

CHILDHOOD AND CULTURE

Our food preferences are deeply shaped by the culture and circumstances we're exposed to in childhood. Yet many of us believe we start with a blank slate when it comes to choosing our adult diet. We often assume that the recipes we see online or the meals our friends enjoy can simply be plugged into our lives. But in reality, the foods we grew up eating are closely tied to our sense of identity, influenced by our local environment, economic factors, heritage, and even religion.

These early experiences don't just shape what we enjoy eating; they also affect how we perceive food on a psychological level. Positive associations with certain foods, often linked to childhood memories, can trigger pleasure responses in the brain. This makes those foods particularly satisfying, even if someone else with similar taste preferences doesn't experience them the same way. That's why we can't just adopt any popular recipe or copy our favorite celebrity's diet and expect it to feel natural.

Instead, we tend to stick with meals that remind us of foods we grew up with, or that align with our cultural background. This doesn't mean we need to eat sugary cereal for breakfast every day just because it was part of our childhood, but it does mean we're more likely to stick with a meal that evokes something familiar like swapping cereal for oatmeal topped with granola. While we're adaptable and can expand our palates to include new foods, recognizing our food heritage helps us understand what gives us joy and is more likely to feel sustainable.

Taste, at its core, is a survival mechanism that helps us identify safe and nutritious foods. But in today's world, this system is often hijacked by highly processed foods engineered to hit the sweet, salty, and savory notes that our taste buds crave. While these flavors are universally appealing, our more nuanced food preferences are shaped by what we were exposed to in infancy and childhood. So, if you struggle with certain flavors or dislike specific foods, it could be a reflection of your early food environment.

EARLY EXPOSURE

Early exposure to a variety of foods during infancy and childhood plays a vital role in shaping our food preferences.[2,3] Studies show that repeated exposure to certain foods can increase a child's acceptance of them and are more likely to develop a taste for them later in life. For example, children introduced to a wide variety of vegetables at a young age are more likely to enjoy and regularly consume them as they grow.[4,5] This highlights the importance of offering diverse foods to children, setting the foundation for a more varied and balanced diet in adulthood.

Introducing a variety of foods early on also helps prevent strong aversions and picky eating, laying the foundation for a diverse diet that is more sustainable and linked to better long-term health, including a reduced risk of chronic disease.

Reflecting on our childhood food experiences can reveal where we might need to rethink old habits and embrace more balanced ones. Understanding the role of early exposure allows us to make informed dietary choices and encourages us to introduce variety to the next generation. Rather than following an overly idealized meal plan you see online, it's more practical to consider your personal history and develop realistic, enjoyable habits.

While early exposure to healthy eating shapes our future, the good news is that we remain adaptable as adults. We can still use our past experiences as a tool to create healthier patterns that align with both our preferences and nutritional needs.

HABIT EXPOSURE

The meals we were introduced to, the eating habits we observed, and the food culture within our family laid the groundwork for our future attitudes toward food. For instance, growing up in a family where shared, balanced meals were valued often leads to a healthier relationship with food. On the flip side, childhood environments marked by food scarcity or rushed meals may create anxiety around eating, potentially leading to overeating or unhealthy habits as an adult.

TRADITIONS AND VALUES

Cultural and personal values heavily influence our food choices. Religious and ethical beliefs shape dietary practices, such as vegetarianism or kosher and halal diets, while others focus on sustainability by choosing locally sourced or organic foods. These values not only affect what we eat but also how we view food and nutrition. For example, someone prioritizing sustainability might prefer plant-based proteins, while another person may favor traditional foods from their cultural heritage, even if they don't fit mainstream health advice.

Cultural preferences are deeply ingrained from a young age. In Japan, the love for umami-rich foods like miso soup is cultivated early, while in India, exposure to a variety of spices fosters a lifelong tolerance for complex, spicy flavors. In Ethiopia, traditional foods like injera and doro wat are staples, and communal meals emphasize the importance of food in social connections. Similarly, Mediterranean cultures focus on fresh vegetables, olive oil, and fish, establishing healthy eating habits that persist into adulthood.[6,7]

Understanding how your values and cultural background shape your food choices allow you to make decisions that resonate with your identity while still meeting your nutritional needs. As much as 70% of our food preferences and behaviors are shaped by the cultural and familial environments, we grow up in.[8,9] Recognizing the influence of these early experiences helps us make more informed and helps steer us away from nonsense—like the idea that we must adapt to a specific popular diet or celebrity nutrition plan. This is bound to fail, because we need to honor our own traditions.

THE CLEAN PLATE CLUB

A common childhood practice many underwent is called the "Clean Plate Club." This is where children (or adults) are encouraged or forced to finish everything on their plates. While this was meant to teach appreciation for food (and perhaps avoid food waste), it often leads to unhealthy eating habits, such as ignoring natural hunger cues and overeating out of obligation. This can foster mindless eating, where food is consumed without enjoying its flavors or textures.

To counter this mentality, it's essential to focus on mindful eating—savoring each bite, eating slowly, and respecting satiety cues. Leftovers can be saved and enjoyed later, reframing them as something to look forward to instead of feeling guilty for not finishing. Those who grew up in food-scarce environments or with restrictive parents may also develop habits of overeating or hoarding food. By recognizing these patterns, we can begin to trust our hunger signals and cultivate a healthier relationship with food.

Our emotional attachment to certain foods often stems from childhood experiences, shaping our preferences and beliefs about what is "good" or "bad." It's freeing to realize that as adults, we have the power to redefine our relationship with food, basing our choices on current knowledge and what works best for us, not outdated habits from our past.

Instead of buying into the myth that we all should be eating the same foods or that everyone can just as easily follow the same popular nutrition advice, we must remind ourselves that our personal exposures and experiences throughout life heavily shape our food choices. Each of these unique experiences can be molded into healthier versions of eating, but they will almost certainly look different.

HEALTH CONDITIONS

Common health conditions like diabetes, heart disease, and food allergies have a big impact on our nutritional needs, requiring specific dietary adjustments to manage symptoms and prevent complications.

The American Diabetes Association reports that about 34.2 million Americans, or 10.5% of the population, have diabetes, underscoring the importance of dietary management to prevent complications like neuropathy and kidney damage. Likewise, those with heart disease often need to follow a low-sodium diet, as high sodium intake contributes to hypertension, a major risk factor for heart disease. The CDC estimates that nearly half of U.S. adults have hypertension, emphasizing the need for sodium reduction in their diets.[10]

Although we already discussed the potential overreach of gluten issues for a majority of the population, those with celiac disease, which affects approximately 1% of the global population, avoiding gluten is essential to prevent damage to the small intestine and issues like malabsorption and nutrient deficiencies. This goes to show just how important knowing your own health conditions is, as many people may not need to remove gluten at all, while others absolutely must get it out of their diet. Such dramatic differences in needs may require testing if you are unsure of where you might land.

Whatever the specific condition may be, the value of adopting a specialized diet is that it can significantly improve health outcomes. This is why a low-fat diet, while not appropriate for everyone, is helpful for certain conditions, like those with gallbladder issues, as it can prevent pain and indigestion.

Consulting a healthcare provider or dietitian ensures that dietary adjustments are not only effective but also nutritionally sound, helping to manage the condition and support overall well-being. While many of us may assume our diets should mirror popular trends, these examples highlight how individualized our needs can be based on unique health circumstances.

As well as common conditions like diabetes and heart disease, there are many other health conditions that would require even more specific dietary interventions, such as:

Phenylketonuria (PKU) – A rare genetic disorder affecting about 1 in 10,000 to 15,000 newborns in the U.S. PKU prevents the metabolism of phenylalanine, an amino acid found in protein-rich foods and artificial sweeteners like aspartame.[11] People with PKU must follow a strict low-phenylalanine diet to avoid severe neurological damage, often relying on special medical formulas for adequate nutrition.

Irritable Bowel Syndrome (IBS) – IBS affects around 10 to 15% of the global population and is characterized by symptoms like abdominal pain, bloating, and altered bowel habits.[12] Managing IBS typically involves identifying and avoiding trigger foods, such as those high in FODMAPs, which are poorly absorbed in the small intestine and can worsen symptoms.

Gout – Gout is a type of arthritis caused by elevated levels of uric acid, which leads to the formation of crystals in joints, often triggering sudden, severe pain. Those with gout need to limit foods high in purines, such as red meat, shellfish, and alcohol, which can raise uric acid levels and cause flare-ups.[13]

Chronic Kidney Disease (CKD) – CKD affects approximately 37 million U.S. adults, leading to a gradual loss of kidney function.[14] Dietary management is key to slowing the disease's progression, requiring limits on sodium, phosphorus, and potassium intake, as well as moderating protein to reduce kidney strain.

Eosinophilic Esophagitis (EoE) – EoE is a chronic immune disease that causes inflammation in the esophagus, making swallowing difficult and leading to food impaction. It is often triggered by specific allergens, so individuals with EoE may need to follow an elimination diet to avoid foods like dairy, wheat, soy, eggs, nuts, and seafood.[15]

GENETICS

To truly honor our unique physiology and backgrounds, it's essential to recognize that genetics plays a significant role in how each of us responds to food. The common misconception is that everyone reacts the same way to food and that struggling with overeating or making poor food choices is a personal, moral failing. In reality, our genetics powerfully influence our cravings, hunger, and even how satisfied we feel after eating.

For many, this can feel frustrating, like something beyond our control. However, understanding these genetic differences can actually be empowering. By acknowledging that our biology may be wired to respond to certain foods differently than others, we can stop blaming ourselves for perceived shortcomings. Instead, we can focus on interventions that are better suited to our individual needs. This shift in perspective allows us to make smarter, more personalized choices that support our health rather than adhering to a universal approach that may not work for us.

FOOD REWARD

Food reward, the pleasure and satisfaction derived from eating, varies widely among individuals, largely due to genetic differences in how our brains respond to nutrients like sugar and fat. For some, a sweet treat triggers a strong sense of pleasure, while others may find fatty foods more rewarding. This variation can significantly influence our food choices, often drawing us toward foods that either support or undermine our health goals.

Research reveals that certain genetic variations make some people more sensitive to the rewarding effects of sugar, leading them to consume more or less sugary foods based on these inherited traits.[16,17,18,19] This underscores the fact that some people may benefit from stricter boundaries, such as using non-caloric sweeteners, while others can enjoy more flexibility. Understanding your unique taste preferences and food reward system can help guide more satisfying and sustainable food choices.

Instead of forcing yourself to eat foods you dislike, focus on finding nutritious options that align with your tastes, making it easier to maintain a balanced, enjoyable diet long-term.

LEPTIN

Leptin, often called the "satiety hormone," helps regulate hunger and fat storage. Genetics play a role in how sensitive we are to leptin, which impacts how we store fat and feel full after eating. Some people might be genetically inclined to store fat in areas like the belly, which can increase the risk of metabolic issues.

Endocrinology studies have shown that people with certain variations in the leptin receptor gene are at higher risk for obesity due to decreased leptin sensitivity.[20,21] This means that some people may benefit from a more personalized diet that addresses their hormonal response to food. For instance, a diet that's lower in certain fats or carbs might work better for people with these genetic traits when it comes to managing their weight. With the growing use of GLP-1 medications, which mimic hormones that help control appetite and blood sugar, we can see how understanding genetics can lead to more personalized and effective ways to manage weight.

GLP-1 MEDICATIONS

GLP-1 (glucagon-like peptide-1) medications have become popular because of their effectiveness in addressing hunger and "food noise," or the constant inner thoughts about food. These medications mimic the action of the GLP-1 hormone, helping regulate appetite, insulin, and glucose metabolism. They are particularly helpful for individuals who have genetic predispositions to intense cravings or an overactive appetite.

Studies show that GLP-1 medications can help reduce body weight by 10 to 15% in individuals who struggle with traditional weight loss methods due to their genetic tendencies.[22,23] Yet, while these medications can be effective, they're not without side effects, like nausea or gastrointestinal discomfort.[24] Additionally, long-term success still depends on maintaining healthy lifestyle changes like diet and exercise. Understanding one's genetic makeup can help in evaluating whether GLP-1 medications are a suitable tool for weight management.

FOOD DEPENDENCY

While sugar alone isn't typically addictive, combining sugar with fat, salt, and certain textures can create a powerful drive to consume specific foods. This is partly due to genetic predispositions, which make some individuals more susceptible to food dependencies, particularly for highly palatable foods with specific combinations of ingredients. This can make maintaining a healthy diet more challenging, as these food combinations often trigger cravings and overeating.

Research has shown that around 20% of people have a variant in the FTO gene, which increases their preference for high-calorie, indulgent foods.[25] For these people, resisting foods like pizza or pastries, which are engineered to be especially rewarding, can be much more difficult. A personalized diet that cuts down on trigger foods and focuses on filling, nutrient-rich options can help manage food cravings and support long-term health. Understanding how our genetics shape our food preferences lets us make smarter, more tailored nutrition choices.

BODY SIZE AND COMPOSITION

Height, weight, muscle mass, organ size, and hormonal variations all play significant roles in determining individual caloric and macronutrient needs. Understanding these differences can guide more informed and effective dietary choices.

HEIGHT AND WEIGHT

Height and weight are key factors in determining how much energy we need. Taller people generally require more calories to sustain their larger skeletal structures and body mass. For example, someone who's 6 feet tall typically needs more calories than someone who is 5 feet tall, even if both have similar activity levels. This is because taller individuals have more cells and a bigger surface area, leading to greater heat loss and a higher energy demand.[26]

Body weight is another important factor in figuring out calorie needs. Someone who weighs 200 pounds will need more energy to maintain their weight compared to someone who weighs 150 pounds. But it's also important to think about what that weight is made up of—whether it's more muscle or fat. Muscle burns more calories when resting than fat, so a more muscular person will have higher energy needs.

Many of my clients focus on reaching a specific weight because they often compare themselves to others. What they probably don't realize is that striving to match someone else's weight, especially when your height, bone structure, or muscle mass differs, is unrealistic and even potentially harmful. Instead of chasing a number, focus on what works for your body. If your current eating habits give you energy, keep your weight stable, satisfy hunger, and are enjoyable, there's no need to change just because of external pressures. Prioritize your health over societal expectations or comparisons to others.

ORGAN SIZE

The size of your organs, especially metabolically active ones like the liver, heart, and kidneys, also affects how many calories you need. Larger organs require more energy to function, impacting overall energy expenditure. Research shows that metabolically active organs, like the liver and heart, make up only about 5-6% of your body weight but can account for up to 60% of your resting energy expenditure (REE).[27]

Two people who weigh the same might have different organ sizes, leading to varying caloric needs (although this is often marginal).

BONE DENSITY, MUSCLE AND FAT

Those with higher bone density need more nutrients like calcium and vitamin D to maintain bone health, while individuals with higher levels of visceral fat are at greater risk for heart disease.

Research from the American Heart Association shows that people with more visceral fat have a 50% higher risk of heart disease than those with subcutaneous fat.[28] For instance, postmenopausal women, who are more prone to osteoporosis, may need a diet rich in calcium and vitamin D, along with weight-bearing exercise, to help maintain bone density and reduce the risk of fractures.

Having more muscle mass is often linked to higher levels of growth hormone and testosterone, which influence how the body uses protein and fat. Those with more muscle mass may have up to 20% higher growth hormone levels, promoting increased protein synthesis and fat metabolism.[29] This means individuals with more muscle may need a protein-rich diet to help maintain and build their muscle mass.

INDIVIDUAL BODIES

The variety in body size and composition shows why personalized nutrition plans are so important. Factors like height, weight, muscle mass, organ size, bone density, fat distribution, and hormones all impact our individual nutritional needs. Following a one-size-fits-all diet is not only unhealthy, but it can lead to undernourishment, overeating, or unbalanced macronutrients, which can harm your health. A tailored approach, based on your body's unique traits, is key to optimizing health and getting the best results.

Standardized diets often miss the mark for different body types, which is why personalized nutrition is so important. By honoring our unique physiology, we can make better food choices, achieve our health goals more effectively, and boost our overall well-being.

UNIQUE HABITS AND SCHEDULES

Meal timing and frequency can vary widely depending on individual work hours, sleep patterns, and daily activities. As we move through different stages of life, our habits evolve, requiring us to adjust our nutrition to maintain balance and health.

TIMING AND SEASONS

Life is constantly changing, and so are our schedules and responsibilities. Whether you're a busy professional, a parent balancing multiple duties, or a retiree with more free time, your daily routine influences your eating habits and nutritional needs. Different seasons of life, such as pregnancy, caregiving, or retirement, also bring unique nutritional challenges. For example, during pregnancy, the body requires more calories, protein, iron, and folic acid to support both mother and baby. On the other hand, retirees may need fewer calories but should focus on nutrient-dense foods to stay healthy as their metabolism slows down.

We don't all experience the 24 hours in a day the same way, as our priorities differ. A working parent may not have the time or energy for elaborate meals daily, and that's okay. The key is finding a balance that works for your life and health. As Danielle Wilksons wisely notes, "A 23-year-old influencer doesn't have the same demands, lifestyle, and stressors as a 36-year-old mom-of-three who works two jobs."[33] Understanding that your nutritional needs evolve with age and life stage helps in making more effective food choices and gives us a better perspective.

AGES AND STAGES

Nutritional needs evolve from infancy to old age, and each stage of life brings unique requirements to support growth, development, and overall health. Research from the National Institute on Aging shows that after age 40, adults lose an average of 1–2% of muscle mass per year without strength training.[34] This muscle loss affects metabolism, making it crucial to adjust dietary intake to prevent weight gain and maintain muscle mass.

Nutritional needs are also heightened during periods of rapid growth, such as adolescence, where increased calories, protein, and essential vitamins like calcium and vitamin D are vital for bone development. In contrast, older adults require fewer calories but more nutrients, such as vitamin B12, to maintain cognitive function and prevent deficiencies.

STRESS AND SLEEP

Beyond schedules, stress levels and sleep quality significantly influence nutritional needs and habits. A study on sleep and obesity found that people who sleep fewer than 6 hours per night are 55% more likely to become obese compared to those who sleep 7–8 hours.[35] This connection collaborates with research showing how sleep impacts hunger hormones, eating habits, and meal timing. It just goes to show how important sleep is for staying healthy and managing weight. In the same way, ongoing stress can lead to emotional eating or skipping meals, which throws off nutrition and can cause weight changes.

ACTIVITY LEVELS

Physical activity levels also play a critical role in shaping nutritional needs. According to the American College of Sports Medicine, those who engage in regular high-intensity exercise may need 1.2 to 2.0 grams of protein per kilogram of body weight, compared to 0.8 grams for sedentary adults.[36] A higher protein intake can enhance satiety and support overall health, making it a valuable tool for those with varying activity levels.

Whether you're an athlete, a weekend warrior, or someone with a sedentary lifestyle, aligning your diet with your activity level is crucial. High-intensity workouts require more carbohydrates and proteins, while a sedentary lifestyle may benefit from nutrient-dense, lower-calorie foods to prevent weight gain. While the average "gym bro" might swear by unseasoned chicken breast and broccoli, it's important to find nutritious and creative options that fit your preferences and lifestyle if this helps you stay on track.

The timing and regularity of meals vary widely depending on individual work hours, sleep patterns, and other daily activities. Daily routines, like meal timing and frequency, significantly influence how our bodies process and utilize nutrients. As we move through different seasons of life, our habits also evolve, requiring adjustments in our nutrition to maintain health and balance.

DIVERSE GOALS

Nutritional needs vary significantly depending on individual goals, lifestyle, and personal values. It's important to think about what food can do for *you* and not get caught up in living someone else's life. Whether you are focused on losing weight, building muscle, managing a chronic illness, or supporting environmental or ethical causes, each goal calls for its own approach, including adjustments in calorie intake, macronutrient balance, and food choices.

Weight Loss – For those focused on weight loss, the primary goal is to create a change in portions or total energy intake—while maintaining enough protein to preserve muscle mass. A common strategy includes incorporating high-protein, moderate calorie foods, along with regular physical activity, to support fat loss without sacrificing lean tissue. Balanced meals that promote satiety and consistency can be key to long-term success.

Muscle Gain – Those seeking muscle gain require a calorie surplus and should consume more calories than they burn daily. This approach is paired with a higher protein intake to support muscle repair and growth. Carbohydrates provide the energy needed for intense workouts, while healthy fats promote healthy hormone production. Similarly, nutrient timing and portion control can optimize muscle-building efforts.

Chronic Illness Management – Those managing chronic illnesses, such as diabetes, heart disease, or hypertension, need a specialized diet that supports overall health while addressing specific medical concerns. For example, people suffering from diabetes benefit from balancing blood sugar levels through a diet rich in whole grains, lean proteins, and fiber while limiting sugars and refined carbohydrates. Those managing heart disease may focus on heart-healthy fats, like omega-3s, and limiting sodium and trans fats to maintain healthy cholesterol and blood pressure levels.

Ethical and Environmental Considerations: Some people prioritize ethical or environmental concerns, choosing a diet that aligns with their values. For these people, a plant-based or sustainable eating approach might take precedence, emphasizing locally sourced foods and organic products or avoiding animal-based products altogether. These dietary choices require careful planning to ensure all essential nutrients are met, such as vitamin B12, iron, and protein, for those following vegan or vegetarian diets.

Pleasure and Survival – Lastly, some people take a more flexible approach, focusing on eating for both pleasure and survival. This often follows the 80/20 rule, where 80% of the diet is made up of nutrient-dense, whole foods, and the remaining 20% allows for indulgence and flexibility. Some may prefer a stricter 90/10 balance, while others might go for a more relaxed 60/40 approach. Although extreme voices may advocate for 100% "clean" eating or complete indulgence, most individuals find a middle ground where they prioritize health while allowing space for enjoyment.

Defining your own success, but aim for concrete and specific targets that align with individual values and lifestyles while remaining flexible enough to adapt to your growing and evolving goals.

FOOD ENVIRONMENT

If I hear one more person on social media say that "inflammation is the root cause of all diseases," I might actually lose my mind. Here's the thing: if we want to truly understand the root cause of our health issues, we have to go much deeper. Inflammation doesn't just appear out of nowhere. It's a symptom, not the source. Inflammation results from poor nutrition, stress, lack of exercise, and other lifestyle factors that are largely dictated by the environment we live in and the social networks we are a part of.

It might be easy to point fingers at inflammation, laziness, or even a lack of willpower, but those are surface-level explanations. If we want real change, we have to dig deeper and address the root causes of what is shaping our habits, our options, and our choices in the first place. That's where the social determinants of health come into play. These are the powerful, often unseen factors that have a profound and lasting impact on nutrition, well-being, and overall health. They shape the food environment and explain why some communities have easy access to healthy, fresh food while others struggle to find anything remotely nutritious.

The truth is that our environment shapes our food choices far more than we might like to admit. The availability of fresh produce, the convenience of processed food, the cost of groceries, and the social norms within our communities all play major roles in what ends up on our plates. If we want lasting improvements in health, we have to start by understanding and addressing these deeper, systemic issues. This is more than a personal choice. It's about the world we live in, the systems we move through, and the obstacles we face every day.

SOCIAL DETERMINANTS OF HEALTH

There's no denying that motivation and discipline are important factors in determining health success. Even so, the reality is that these factors are not the reason for the widespread health issues occurring throughout the world. It's actually because of the social determinants of health, factors like income, education, neighborhood conditions, and social support. These are key to understanding the disparities in nutrition across different populations. These determinants impact what food is available, affordable, and desirable, creating significant differences in dietary quality and health outcomes.

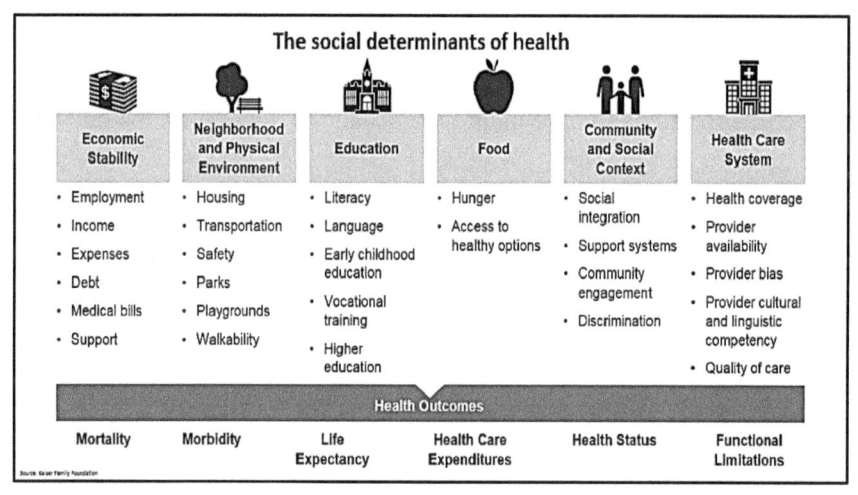

The social determinants of health					
Economic Stability	**Neighborhood and Physical Environment**	**Education**	**Food**	**Community and Social Context**	**Health Care System**
• Employment • Income • Expenses • Debt • Medical bills • Support	• Housing • Transportation • Safety • Parks • Playgrounds • Walkability	• Literacy • Language • Early childhood education • Vocational training • Higher education	• Hunger • Access to healthy options	• Social integration • Support systems • Community engagement • Discrimination	• Health coverage • Provider availability • Provider bias • Provider cultural and linguistic competency • Quality of care

Health Outcomes					
Mortality	Morbidity	Life Expectancy	Health Care Expenditures	Health Status	Functional Limitations

Source: Kaiser Family Foundation

Income and Economic Constraints – Economic limitations can make it difficult for families to afford nutrient-dense foods, such as fresh fruits, vegetables, and high-quality proteins. Families and individuals on lower incomes often budget heavily and have to purchase cheaper, calorie-dense processed foods, which lack essential nutrients. According to reports, 12.8% of U.S. households experienced food insecurity in 2022.[37] This insecurity forces families to make difficult choices, such as opting for lower-cost processed foods or skipping meals altogether. Such diets are linked to higher rates of obesity, malnutrition, and diet-related diseases like diabetes.

Education and Awareness – Education is another key factor shaping dietary choices. Those with higher education levels tend to have good health literacy, like the ability to understand nutrition labels and the long-term benefits of a balanced diet. This access to information can lead to more health-conscious food choices. Those with limited education, on the other hand, might not fully grasp the consequences of poor dietary habits or how to make healthier substitutions. Without basic nutritional education, it becomes significantly harder to navigate the complex world of modern food marketing and make informed decisions.

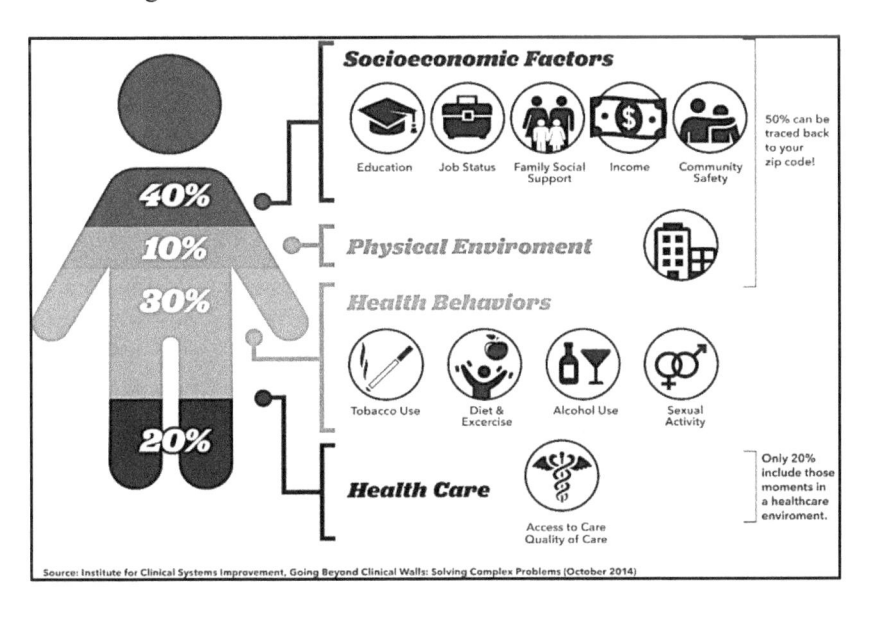

Source: Institute for Clinical Systems Improvement, Going Beyond Clinical Walls: Solving Complex Problems (October 2014)

Neighborhood and Food Deserts – Living in a food desert, a neighborhood with limited access to affordable, healthy food options, poses a major barrier to maintaining a balanced diet. About 23.5 million Americans reside in food deserts, where fast food and convenience stores are more prevalent than grocery stores offering fresh produce.[38] Without access to fresh fruits, vegetables, and lean proteins, those living in a food desert may rely on processed and prepackaged foods. This increases their risk of developing chronic diseases. Similarly, this geographical divide is one of the clearest examples of how the social determinants of health directly influence nutritional outcomes.

Transportation Access – Access to reliable transportation is another major determinant of food security. For those without a car or access to public transport, reaching stores that offer healthy food options can be a big challenge. Because of this, people might shop at nearby convenience stores, which have limited or unaffordable fresh produce and healthy items. A study revealed that students with fast-food restaurants near their schools (within half a mile) ate few fruits and vegetables and more soda, increasing their risk of being overweight compared to peers without these proximity issues.[39]

Healthcare Access and Quality – People who lack health insurance or have limited access to health care may miss out on crucial screenings and dietary advice for managing chronic conditions. About 1 in 10 people lack health insurance in the U.S., making it difficult for them to access the resources needed for healthy eating.[40] It should also be mentioned that healthcare systems tied to employment status create disparities in the quality of care, further exacerbating health inequities.

Food Scarcity and Obesity – Although it might sound strange, food scarcity can actually lead to obesity. Hypercaloric processed foods are more affordable and accessible in low-income areas. This can cause overconsumption of empty calories and nutrient-poor meals. These unhealthy eating patterns are reinforced by aggressive marketing aimed at vulnerable populations. Even those who desire to make healthier choices find it difficult to afford or access nutritious foods. A staggering 80% of Americans report feeling financially unable to consistently make healthier purchasing decisions.[41]

STRATEGIES FOR FOOD ACCESS

To address the gaps in access to nutritious food, several strategies can help bridge the gap between fresh, healthy food options and those facing barriers. While these options will not fix the deeper issues at hand, they can give individuals a meaningful shift in health.

- **Fresh vs. Frozen and Canned Produce** – While fresh produce is ideal, frozen and canned fruits and vegetables can provide the same essential nutrients, especially in areas where fresh options are scarce or expensive. Selecting low-sodium canned vegetables or unsweetened frozen fruits can help people maintain a healthy diet when fresh options aren't feasible.

- **Growing Food** – Community gardens and home gardening initiatives can be powerful solutions in areas with limited access to fresh produce. These programs not only provide nutritious food but also foster community engagement and educate people on sustainable eating practices.

- **Creative Meal Planning** – For those with limited access to healthy food, creative meal planning can make a significant difference. Meals based on whole grains, legumes, and frozen vegetables can improve dietary quality, even when fresh options are hard to come by.

- **Relationships and Social Dynamics** – The people we surround ourselves with also play a critical role in shaping our food choices. Family, friends, and workplace environments can either support or sabotage healthy eating habits.

- **Family and Household Influence** – Household dynamics can significantly influence food choices. If a family member consistently opts for takeout, it can be harder to maintain healthy eating patterns. On the flip side, having a partner or roommate who prioritizes nutritious meals and exercise can encourage healthier habits.

- **Workplace Environment** – Workplaces can be filled with tempting, unhealthy foods, like free snacks in the break room or vending machines stocked with indulgent foods. This might contribute to mindless eating and poor choices. Creating a healthier workplace food environment can make it easier for employees to make nutritious decisions throughout the day.

- **Childhood Nutrition** – Parents and caregivers have a significant influence on children's dietary habits. Educating parents about the importance of balanced nutrition and providing them with access to healthy foods can set the foundation for a lifetime of healthy eating habits.

THE BIGGER PICTURE

The social determinants of health and the food environment play crucial roles in shaping our dietary habits and overall nutrition. While personal responsibility matters, the larger systemic issues cannot be overlooked. This should not take away the need to empower individuals and families to still make meaningful changes, but we can't ignore something that is such a huge part of the equation. Instead of choosing to either address the social determinants of health through societal and policy changes or address our individual responsibility, we should encourage both solutions as they allow us to make a difference now and in the long run.

MENTAL HEALTH

Stress, anxiety, depression, and other mental health conditions can alter not only how we feel but also what and how we eat. Recognizing this relationship is crucial because food can become both a cause and a consequence of mental health struggles. While physical health gets a lot of attention in diet choices, mental well-being plays just as big a role in shaping our eating habits and nutritional needs.

Stress and Eating Habits – Significant stress can trigger emotional eating. Reaching for high-calorie comfort foods like sweets, chips, or fast food to soothe difficult emotions. While this may offer temporary relief, it often leads to poor dietary choices that can worsen physical health and, ironically, increase stress. This can create a vicious cycle: stress leads to unhealthy eating, which causes more stress, creating a loop that can be difficult to break.

Mental Health Conditions and Nutrition Deficits – Mental health conditions like depression and anxiety can lead to a loss of appetite, resulting in inadequate nutrient intake. When mental health diminishes, basic self-care practices like meal preparation or regular eating can become overwhelming, leading to deficiencies in key nutrients like iron, vitamin D, or omega-3 fatty acids. These deficiencies can further exacerbate mental health issues, making recovery even more challenging. This interconnectedness between mental health and nutrition underscores the need for a holistic approach to both.

EATING DISORDERS

Eating disorders, such as anorexia nervosa, bulimia nervosa, and binge eating disorder, represent extreme disruptions in eating habits that are closely linked to mental health. Each condition affects the body in its own way, so the nutritional strategies to treat them must be carefully tailored. Many people wrongly assume eating disorders are driven solely by a desire to be thin, but they're complex mental health conditions that require very different and nuanced treatment approaches.

Restrictive Eating Patterns (Anorexia Nervosa) – Anorexia is characterized by extreme food restriction and an intense fear of gaining weight. This can have serious consequences, like malnutrition, muscle loss, heart problems, and weakened bones (osteoporosis). Many people with anorexia avoid entire food groups, which further exacerbates nutrient deficiencies, particularly in calcium, iron, and essential fats. Treating this condition requires careful re-feeding strategies to restore health, but the psychological aspect is just as important. Without tackling body image and fear around food, recovery is difficult.

Binge-Eating and Emotional Eating – Individuals with binge-eating disorder (BED) eat large amounts of food in a short period, often as a way to cope with emotions like sadness, loneliness, or boredom. Unlike those with anorexia, people with BED may not restrict food but struggle with an overwhelming lack of control around eating. Dealing with emotional triggers and learning healthier coping mechanisms are key components of treatment.

Purging and Nutrient Loss (Bulimia Nervosa) – Bulimia involves cycles of binge eating followed by purging, laxatives, excessive exercise, or strict dieting. This can result in serious physical consequences, such as electrolyte imbalances, dehydration, and long-term damage to the digestive system. Individuals with bulimia can often maintain a normal weight, making it harder to recognize the severity of the disorder. Nutritional therapy aims to restore balance, but like anorexia and BED, the psychological aspects must also be addressed.

PERSPECTIVE

Food is rarely just about eating. It can symbolize control, comfort, fear, joy, or even punishment. Understanding these symbolic meanings is critical in supporting recovery—even for those without an eating disorder.

Symbolic Meanings of Food – For someone recovering from anorexia, eating a donut might symbolize triumph over the fear of indulgence. For someone else, a donut may represent a step in the wrong direction as they have decided against emotional eating triggers right now. Recognizing the symbolism attached to certain foods helps tailor treatment to each individual's emotional needs.

Food as Joy and Balance – Many people work on finding a balance between enjoying food for pleasure and staying healthy. Making room for joy in food choices, whether it's through a favorite treat or a nourishing meal, is key to developing a positive relationship with food.

Understanding the profound impact mental health has on nutrition choices is essential for anyone looking to make meaningful improvements in their diet. Whether it's managing stress, overcoming an eating disorder, or simply finding a balanced approach to food, mental health plays a critical role. By addressing both the psychological and physical aspects of nutrition, we can create healthier, more fulfilling relationships with food and improve overall well-being.

BUT WE ARE STILL HUMAN

While we all have our unique nutritional needs, it's essential to remember that, at the core, we're all human and share more similarities than differences. Our bodies, despite variations in genetics, taste preferences, and lifestyle choices, require the same core nutrients, like carbohydrates, proteins, fats, vitamins, and minerals, to maintain proper functioning. These nutrients help power key processes like energy production, immune function, muscle repair, and brain health. The recommended intake for these nutrients typically falls within similar ranges for most people, underscoring the shared biology that connects us.

So, while this chapter is all about discovering how unique we can be, there are some universal truths when it comes to nutrition. For example, diets overly reliant on processed foods, extreme calorie restriction, or excessively high intakes of one macronutrient (like fat or protein) often neglect the balance our bodies need to thrive. Just because a certain approach works for one individual or appears trendy doesn't mean it's beneficial for most people or even healthy in the long term.

The idea that our uniqueness justifies extreme or unbalanced diets can be harmful. While everyone's body reacts differently to certain foods, it's a mistake to think that some of the most fundamental nutrition principles don't apply to everyone. The "everyone is different" argument shouldn't be used to dismiss well-established recommendations.

UNDERSTANDING YOUR UNIQUE NEEDS

While we share basic nutritional needs, our individual eating patterns are shaped by personal preferences, cultural influences, daily routines, and even social dynamics. Some people may thrive on eating smaller, more frequent meals throughout the day, while others feel most satisfied sticking to three larger meals. There isn't just one perfect approach to when or how often we eat, but there are foundational principles that can guide each of us toward healthier eating patterns.

Intermittent fasting, vegetarianism, and ketogenic diets are just a few examples of popular eating approaches that cater to individual preferences, lifestyles, and health goals. However, while these eating patterns may

CHAPTER 8: UNIQUE

vary, the key to success lies in how well they meet our body's need for essential nutrients. A well-executed vegetarian diet, for instance, can be just as balanced and nutrient-dense as a diet that includes meat, as long as attention is paid to getting enough protein, iron, and other key nutrients. Similarly, intermittent fasting might work wonders for some people in terms of managing hunger or weight, but it won't suit everyone, especially those who prefer consistent energy from regular meals and snacks.

Finding an eating pattern that works for you involves more than just meeting your nutritional needs; it also needs to feel sustainable and enjoyable. An eating style that fits naturally into your life is more likely to become a long-term habit rather than a short-lived diet. For instance, someone who enjoys larger, heartier meals might struggle with intermittent fasting, which limits meal times, while another person who prefers light, frequent snacks may find the traditional three-meal-a-day structure unsatisfying.

What's most important is ensuring that your chosen eating pattern not only fits your lifestyle but also aligns with your body's needs for essential nutrients. Whether you're drawn to vegetarianism, intermittent fasting, or any other dietary approach, it's vital to ensure that your diet remains balanced and nutrient-dense. This is how you can maintain both physical health and enjoyment, creating a harmonious relationship with food that promotes long-term well-being.

Ultimately, understanding your unique needs within the framework of human biology allows you to create an eating plan that nourishes both your body and your lifestyle.

WHERE DID THIS NONSENSE COME FROM?

Why do we get it so wrong when it comes to determining our own nutritional needs?

OVEREMPHASIS ON THE WRONG QUALITIES

Do women really need different multivitamins from men? While it's true that some nutrients are more critical for women, like iron, due to menstruation, many of the other differences in multivitamins are based on averages linked to size or activity levels, not gender. The idea that men and women have vastly different nutritional requirements is often exaggerated, leading to marketing tactics that sell products based on gender stereotypes rather than actual needs.

For example, pink-packaged protein powders marketed to women don't provide a different benefit simply because of the packaging. In reality, the nutritional needs of an active woman might be more aligned with an active man's needs than with a sedentary woman's. When choosing supplements, it's essential to focus more on individual factors like lifestyle, physical activity, and specific health goals rather than overgeneralized categories like gender. This overemphasis on irrelevant qualities distracts from the real determinants of health and nutrition.

ATTRIBUTION ERROR

Attribution error happens when we attribute success or failure in nutrition to personal discipline or the inherent qualities of a diet, ignoring broader influences like genetics, environment, and metabolism. For example, someone might believe that their weight loss success is solely due to their strict adherence to a certain diet, without considering other factors like how their environment may have contributed.

This mindset can lead to overgeneralizing the effectiveness of a diet, pushing people to assume that what worked for them should work for everyone. However, nutrition is much more complex and individualized than that. Success on a diet often depends on factors beyond just willpower or the quality of the diet itself. It's about how well the approach aligns with one's unique circumstances.

STATUS QUO BIAS

Status Quo Bias is the tendency to prefer things to stay the same, even when those things may no longer be serving us. In nutrition, this bias can show up when someone sticks to familiar eating habits or a diet they've followed for years despite changes in their body's needs. For instance, as we age, our activity levels might change, and our nutritional requirements evolve, yet many people resist adjusting their diets to reflect these changes.

This bias can lead to stagnation in dietary habits, which might result in weight gain, nutrient deficiencies, or other health issues. Recognizing the need for change and adapting to evolving nutritional needs is crucial for maintaining long-term health, especially as life circumstances shift. Personalizing our diet requires making changes over time.

FALSE CONSENSUS BIAS

The *False Consensus Bias* is the tendency to overestimate how much others share our own beliefs and behaviors. In nutrition, this manifests when people assume that their way of eating, whether it's vegan, low-carb, or paleo, is the best approach for everyone. This bias fuels the spread of generalized diet advice, often ignoring the fact that people have diverse nutritional needs based on their genetics, lifestyle, and preferences.

For example, someone who thrives on a ketogenic diet might believe that everyone should adopt it, even though this eating style may not suit someone with different preferences or health conditions. False consensus can contribute to the proliferation of one-size-fits-all diets that don't take individual variation into account, leaving many people feeling frustrated when those diets fail to deliver the promised results.

HOW TO FOCUS ON YOUR OWN NUTRITION

1. **Acknowledge and Reflect on Childhood Influences** – Reflect on how your upbringing, cultural practices, and early food experiences have shaped your current eating habits. Identify which of these align with your present health goals and which may no longer serve you. Gradually introduce new foods and practices that better support your health while still respecting your cultural heritage and personal preferences.

2. **Tailor Your Diet to Your Body Composition** – Recognize that your height, weight, and muscle mass directly affect your energy and nutrient needs. Use tools like body composition assessments to get a clearer picture of what your body requires, adjusting your diet to support your specific needs. For example, this might mean increasing protein for muscle maintenance or tweaking your calorie intake based on your activity level.

3. **Align Your Diet with Your Habits and Environment** – Consider your daily routines, including work hours, sleep patterns, and physical activity, to create a meal plan that fits your lifestyle. Adjust factors like meal timing and frequency to optimize energy levels and digestion. Be flexible and adapt to life changes like pregnancy, aging, or seasonal shifts, making necessary adjustments to ensure your diet remains supportive of your current needs.

4. **Set Clear, Personalized Goals** – Identify specific nutrition goals, such as weight loss, muscle gain, or managing a health condition and develop a tailored plan to achieve them. Regularly reassess these goals and make changes to your diet as needed to stay aligned with your health objectives.

5. **Improve Food Access and Support Healthy Eating** – Actively work to improve your access to nutritious foods, whether through sourcing local produce, growing your own food, or finding reliable ways to get fresh options in your area. Engage with your community to foster a supportive environment for healthy eating. Recognize the socioeconomic challenges that might limit access to quality food and advocate for systemic changes, like improved food policies, to benefit not just yourself but others in your community as well.

Focusing on your unique nutrition needs helps you build a personalized, sustainable approach to health, but it's essential to stay grounded in the bigger picture. Up next, we'll explore the core fundamentals of nutrition—principles that remind us not to miss the forest for the trees while striving for individual goals.

CHAPTER 9: FUNDAMENTALS

"In a world of constant change, the fundamentals are more important than ever."

— **Jim Collins**

Now that we've debunked much of the nutrition misinformation, it's time to shift our focus to the core truths and what we do know about good nutrition. This chapter isn't about trendy diets or rigid rules; it's about the essentials that form the foundation of a healthy diet. With these basics, you'll be better equipped to navigate the complex and often overwhelming world of food and health.

We'll explore the fundamental building blocks of nutrition, from the role of carbohydrates and fats to the truth about protein needs. We'll also address some of today's most debated topics and find out what you really need to be healthy. Whether you're new to understanding nutrition or want to refine your approach, this chapter will arm you with the essential knowledge you need to create a nourishing, sustainable way of eating.

WHAT ARE THE FUNDAMENTALS OF NUTRITION?

Understanding the fundamentals of nutrition is like laying the blueprint for lifelong health. This is not about strict rules but rather core principles that guide you toward making informed, beneficial choices for your body.

At its core, nutrition involves two essential processes:

1. **The Creation and Consumption of Food** – This encompasses everything from selecting, preparing, and eating your food. It's about making conscious, informed choices about what you put into your body, recognizing that food is more than just fuel; it's a source of nourishment that can either support or harm your health.

2. **Digestion and Metabolism of Nutrients** – Once you consume food, your body breaks it down into proteins, fats, carbohydrates, vitamins, and minerals. These nutrients are then absorbed and used to maintain energy, support bodily functions, and promote overall well-being.

WHY IS GOOD NUTRITION IMPORTANT?

Good nutrition isn't just about feeling full or eating "healthy"; it's about optimizing your body's capabilities, reducing health risks, and ultimately improving the quality and longevity of your life.

Enhances Functional Capabilities – Proper nutrition provides the energy and strength needed for everyday activities whether it's physical exercise or mental tasks. It supports your immune system, speeds recovery from illness, and maintains overall body functionality.

Reduces Health Risks – A balanced diet can lower your risk of chronic conditions like heart disease, diabetes, and obesity. By giving your body the right nutrients, you support its natural defenses, helping it stay healthy over the long term.

Improves Quality and Quantity of Life – Good nutrition not only adds years to your life but improves the quality of those years. A nutritious diet leads to better mental health, more energy, and a greater sense of well-being, enabling you to live life fully and actively.

THE IMPORTANCE OF HEALTHY *THEMES* IN NUTRITION

When thinking about good nutrition, focus on overarching principles or healthy themes. Themes provide a flexible framework that can be tailored to meet individual needs and preferences, all while still supporting overall well-being.

Key Themes:

1. **Adequacy and Balance of Nutrients** – Incorporate a wide variety of foods to ensure you're getting all essential macronutrients (carbohydrates, proteins and fats), micronutrients (vitamins and minerals), and non-nutrient components (antioxidants, polyphenols, etc.). Instead of following restrictive diets that eliminate entire food groups, focus on achieving a healthy balance that fits your body's needs and lifestyle.

2. **Timing and Portions** – While you certainly don't have to track calories, it's important to ensure you're not under or overeating for your energy needs. Developing a regular eating schedule that aligns with your exercise routine and sleep patterns can help you better tune into your hunger and fullness cues, giving your body the right portions and types of food it needs to thrive.

3. **Whole Foods** – Whole foods like fruits, vegetables, whole grains, nuts and seeds, legumes, healthy fats and lean proteins should form the basis of your diet. These are nutrient-dense and minimally processed, providing the nutrients and energy your body needs.

4. **Outlook and Mindset** – Stop comparing your nutrition to what you see on social media or to those with different health needs. Start focusing on enjoying food and understanding that your body thrives on nutrient-rich foods while still benefiting from the joy of indulgent choices. By removing the noise of diet fads and embracing the joy and social connection that food brings, you can create a healthier, more fulfilling relationship with eating.

PERSONALIZING NUTRITION WITHIN THESE THEMES

While these foundational principles apply to everyone, how you put them into practice is entirely up to you. This flexibility allows you to shape a diet that fits your preferences, lifestyle, and health goals. The key is to make choices that work for you while still following these broad, beneficial guidelines. Nutrition is both a science and an art: this chapter covers the science, but the real transformation happens when you start experimenting and personalizing this knowledge to suit your own needs. First, let's look at the themes that cultivate fundamentally sound nutrition.

ADEQUACY AND BALANCE OF NUTRIENTS

At the core of any healthy diet are the essential building blocks known as *macronutrients* and *micronutrients*. These nutrients are the foundation of nutrition, providing the energy and vital components our bodies need to function, grow, and thrive. Understanding the role of macronutrients and micronutrients is crucial for creating a balanced diet that supports overall health.

MICRONUTRIENTS

While macronutrients are needed in larger amounts, micronutrients, such as vitamins and minerals, are equally important, even though we require them in smaller quantities. These nutrients play a variety of critical roles, including supporting metabolism, immune function, bone health, and the prevention of chronic diseases.

Vitamins are natural substances our bodies can't produce enough of by themselves; therefore, they are attained through the food we eat. They are categorized as either water-soluble (such as vitamins B and C) or fat-soluble (vitamins A, D, E, K). Each vitamin has specific functions, like vitamin D, which absorbs calcium and is responsible for bone health, or vitamin C's importance in immune function and collagen synthesis.

Minerals are inorganic elements that also must be obtained through food. This includes some such as calcium and magnesium, which are needed for bone health and muscle function, and trace minerals like iron and zinc, which are crucial for oxygen transport and immune function.

A diet rich in a variety of fruits, vegetables, whole grains, and lean proteins ensures that we get the broad spectrum of micronutrients necessary for optimal health. Some foods do have impressive nutrient density, meaning they carry a lot of micronutrients compared to their total calorie content.

Foods like berries, leafy greens, fish and seafood, potatoes, seaweed, lean meat, bell peppers, mushrooms, alliums, citrus fruits, nuts and seeds, dairy products and legumes are some particularly great foods to increase micronutrient intake. To simplify these foods even further for practical effect, it can help to make sure that you are engaging with a variety of food groups on a daily basis. If most of your meals contain at least one fruit or vegetable, one protein option, one carbohydrate from whole grains or legumes, and one healthy fat, you are likely getting the diversity of micronutrients you need.

The following is a list of some common American dishes that work well for patients and clients with whom I often work with. However, the point of showing these examples is to show the range of food groups that should be included during each day for micronutrient needs. It's not intended to show what types of meals are necessarily best, just a helpful reference point.

BREAKFAST EXAMPLES:

- A breakfast bowl of oatmeal with milk or yogurt, topped with blueberries and almonds.
- An omelet with mushrooms, bell peppers, and spinach with a side of whole grain toast with peanut butter.

LUNCH EXAMPLES:

- A salad bowl with leafy greens, grilled chicken, quinoa, beans or edamame, and balsamic vinaigrette.
- A sandwich with whole grain bread that includes avocado, a slice of cheese, tomato, turkey, and mustard.

DINNER EXAMPLES:

- Salmon cooked in EV olive oil, some rice or quinoa on the side, along with broccoli or carrots.
- A main protein (lean beef, shrimp, or tofu) alongside a fiber-rich carb like potatoes or whole grain pasta with marinara sauce, onions, and some grated parmesan cheese.

There are so many other cultural combinations that include these food groups as well. A great example is how several cultures incorporate beans as nutritious staple food, but do so at breakfast or within a main dish like chilaquiles. A pretty common theme among different food cultures that offers micronutrient diversity is the classic combination of a *protein wrapped in carbs and paired with fat*. Whether it's tacos, gyros, ravioli, sushi, dumplings, or a sandwich, this often helps meet nutrition goals very well. Many of these foods have become demonized, but when eaten in appropriate amounts and prepared well, they are great foods to have in your diet.

A key takeaway from these types of meals is that you must find the ones that work best for you and use ingredients and cooking techniques that emphasize nutrient density. If weight management, specifically losing weight, is challenging for you, choosing foods with less added sugar and oil can support a healthier weight as well.

CHAPTER 9: FUNDAMENTALS

Sometimes, certain populations have nutrient needs that make it very challenging to eat enough food or obtain all of the vital nutrients needed for growth or health maintenance. In these cases, fortified foods or supplements, while not necessary, can be useful for pregnant women, older adults, children, and those with dietary restrictions or specific medical conditions.

Micronutrients support the intricate biochemical processes that keep us healthy, and understanding and balancing these essential nutrients is key to building a strong foundation for a nutritious diet. Although not considered micronutrients, we should also consider the role of *phytonutrients* and other compounds from whole foods that lead to better health outcomes. Diversity of colorful foods and different food groups can accomplish this goal.[1,2] If our foods are all one color, we would likely benefit from adding in different color foods as these various pigments indicate distinct compounds like phytochemicals that can perform different functional capacities in our bodies.

MACRONUTRIENTS

Macronutrients are the nutrients we need in larger quantities. They are the primary source of energy for our bodies. There are three main types of macronutrients: proteins, carbohydrates, and fats.

PROTEINS

Proteins are essential macronutrients that play a critical role in building and repairing tissues, producing enzymes and hormones, and supporting immune function. Proteins are composed of smaller units called amino acids, often referred to as "the building blocks of life." There are 20 different amino acids that form proteins in the human body, nine of which are essential and must be obtained through our diet, as the body cannot produce them on its own.

PROTEIN-RICH FOODS

To ensure a balanced intake of all essential amino acids, it is important to include a variety of protein sources in your diet. While animal-based proteins have enough of the essential amino acids per serving, plant-based proteins are still effective at improving protein intake and are strongly tied to healthy metabolic outcomes. Depending on your own goals, mixing up the types of protein sources is important.

Below are some top protein-rich foods from both animal and plant-based sources.

ANIMAL-BASED PROTEINS

1. **Chicken Breast**
2. **Fish (Salmon, Tuna)**
3. **Eggs**
4. **Greek Yogurt**
5. **Beef**
6. **Turkey**
7. **Cottage Cheese**
8. **Pork Tenderloin**
9. **Shrimp**
10. **Milk**

PLANT-BASED PROTEINS

1. **Lentils**
2. **Tofu and Tempeh**
3. **Chickpeas**
4. **Beans**
5. **Edamame**
6. **Quinoa**
7. **Chia Seeds**
8. **Pistachios**
9. **Hemp Seeds**
10. **Protein Powder (whey protein powder is a great animal-based option as well)**

*A quick word on soy, which is a popular plant-based protein. It's a pretty common myth that soy products negatively affect hormones, thyroid, and other metabolic processes. These are simply untrue, and soy foods are as beneficial as they come, providing a well-rounded source of nutrition.[3-8]

FINDING A BALANCE

Protein-rich foods are popular for a reason. We want plenty of this amazing nutrient, and it can be hard to overdue protein no matter what your individual goal may be. However, while protein is crucial for maintaining muscle and overall health, it's important not to get too carried away because, as noted earlier, we eat foods, not nutrients. So, when we continue to emphasize more and more protein consumption, the potential problem becomes either forcing too much food into our diet or including protein-rich foods that are also calorically dense or have components that we want to limit. Instead of focusing on eating large quantities of food to meet protein goals, include one protein-*rich* source at each meal without allowing it to push out other healthy options on your plate.

Protein should always be a staple in our diets, but we must also understand that choosing a variety of protein-rich foods that are prepared in a healthier way can be just as important.

To determine your minimum daily protein needs, it's a pretty safe bet that the average person wants to aim for at least half their body weight in grams of protein. So, a 200-pound person might shoot for 100 grams per day, but this will again depend on individual needs.

CARBOHYDRATES

Carbohydrates are our body's preferred energy source because they can be quickly used and are the only fuel that can produce ATP in the absence of oxygen. They break down into glucose, which fuels our brain, muscles, and other tissues.

Carbohydrates can be found in foods like grains, fruits, vegetables, legumes, nuts, seeds, and even dairy. Complex carbohydrates, such as those in whole grains and vegetables, provide a slower release of energy, while simple carbohydrates, like those in sugary snacks and drinks, offer quick sources of energy.

COMPLEX CARBS

Carbohydrates are abundant in many foods. This makes it easy to incorporate them into a balanced diet. Some common sources include:

Grains – Foods like bread, pasta, rice, and oats are rich in carbohydrates, particularly complex carbohydrates that offer sustained energy.

Fruits – Apples, bananas, berries, and oranges provide not only carbohydrates but also essential vitamins, minerals, and fiber.

Vegetables – Potatoes, corn, peas, and squash are excellent sources of carbohydrates, especially when consumed in their whole, unprocessed forms.

Legumes – Beans, lentils, and chickpeas are high in carbohydrates and offer a good amount of protein and fiber.

FIBER

Fiber is a type of complex carbohydrate. Although it's not broken down by our enzymes to be used as a source of energy, it does play a crucial role in maintaining overall health and wellness, offering numerous benefits such as:

Cholesterol Reduction – Fiber helps reduce cholesterol levels by binding to bile in the digestive system. Since bile is made of cholesterol, this binding prevents its absorption, prompting the body to use more cholesterol to produce additional bile. This process effectively lowers blood cholesterol levels.[9]

Gut Health and Microbiome Support – Fiber is essential for a healthy gut microbiome. Different types of fiber from various plant foods promote a diverse and balanced bacterial population in the gut. This diversity helps keep harmful pathogens at bay and supports overall gut health.[10]

Reduced Inflammation and Cancer Risk – By adding bulk to stool and improving gut transit time, fiber reduces the workload on the gastrointestinal tract. This can decrease inflammation and lower the risk of colon cancer.[11]

Improved Insulin Sensitivity – Fiber increases the production of short-chain fatty acids in the gut, which can enhance insulin sensitivity and support other metabolic processes.[12] It can also help slow down the release of sugar into the bloodstream.

Longevity – Research has shown that for every 10-gram increase in daily fiber intake, there is a corresponding 10% reduction in overall mortality risk.[13]

While fiber offers numerous health benefits, it's essential to introduce it into your diet gradually. Rapidly increasing your fiber intake can cause side effects like bloating, gas, and digestive discomfort. To minimize these issues, start by slowly incorporating fiber-rich foods, giving your digestive system time to adapt. This approach allows you to reap the full benefits of fiber without experiencing unwanted side effects.

As a general guideline, aim for at least 14 grams of fiber per 1,000 calories consumed, though the benefits continue to increase with even higher amounts. When selecting carbohydrate-rich products, look for a fiber-to-total-carbs ratio of 1:10 or lower, with ratios closer to 1:8 or even 1:5 being ideal.

FIBER-RICH FOODS

1. Lentils (Legume)
2. Chia Seeds (Seed)
3. Black Beans (Legume)
4. Raspberries (Fruit)
5. Quinoa (Whole Grain)
6. Oats (Whole Grain)
7. Almonds (Nut)
8. Broccoli (Vegetable)
9. Sweet Potatoes (Root Vegetable)
10. Pears (Fruit)

ARE SUGAR AND CARBS A PROBLEM?

Sugar is the basic building block of all carbs, so it's important to understand its role in a balanced, realistic context. When we talk about sugars, we're usually referring to their simplest forms, like glucose and fructose. Whether it's honey, maple syrup, or agave nectar, all these sweeteners are chemically similar to table sugar; once ingested, your body processes them in the same way. However, the effect of sugar on your body largely depends on the food matrix in which it's consumed. Whole foods, which provide fiber, vitamins, and other nutrients, have a different impact on satiety and health outcomes compared to foods with added sugars, where the sugar exists on its own or has been extracted from its original source.

Interestingly, despite a reduction in sugar consumption in recent years, obesity rates continue to rise, indicating that sugar alone isn't the sole culprit of the rise in obesity. Research shows that varying levels of sugar intake can result in similar outcomes for weight loss.[14] Additionally, some of the leaner countries in the world consume diets high in carbohydrates, challenging the notion that carbs or sugar are inherently fattening.

Take pasta, for example, often vilified as a "bad carb." Despite its reputation, pasta can be part of a healthy diet when consumed in appropriate portions and paired with nutrient-dense foods.

The Glycemic Index (GI), a tool developed in 1981 to measure how quickly foods raise blood glucose levels, has contributed to the demonization of certain carbs even though it has pretty big limitations—it doesn't account for the overall quality or nutrient density of foods and may not be as useful for the average person despite popular use in nutrition circles.[15]

While moderating intake of simple sugars added to our foods is a helpful way of improving overall health, removing it is not a dietary silver bullet. Studies on overfeeding show that 98% of adipose tissue actually comes from fat sources, while only 2% comes from sugar, as the body prefers not to convert sugar to fat unless necessary.[16] The key is to balance your overall energy intake and focus on the broader context of your diet rather than fixating on sugar content alone. That said, foods extremely high in added sugars do pose a problem, so it's important to understand how to moderate or reduce them in your diet.

One of the easiest ways I have seen this done is by removing and replacing drinks like soda with alternative options that have little to no sugar in them.

IS SUGAR ADDICTION REAL?

I've heard so often that people feel they are addicted to sugar. While it's certainly a tempting ingredient within our favorite sweet treats, it's also not really an addiction in the way you may think it is. Let's put it this way: you don't see people eating sugar straight from the bag; instead, they consume it through pastries, soda, and other desserts where additional factors like saltiness, fat content, and mouthfeel play a significant role, too.[17,18,19] Believe it or not, the fizziness of soda and the perfect blend of textures and flavor combinations in desserts is actually more compelling than the sweetness of sugar on its own. Overconsumption of these foods isn't driven by sugar alone, but by the combination of these sensory factors, creating a challenging dependence.

When it comes to the love of sugar or any nutrient within food, it's not classified as an addiction in the same way we categorize addiction to alcohol or drugs. While you may feel an uncontrollable "addiction" to sugar, it's more accurate to view this as a *dependence* on multiple hyperpalatable elements within ultra-processed foods.[20] This distinction helps separate food dependence from stronger addictions, allowing for more effective coping strategies. Given that individuals vary in their dopamine responses to food, the intensity of this experience can differ too, making it harder for some to manage.[21]

Both sugar and other sources of carbs are a wonderful part of food, but can overstimulate us thanks to our creative, but tempting food innovations. Either way, we need a healthy relationship with carbs and sugar that allows us to put boundaries on certain foods but still use them to support our overall health.

FATS

Fats are an essential part of the diet, playing crucial roles in energy production, nutrient absorption, and cell function. They provide a concentrated source of energy, support cell structure, help absorb fat-soluble vitamins (A, D, E, K), and are necessary for hormone production. Among the different types of fats, omega-3 and omega-6 fatty acids stand out as essential fats that our bodies cannot produce on their own. Therefore, they must be obtained through our diet, similar to the essential amino acids. However, not all fats are created equal, and their effects on health can vary significantly depending on the type and quantity consumed.

TYPES OF FATS

1. **Saturated Fats** – Found in foods like butter, lard, coconut oil, and fatty cuts of meat, saturated fats can provide the body with energy and may positively influence testosterone production. However, they have been shown to increase levels of LDL cholesterol, which can raise the risk of

heart disease. Consuming high amounts of saturated fat over time can also worsen metabolic health, especially when making up a large percentage of total daily fat or calorie intake. However, the context of food matters. For example, full-fat dairy products like yogurt and cheese may have less harmful effects compared to more processed sources like butter.[22] The same goes for cacao and dark chocolate, which do have saturated fat but offer fewer adverse effects thanks to many polyphenols and other compounds in them.[23]

2. Trans Fats – Trans fats are known to be highly detrimental to health, significantly raising the risk of heart disease by increasing LDL cholesterol and decreasing HDL cholesterol. Fortunately, trans fats have been largely banned from the food supply in the U.S., reducing their presence in processed foods.[24]

3. Unsaturated Fats

Monounsaturated Fats – Found in olive oil, avocados, and nuts, these fats are heart-healthy and can help reduce chronic inflammation and improve cholesterol levels.

Omega-3 Fatty Acids – These fats are known for their anti-inflammatory properties and play a key role in brain function, heart health, and reducing the risk of chronic diseases. The three main types of omega-3s are ALA (found in plant oils), EPA and DHA (both found in marine sources). Consuming a diet rich in omega-3s can support cardiovascular health, reduce inflammation, and promote mental well-being. This is a nutrient that is often under consumed, so increasing your intake is almost certainly a great idea.

Omega-6 Fatty Acids – Omega-6 fats are also essential, supporting skin health, bone metabolism, and the body's inflammatory response. While omega-6s are necessary, it's important to balance their intake with omega-3s, as many people are currently consuming enough omega-6s and missing out on adequate omega-3s.

10 Whole Food Sources of Fats

1. **Fatty Fish (e.g., Salmon, Mackerel, Sardines)**
2. **Chia Seeds**
3. **Walnuts**
4. **Flaxseeds**

5. **Hemp Seeds**
6. **Edamame (Young Soybeans)**
7. **Eggs**
8. **Almonds**
9. **Pumpkin Seeds**
10. **Avocado**

Incorporating these whole foods into your diet can help ensure you get a balanced intake of essential fats, promoting overall health and well-being. These foods not only supply necessary omega-3 and omega-6 fatty acids but also come packed with other vital nutrients that support a healthy, balanced diet.

REFINED AND CONCENTRATED FATS

Refined and concentrated fats, such as butter, ghee, coconut oil, palm oil, lard, olive oil, avocado oil, vegetable oils, seed oils, and peanut oil, are commonly used in cooking and in many processed foods. These fats are calorie-dense and should be consumed in moderation, as overconsumption can cause excess calorie intake and weight gain. While typically not as favorable as fat in the context of whole food, the concentrated versions used in food create a much better culinary outcome and can still provide nutritional benefits. But how do we choose between these refined sources?

SEEDS OILS

In recent years, seed oils have become a hotly debated topic in the realm of nutrition, often criticized on social media and within certain health circles. Because they are ubiquitous in our food supply, many have questioned whether or not we should avoid them.

The voices that do think we should remove seed oils are usually concerned about the production process of these oils and the potential for polyunsaturated fats to threaten our health. Those who believe polyunsaturated fats are a poor choice for cooking and food products often promote saturated fats, like butter, as a smarter health choice.

CHAPTER 9: FUNDAMENTALS

Now, we already know that nutrition is rarely as black-and-white as choosing between a seed oil or butter and having some of both is entirely reasonable. But there are some helpful facts to consider that can bring clarity to the average person who is trying to decide which source of fat they want in their foods.

First, it's important to understand that seed oils are not *necessary* for a healthy diet. While we do need some dietary sources of omega-6 and omega-3, they don't need to come from seed oil. You can absolutely limit or avoid seed oils and will likely thrive if all other areas of nutrition are covered.

Alternatively, you can also include them in moderation, as most people do, without completely derailing your health. So, the intensity of the debate that surrounds these fats often overshadows the more nuanced reality of dosage, processing, and individual dietary choices.

So, how do seed oils stack up? After all, this can help us decide if we can use them in our cooking and food choices. Seed oils, which are derived from vegetables and other plants, provide a strong dosage of omega-6. Although often misattributed to inflammation and poor health, these do not inherently cause obesity or inflammation when consumed as part of a balanced diet.[25,26,27,28]

Most studies examining these oils even use them straight from store shelves, so it's a very practical outcome and a good reminder that we do not have to fear them if we don't overuse them. The real issue with these seed oils comes from excessive calorie intake. And since we have already touched on our collective overconsumption of calories, which can be problematic, it makes sense that a lot of these calories come from these oils (which happen to be the bulk of added fat in foods because they are less expensive).

Seed oils are also potentially less healthy when compared to some other, less processed oils like extra virgin olive oil, as processing does strip away compounds that would improve health, like polyphenols.

So, instead of falling for the trap that seed oils are inherently bad, remember that any high calorie food can be overconsumed more easily and if you have the option to upgrade to extra virgin olive oil, this would likely improve your health.

It makes sense that we should be conscious of overusing them and switching them out for more whole food fats, but in general this a great example of nutrition nonsense as people are always trying to find that ONE food or nutrient to blame, even though there are so many factors to consider.

UNSATURATED FAT AND SATURATED FAT

Seed oils and olive oil are examples of predominantly unsaturated fat sources, while foods like butter and coconut oil are examples of predominantly saturated fats. Although we touched on them earlier, which of these would benefit us more when it comes to preparing our meals?

When looking at the highest quality comparisons of matched energy intake across converging lines of evidence, it's fairly unanimous that polyunsaturated fats lead to better outcomes compared to saturated fats.[29-39] This is because they are consistently associated with better heart health, reduced inflammation, and improved metabolic outcomes (feel free to sift through the mounds of studies I have compiled).[40-55] If this comes as a surprise to you, it might be because the *loudest* and most *extreme* voices provide some of the most *misguided* advice.

So, while both of these fats can and do make up different healthy foods in our diet, when it comes to selecting them on a regular basis, you will likely improve your health by swapping saturated fats for unsaturated ones.

Why? Well, mechanistically speaking, this is because saturated fats downregulate LDL clearing in the liver by reducing the activity of LDL receptors on liver cells. They can also increase ApoB-containing lipoprotein production. Meanwhile, unsaturated fats do much of the opposite—they upregulate LDL receptors in the liver and decrease triglycerides, which reduces the amount of lipoprotein remnants. Simply put, a high saturated fat diet is less ideal compared to a diet that swaps them out for unsaturated fats.[56-63]

But this is no reason to remove saturated fat from the diet. Just as with sugar or processed oils, it's smart to set a limitation on saturated fat without fearing it, as it can also provide energy, taste, and culinary benefits. Because while it may be smart to moderate butter usage, life would be no fun without it. Plus, with so many other lifestyle factors at play, it's not worth losing sleep over.

BUT I FEEL FINE NOW

One of the central misconceptions when it comes to fat is the impact it can have on heart disease. Heart disease is typically not something that results in major adverse events until much later in life. It takes many decades for our resilient and flexible bodies to be worn down by a bad diet to the point where we see strokes and heart attacks.

So, although you may see a fit influencer promoting the use of a certain food or nutrient like saturated fat in all their meals at a relatively young age, they cannot *feel* the slow process of heart disease developing, and it won't often result in death at a young age, but it's often the difference between living to the age of 75 instead of 85. This difference seems to be hard for most of us to comprehend, especially younger influencers who think they will be invincible forever.

To attenuate these risks later in life, the best nutrition approach is to improve your body's lipid profiles, specifically the amount of LDL cholesterol in your blood. Although many voices love to push back on the narrative that we shouldn't concern ourselves with our cholesterol, improving this metric will absolutely improve your long-term health risk. Your LDL cholesterol is an *independent* risk factor for heart disease, which you can reduce by increasing fiber, replacing saturated fat with unsaturated fat, eating the appropriate number of calories and including more exercise.[64-71]

FATS AND YOUR HEALTH

With so much talk about healthy or unhealthy fats, the truth is that while multiple types of fat can fit into the context of a healthy diet, it can actually matter quite a bit if you are looking to make a sizable shift in future cardiovascular and metabolic health.

The right choice can actually be one of the most important things you can do to reduce the risk of cardiovascular disease outside of quitting smoking and exercising more. So, by replacing heavily saturated fat foods with more unsaturated fats, most people will improve blood lipids, namely *LDL cholesterol*. Reducing LDL cholesterol is a significant way to lower the likelihood of heart disease.

Although many voices love to push back on the narrative that we shouldn't concern ourselves with our cholesterol, improving this metric will absolutely improve your long-term health risk. Specifically, your LDL cholesterol is an independent risk factor for heart disease, which you can reduce by increasing fiber, lowering saturated fat intake, and including more exercise.[65-72]

Incorporating fats into your diet in a balanced way involves choosing the right types of fats, using them appropriately in cooking, and being mindful of portion sizes. Prioritizing unsaturated fats from sources like olive oil, fish, and nuts while limiting saturated fats from sources like butter and lard can help support overall health. Remember, the key is not just the type of fat but also how much and how it is used.

SO, DO I CHOOSE MORE CARBS OR FAT?

Now that the importance and nuances of certain types of carbohydrates and fats in the diet have been discussed, it may raise the question of whether one of these macronutrients should be *emphasized* more than the other in order to reach certain weight goals or improve health. But time and time again, in controlled studies, both low-carb and low-fat diets have shown very similar effectiveness in controlling body weight.[72]

Looking at real-world results, it's clear that personal consistency is the key factor, not whether someone focuses on or limits carbs or fats. Either approach can work for weight loss, but success ultimately depends on the individual.

Blaming carbs or fat doesn't make sense when they can both contribute to excess energy intake. The low-fat movement, which led to an increase in refined carbohydrates as their replacement, produced poor results.

The current low-carb trend isn't faring any better. Despite a decline in sugar consumption over the past 20–25 years, obesity and related health issues continue to rise.[73] Truthfully, it's not carbs or fats that matter most for weight outcomes. Instead, it's adherence, overall caloric intake, and individual differences that are the main mediators determining success.[74] Excessive intake of either macronutrient can be problematic, but setting healthy boundaries without removing any one nutrient completely is the best approach.

HYDRATION

Water, often overlooked as a macronutrient because we need it in large quantities, is essential for survival. Proper hydration maintains bodily functions. While drinking plain water is vital, a significant amount of hydration can be gained from water-rich fruits and vegetables as well. Despite common beliefs, even beverages like tea, coffee, and milk contribute to overall hydration.

Even though the importance of drinking water is well known, many people either overestimate or underestimate their water needs.[75,76] A more tailored approach is to drink half your body weight in ounces of water per day, and then adjust for factors like temperature, sweat levels, health conditions and exercise.

While knowing how much water you might personally need is great, it's also important to remember that you do get fluids from water-rich foods and other beverages, so many of us may not need to force ourselves to drink gobs of water each day to meet our needs.

DO YOU NEED ELECTROLYTES

Electrolytes are absolutely necessary for various bodily functions, including maintaining hydration, but most adults can actually get enough electrolytes through their diet alone.

The human body has homeostatic mechanisms that prevent excessive sodium excretion when electrolyte levels are low, making additional electrolyte supplements unnecessary for most people. Popular hydration powders often contain high levels of sodium, which is linked to elevated blood pressure, which is one of the most significant risk factors for cardiovascular disease, which, in turn, is the world's leading cause of death.[77]

The common electrolyte products that we are constantly being told are essential for health are marketed everywhere. But the truth is that these are only necessary in specific contexts, like prolonged sports activities or specific medical conditions like POTS. For the general population, especially those who don't engage in heavy sweating or intense workouts, simply consuming a balanced diet rich in fruits and vegetables is a much more effective (and economical) way to maintain electrolyte balance. These foods naturally provide a combination of water, electrolytes, and other vital nutrients. Also, contrary to popular belief, muscle cramps are not typically caused by a lack of electrolytes, so taking more supplements likely will not help solve this issue.[78]

Research indicates that athletes who experience cramping often have similar levels of hydration, mineral content, and sweat composition as those who do not cramp.[79-81] The primary cause of cramping may be neuromuscular fatigue or the overuse of muscles that are not adequately prepared for sudden or intense activity. While taking an electrolyte mix from time to time might be nice for specific regimens, like working out, it's vastly overhyped for the average daily routine. But if you are going to use some electrolytes for a workout and you want a cheaper option, just put a pinch of salt in your water to save your time and money.

Also, just to put it out there, specialty salts like Himalayan pink salt or Celtic Sea salt do not offer magical health benefits. Nutritionally, these salts are also just made up of sodium and chloride, so choose your salts based on preference rather than marketing myths.

TIMING AND PORTIONS

When it comes to meal frequency, simplicity often leads to better adherence and overall success. While there's flexibility in how many times you can eat each day, the traditional three meals a day approach tends to strike the best balance for most people. Eating three meals a day aligns with societal norms, making it easier to maintain consistency and avoid unnecessary complications. This approach supports stable blood sugar levels, consistent energy throughout the day, and prevents the extremes of under-eating or overstuffing.

Spacing your meals 4–6 hours apart allow your body to properly digest food and rest between eating. Although fasting can be a preferred method for some people, I think the simplest and most natural fasting period is the time you spend sleeping.

It may also help if you give your body about two hours between your last meal and bedtime, as this can promote better sleep and ensure you wake up ready for breakfast. This first meal of the day can be a great opportunity to include a balance of protein, fats, and carbohydrates, setting a strong foundation for your day. Whether you prefer to eat breakfast right away or after some morning activities, it's essential to fuel your body like an athlete preparing for a performance—focused on nutrition that supports your energy, digestion, and overall well-being.

SNACKING

Snacking may seem like a small part of your dietary routine, but it can play a significant role in achieving your health goals. The approach to snacking should be highly personalized based on your individual needs, preferences, and objectives.

For example, if you're recovering from an eating disorder, incorporating 1–3 snacks daily might be crucial to avoid undereating, maintaining a healthy weight and stabilizing your eating patterns. On the flip side, if you struggle with grazing too often throughout the day, setting specific meal and snack times can help prevent overeating.

Snacking can also be essential for those who are growing or pregnant, because increased nutrient and energy needs can be challenging with just 2-3 meals. On the other hand, if you prefer larger meals, snacking might interfere with your ability to recognize and respond to hunger cues during mealtimes.

While snacking and meal frequency should be flexible and adaptable to your lifestyle, having a personalized and structured plan can increase your chances of success. Rather than just discussing what works for you, take the time to write down your ideal meal routine and start implementing it today.

WHOLE FOODS

By prioritizing healthy options in meals every day, you can hit nutrient goals that help limit foods that may not be as health promoting. But by consistently meeting these targets you can be sure that indulgent food choices can fit in alongside these meals in a more intuitive way while still getting maximum nutrition support for your brain and body. Here are the themes that we know offer quality nutrition support:

FRUITS AND VEGETABLES

Daily Goal – Aim for 5–6 servings per day.

Visual Guide – The "1-2-3 Rule" can simplify this: one serving at breakfast, two at lunch, and three at dinner/dessert.

Examples:
- **Breakfast** – A cup of berries.

- **Lunch** – Salad greens with cucumber.
- **Dinner** – Sweet potato, broccoli, and a nectarine with dessert.

WHOLE GRAINS

Daily Goal – Opt for whole grains over refined grains as this can boost protein and fiber intake. Including one at each meal or snack can help you get enough fiber and micronutrients from this food group.

Example Swaps:

- Replace sugary oat packages with homemade overnight oats.
- Choose whole grain breads and tortillas.
- Limit added sugars and salt in your grain choices.

LEAN PROTEINS

Daily Goal – Should be based on your size and activity goals. But including a protein-rich option at each meal that gets you 15–30 grams at a time is ideal.

Visual Guide – Animal based foods will be about the size of the palm to accomplish this serving and plant-based foods may be roughly about one cup worth. Diversify protein by incorporating a variety of lean meats, fish, beans, and plant-based proteins. Try adding beans or lentils to soups and salads for an extra boost of protein and fiber.

DAIRY/DAIRY ALTERNATIVE

Daily Goal – Unless you are confidently meeting calcium and vitamin D goals each day, 2–3 cups of dairy per day would be beneficial. Don't limit yourself to just milk as options like Greek yogurt, cheese, or kefir can end up in a variety of recipes.

Example Swaps:

- Choose low or non-fat options without added sugars if your goal is to moderate energy intake. If not, full fat dairy does not need to be feared.
- Use milk or fortified plant-based alternatives to meet needs for vitamin D, calcium, and B12.

HEALTHY FATS

Daily Goal – Incorporate healthy fats like fish, avocados, nuts, and seeds.

Cooking Oils:

- Use extra-virgin olive oil, avocado oil, chia oil, sesame oil, peanut oil, or canola oil in moderation.
- Limit frying and choose oils based on freshness and cooking purpose.

Example Swaps:

- Use vinaigrettes made with olive oil or tahini instead of cream-based dressings.
- Substitute chips or processed snacks with nuts or seeds.
- Spread avocado on toast instead of butter.

COOKING TECHNIQUES:

1. Use herbs, spices, garlic, and lemon juice to reduce the need for salt.
2. Cook with less oil by using an air fryer or oven, which allows you to achieve great taste while being more sustainable.
3. Techniques that often increase nutrition quality that you may want to try out include: fermenting, steaming, pressure cooking, marinating meats with citrus or vinegar bases, microwaving, and slow cooking.

OUTLOOK AND MINDSET

A person's perspective on nutrition can make all the difference in their success. Because of this, it's important not to get discouraged by occasional overeating or setbacks. The best response is to return to healthy habits as quickly as possible, starting with your next meal. Shift your focus away from the fleeting satisfaction of indulgent eating to the lasting joy that comes from nourishing your body with all foods. Remember, nutrition isn't a quick fix; it's a lifelong journey.

Avoid falling into the trap of thinking that nutrition alone can cure all your problems, like cancer and genetic medical conditions. While good nutrition absolutely plays a huge role in overall health, it's not a panacea. Instead, think of it as a foundation that supports other aspects of your well-being. Recognize that a nutrition journey is often slow and steady, requiring patience and persistence. Unlike the fast-paced, chaotic pursuit of success in many areas of life, nutrition is about making consistent, positive choices over time.

Finally, find sources of joy and fulfillment beyond weight loss and body image. If your happiness hinges solely on these aspects, you'll find it difficult to maintain satisfaction, as they are finite and often trivial in the grand scheme of things. Embrace the ambiguity and imperfection in your nutritional journey and focus on the long-term benefits rather than short-term results. By doing so, you'll cultivate a healthier, more sustainable relationship with food and your body.

PRIORITIES AND PILLARS

Before worrying about the minutiae of nutrition, it's essential to get the basics right. Establish a regular eating pattern that suits your lifestyle, ensuring you have stable energy throughout the day by balancing your macronutrients and diversity of food groups. Prioritize getting enough protein and fiber, which are crucial for muscle health and digestion, and make sure you include essential fats in your diet for brain and hormone function.

While occasional indulgences should be part of the plan, limit foods high in added sugars, saturated fats, and salt, and avoid making ultra-processed foods a staple of your diet. Instead, focus on whole foods like fruits, vegetables, lean proteins, whole grains, nuts, seeds, legumes, and healthy beverages like water, tea, and dairy or dairy alternatives.

Remember, nutrition is only one piece of the puzzle. A healthy diet cannot compensate for a sedentary lifestyle, poor sleep habits, chronic stress, or unhealthy relationships. To truly thrive, you need to balance good nutrition with regular physical activity, adequate sleep, stress management, and strong social connections. These are the pillars of a healthy lifestyle, and when they're all in place, they support and reinforce each other, leading to better physical and mental health.

WHERE DID THIS NONSENSE COME FROM?

The fundamentals of nutrition have been constant for quite some time, but because of an overwhelming barrage of bad information, many of us have questioned the basics outlined above. There are a few unfortunate reasons why.

BRANDOLINI'S LAW (THE BULLSH*T ASYMMETRY PRINCIPLE)

Brandolini's Law emphasizes the disproportionate effort required to debunk misinformation compared to the ease of spreading it. Consider the common misconception that carbohydrates are inherently fattening and should be minimized in any healthy diet. This idea has permeated social media, often accompanied by anecdotes and unverified success stories from low-carb diets. However, explaining the complexity of how carbohydrates function as the body's primary energy source and the importance of distinguishing between refined sugars and whole grains requires nuanced, evidence-based discussion.

While it might take only seconds for someone to believe a post that claims that "carbs make you fat," it takes significantly more time and effort to deeply educate people, thus allowing the falsehood to proliferate more rapidly than the truth.

Inaccurate information is easily picked apart when long-form discussions take place, but most of the content we are exposed to now is short and oversimplified. It's significantly faster and easier to churn out 100 videos of myths than it is to explain why each of these is wrong. By the time someone gets around to busting a popular myth, ten more have been created in its place.

THE AFFECTIVE FALLACY

The Affective Fallacy occurs when emotional responses to certain foods dictate beliefs about their health impacts, often overriding scientific evidence. This fallacy illustrates how powerful emotions can lead to misinformed nutritional choices, reinforcing outdated or overly simplistic notions about diet. Here are two popular nutrition examples:

CHAPTER 9: FUNDAMENTALS

BACK AND FORTH ON EGGS

We've already discussed eggs several times, but that's because they have stirred up so much debate and confusion in recent years, with emotions often driving public perception. For years, eggs were demonized due to their cholesterol content, which led many to avoid them out of fear of raising their blood cholesterol levels and increasing heart disease risk.

But recent research has shown that for most people, dietary cholesterol from eggs has a minimal impact on blood cholesterol levels.[82] Unless you have familial hypercholesterolemia or have the genetic trait that makes you a hyper absorber of cholesterol, eggs can absolutely be a daily part of a healthy diet.[83] In fact, eggs are one of the more nutrient-dense foods, rich in high-quality protein, vitamins, and minerals.

ARTIFICIAL SWEETENERS

Many people steer clear of artificial sweeteners due to fear cultivated by stories about artificial sweeteners causing cancer or other severe health issues that circulate widely.

However, extensive research, including studies by the National Cancer Institute, has shown that artificial sweeteners like aspartame and sucralose are safe for human consumption within established limits. Despite this, the fear persists, causing many, in some cases, to revert to consuming more sugar.

Interestingly, using non-nutritive sweeteners like aspartame or stevia can also have practical benefits. For example, swapping regular soda for diet soda can result in significant weight loss (up to 6 kg) by reducing calorie intake without sacrificing the sweet taste many people crave.[84] Research also indicates that these sweeteners don't raise insulin levels, countering a common myth.[85]

Stevia, often marketed as a "natural" alternative, does not appear to significantly alter gut health, though the long-term effects are still uncertain.[86] While these are not at all essential in anyone's diet, including them occasionally can be safe in moderation and may aid in weight management. I think it's also very reasonable to limit or avoid non-caloric and artificial sweeteners too though, as you may not be comfortable using them. Also, for some of the population, like myself, side effects like gas or bloating can be annoying.

ARGUMENT FROM INERTIA

The *Argument from Inertia*, which essentially relies on the idea of "staying the course, explains why people often cling to outdated or incorrect nutritional beliefs, even when presented with new evidence. Here are 3 common examples that throw off our fundamental choices with food:

1. The Fear of Fruit Sugar – Some diet trends promote the idea that the sugar in fruit contributes to weight gain and metabolic disorders. However, research has shown that the naturally occurring sugars in whole fruits are not a problem as they come packaged with fiber, vitamins, water, and antioxidants that support digestion and overall health. Unfortunately, many people still avoid fruits due to the outdated belief that all sugar, regardless of source, should be eliminated from the diet.

2. Eating Small, Frequent Meals to Boost Metabolism – The belief that eating small meals throughout the day boosts metabolism and helps with weight loss has been widely accepted for years. However, newer studies suggest that the total number of calories consumed, rather than meal frequency, is what matters for weight management. Despite this, many people still follow the outdated advice to eat frequent small meals, even though the number of meals you need to manage weight properly depends entirely on your personal choices.

3. All Red Meat is Bad for Health – While processed red meat is linked to an increased risk of heart disease and cancer, recent evidence shows that low to moderate consumption of unprocessed red meat in a *balanced* diet, especially alongside plenty of vegetables and fiber, can be part of a healthy lifestyle. It also takes some nuance to figure out what dosage might be appropriate and how to avoid charring meat, which can increase the risk of carcinogens. Yet, many people still believe that all red meat should be avoided entirely, clinging to older ideas that promote extreme restrictions without distinguishing between dosage, processing, fat content, and other dietary factors.

These examples further illustrate how deeply ingrained beliefs can persist, even when newer and more accurate information becomes available.

GUILT BY ASSOCIATION

Guilt by Association is a cognitive fallacy where people dismiss valid nutrition advice simply because it's tied to a group or ideology they dislike. This bias can lead to missed opportunities for better health. For example, some individuals reject the benefits of plant-based diets because they associate them with extreme environmental activism or animal rights movements they don't support. This prejudice prevents them from recognizing the proven health benefits of incorporating more plant-based foods, such as fruits, vegetables, and legumes, into their diet, which can reduce the risk of chronic diseases and improve overall well-being.

The same bias applies to omega-6 fats, such as those found in seed oils. Seed oils are often demonized because they are commonly used in processed foods, which are generally unhealthy. However, the negative health effects of processed foods are not directly due to the nutrient profile of seed oils themselves. These oils, when consumed in moderation and as part of a balanced diet, can provide essential fatty acids and antioxidants that support good health. By allowing negative associations to cloud their judgment, people may hyper fixate on the wrong areas of nutrition.

HOW TO FOCUS ON THE NUTRITION FUNDAMENTALS

1. **Focus on Food Themes and the Nutrients will Follow** – Remember, we choose foods, not individual nutrients, at each meal. Within each food theme outlined above, choose which foods you prefer and will consistently eat long-term.

2. **Prioritize Whole Foods Over Processed Foods** – Aim to fill your plate with whole, unprocessed foods like fruits, vegetables, whole grains, lean proteins, and healthy fats. These whole and minimally processed foods can also improve gut health because of the diversity of fibers and compounds within the foods that support gut health. People who consume high-fiber diets have a more diverse gut microbiome, which is associated with better overall health outcomes. On the flip side, low-fiber diets were linked to decreases in microbiome diversity, leading to negative health effects.[87]

3. **Develop Consistent Meal Planning Habits** – Write down the number of meals and snacks you aim to eat every day and even the times that you will likely eat. Planning a routine and following it, even within a similar time window each day, can stabilize hunger and fullness hormones and increase the likelihood that you will eat the appropriate amount of food each day.

4. **Focus on Overall Health, Not Just Disease Prevention** – Instead of fixating on avoiding a million different diseases, adopt a holistic approach to health. A balanced diet rich in nutrients and staying physically active can reduce the risk of various health issues, from cardiovascular disease to diabetes, while also supporting overall well-being.

5. **Understand That Nutrition Is Just One Piece of the Puzzle** – A healthy lifestyle encompasses more than just diet. Prioritize other factors such as reducing stress, limiting alcohol and tobacco use, and getting regular check-ups to know your health numbers, like blood pressure and cholesterol levels. By addressing all aspects of your health, you'll create a strong foundation for long-term well-being.

To embrace the foundations of good nutrition, it's essential to bridge these ideas with actionable steps that integrate seamlessly into daily life. In the final chapter we'll look at strategies to help you translate these fundamentals into lasting habits.

CHAPTER 10: FORWARD

"Knowledge is not power until it's applied."

— **Dale Carnegie**

One of the most pervasive myths in nutrition is the belief that if there was just more information and knowledge, we would all be better off. In actual fact, the opposite is often the case. We are actually overrun with so much information and misinformation that it obscures what we likely already know. The basics, many of which are outlined in the previous chapter, provide the framework we need, and any more knowledge is likely just fluff.

The real challenge, then, is not just finding the right quality information but also translating this knowledge into meaningful action. Implementing healthy habits is often complicated by obstacles like financial constraints, hectic schedules, mental health struggles, physical limitations, and environmental factors. For many, overcoming these barriers can feel like an uphill battle. Putting good information into practice is where most people fall short when it comes to proper nutrition.

But regardless of the number or scale of your challenges, some form of progress is always possible. The key is to focus on making practical decisions that improve your nutritional health. This final chapter is designed to empower you to take decisive steps toward better health.

HOW DO WE MOVE FORWARD?

Think of your approach to nutrition like the systems in your home. Whether it's electricity, plumbing, or heating, we rely heavily on many of these systems, yet they go unnoticed on most days. Your nutrition habits should eventually behave in the same way, as a nearly invisible foundation that requires simple maintenance over time. If you invest in establishing sustainable, strong habits upfront, you won't have to start over and build in a new infrastructure every time; you can just make minor tweaks to proven systems.

By putting in a lot of effort early to create a sustainable plan, you can confidently manage your nutrition with less total effort over time. And the creation of these good habits coincides with the removal of bad habits. This is important because instead of just forcing yourself to stop the urge to crash diet or try another monthly juice cleanse, the presence of healthy nutrition goals will eliminate the need for any of these band-aid solutions that won't last. The new dietary plan that you come up with should be one that lasts, and this requires looking at your own nutrition identity.

LEANING INTO A BETTER NUTRITION IDENTITY

As you move forward in your health journey, it's crucial to recognize that lasting change requires more than just a surface-level adjustment of habits. It's about cultivating a deeper identity that aligns with your goals and values. This identity serves as your anchor, protecting you from the allure of quick fixes, fad diets, and nutrition myths that promise fast results but never deliver lasting change. This identity is not one that holds firm to extreme nutrition beliefs, but is one that you can lean on as a reminder of a more reasonable pursuit: holistic health.

A strong nutrition identity does more than just guide your choices; it grounds you. When you have a clear sense of who you are and what you value in terms of health and well-being, you're less likely to be derailed by the constant barrage of conflicting information. Without this strong identity, it's easy to be swayed by the latest diet trend or extreme solution. But with a clear vision, you can filter out the noise and stick to a path that serves your long-term health.

While it's true that identities can be shaped by bad habits just as easily as good ones, the hope is that throughout this book, you've learned to cultivate traits that empower you to choose wisely. Establishing core beliefs and objectives, which is your own personal "nutrition identity," will be like the small, often unnoticed rudder that steers your ship in the right direction. It may provide seemingly small, consistent actions, but over time, this push in the right direction will create monumental changes.

To help you create and solidify a solid nutrition identity that helps you navigate the complexities of nutrition, let's explore four foundational traits.

CHAPTER 10: FORWARD

FOUR TRAITS

To build a strong and lasting nutrition identity, focus on these four foundations: the stories you believe, the habits you perform, the environment you're in, and the relationships you nurture. These four elements (which are adapted from a John Mark Comer sermon geared towards making a shift in your spiritual identity) are also very applicable to the transformation of other areas in your life, including your relationship with food.[1]

1. **Stories** – The beliefs you hold about food and health shape your approach to nutrition. Identify and challenge false narratives that might be holding you back and *replace* them with truths that align with evidence-based health practices.

2. **Habits** – Small, consistent actions have a powerful cumulative effect. Focus on creating daily habits that promote balance and well-being. These habits form the backbone of your new identity and drive your long-term success.

3. **Environment** – The spaces you inhabit, both physical and digital, can support or hinder your progress. Surround yourself with environments that encourage healthy choices, whether that's stocking your kitchen with nutritious options or curating a social media feed filled with positive influences.

4. **Relationships** – The people in your life affect your mindset and habits. Cultivate relationships with those who support your health goals and share your values. A strong support system will reinforce your identity and help you stay on track during challenging times.

By focusing on these four pillars: stories, habits, environment, and relationships, you can create a solid foundation for your nutrition identity.

1. STORIES YOU BELIEVE

Do you make drastic changes every time you see a new nutrition documentary? Are you constantly swayed by marketing efforts that tell you to restrict meat or fruit in your diet? Do you give up perfectly healthy foods like beans and rice because someone made an emotional appeal about the downsides of carbs? If you have stronger, more reliable perspectives and stories, wild myths will be less likely to rewire your belief system. It often helps me to remember the bigger picture—there are many diverse diets around the world that promote similar levels of health. This includes many cultures that utilize all kinds of foods that are continually demonized in America. Just because some influencer mistakenly thinks bread is the boogeyman in nutrition, doesn't mean this false revelation will suddenly start hurting the 80% of the world that eats bread every day. Similar to the ways in which we moved on from childhood stories like Santa and the Tooth Fairy, it's time to move on from irrational nutrition myths like these.

The narratives and beliefs you hold are the foundation of your identity. They influence how you perceive food, health, and your functional capabilities. If you believe you are someone who makes mindful, informed choices about food, this "story" you internally repeat about yourself will guide your actions even in the face of temptation or confusion. Conversely, if you hold onto negative or disempowering beliefs, such as thinking that healthy eating is too difficult or that you're inherently doomed to fail, it can undermine your efforts.

If you are caught up in news cycles about the terrible food system and spend all of your efforts worried about this, you will waste valuable time and mental energy that can be redirected toward better personal habits. You hold a lot of power by choosing to believe in a healthier mindset toward food and can block out the voices that choose to demonize food and promote nutrition myths. Whether you are performing positive self-talk or reminding yourself of the bigger picture in nutrition, this type of "storytelling" with yourself is not necessarily an easy task. It takes practice and won't be a perfect solution for everyone. But it does play a pivotal role in your nutrition identity.

2. HABITS YOU PERFORM

Your daily habits are the building blocks of your identity, and you can build this up through small actions you repeat every day. For example, consistently choosing whole foods over processed snacks, staying hydrated, and incorporating regular physical activity into your routine are habits that *reinforce* the identity of someone who prioritizes health. These habits don't just happen overnight; they are cultivated through intentional practice. By focusing on establishing and maintaining healthy habits, you solidify your identity as someone who is committed to their well-being.

BAD HABITS TO WATCH OUT FOR:

Skipping Meals Regularly – This can lead to improper nutrition or a cycle of under and overeating that makes you feel out of control. Both of these can result in low energy and a vicious pattern of trying to get back on track.

Always Eating in Front of Screens – This might encourage mindless eating and makes it difficult to recognize your hunger and fullness cues. It can also distract you from the joy of eating and sharing a meal with loved ones.

GOOD HABITS TO CULTIVATE:

Meal Planning and Prepping – Preparing meals or recipes in advance reduces decision fatigue and ensures healthy options are readily available. Creating a grocery list before going to the store also helps improve shopping and subsequent eating habits.

Mindful Eating – Pay full attention to the different qualities of your food, savor each bite, and recognize what foods promote the best health outcomes for yourself.

3. THE ENVIRONMENT YOU LIVE IN

The environment you surround yourself with plays a big role in shaping your identity. This includes not just your physical environment, such as the foods you keep at home and the places you frequent, but also the kind of information you're exposed to, like the media you consume and the sources you trust for health advice. An environment that supports healthy choices makes it easier to maintain your identity, while a toxic or unsupportive environment can hinder your efforts. Curating an environment that aligns with your health goals helps reinforce your identity and keeps you on track.

Home Environment – Always stocking your fridge and pantry with nutritious options will make it that much easier to eat well. Creating a pleasant eating space is also important if you want to value meal times with family or eat more mindfully.

Workplace Environment – If you know that snacks available at work are constantly making it hard to stay on track, you may need to bring your own snacks to replace these options or set specific, but sustainable boundaries for yourself.

Social Environment: Surround yourself with like-minded individuals who encourage your healthy habits. As mentioned in previous chapters, you may also need to be wary of joining certain health circles that seem more like a nutrition cult.

Our environments can sometimes overpower our desire for certain nutrition goals. Recognize the need for different strategies in different environments, whether it's navigating fast food menus wisely or limiting the negative content or comments in your life. We can't always choose many of the environments we are a part of, but we can do our best to pick out supportive people and set up smart boundaries within these places that help us thrive.

4. RELATIONSHIPS YOU HOLD

The people you interact with regularly, whether it's family, friends, or work colleagues, shape your behaviors, beliefs, and attitudes toward health. Surrounding yourself with helpful, like-minded individuals who share your values can introduce positivity and keep you motivated.

Be careful of relationships that are unsupportive or encourage unhealthy behaviors, though, because these can pull you away from your goals. Cultivating positive relationships that align with your health identity is essential for long-term success.

Family Influence – Reflect on the eating habits you inherited from your family and decide which ones may be harmful and which ones serve you well.

Partner Influence – Communicate your health goals with your spouse or partner and work together to support each other's nutrition plans.

Friendships and Social Circles – Ask for help from friends that you know will keep you accountable and give you sound advice and support.

Colleagues and Workplace Dynamics – Create a supportive lunch culture and avoid peer pressure to conform to unhealthy eating habits.

Online Communities and Social Media – Curate your digital environment by unfollowing sources of information that are clearly not providing useful nutrition advice.

CHAPTER 10: FORWARD

These four foundations that can form a more legitimate nutrition identity can help you overcome a majority of the nutrition nonsense you encounter. These pillars can empower you to make choices that truly benefit your well-being. And remember, you cannot do this alone; social capital is essential. Just as your identity guides your health choices, a well-thought-out plan ensures that those choices are clear and effective.

REMOVE AND REPLACE THE NONSENSE

Bringing awareness to so much of the nutrition nonsense in the world may feel good, but it won't do much for you if you aren't able to fill it in with something credible. You need to seek out reliable experts and communities who offer clear, evidence-based guidance. Because the world of nutrition is constantly evolving—with new trends and studies popping up almost daily—it's unrealistic to expect the average person to sift through all this information on their own. Instead, find those trusted individuals who can spend time in this area and whose efforts actually benefit your mental and physical health.

One person may not be enough, as no single expert is immune to mistakes. Having a few go-to sources ensures balance, as they can effectively "fact-check" each other. These voices should consistently provide practical, evidence-based insights by taking a balanced approach and avoiding falling into the traps of fad diets or sensationalist trends. This is where the chapter on expertise can be put into practice.

You may find certain professionals who resonate well with you. Just as long as they meet most of the criteria for expertise we've covered earlier, then you can put more stock into what they regularly advise. Just be cautious of the red flags we've discussed throughout this book as no one will ever get it right 100% of the time.

ALWAYS ACKNOWLEDGE BIAS

There are countless reasons why we often get nutrition wrong, and much of it has to do with our own biases. Sometimes, we're so desperate for a quick fix that we'll try any fad diet, no matter how irrational. Other times, we reject all processed foods because we're frustrated with food corporations, only to later realize that not all processed foods are harmful. Cultural norms also play a role. We've been conditioned to obsess over weight rather than focus on healthy habits. This is what helped me in my own weight journey—focusing on getting healthier, not lighter.

Additionally, we tend to be drawn to online influencers who look good or have a charismatic presence, and this appeal can cloud our judgment when it comes to their health advice. Often, the issue isn't even the facts but how they're presented; misunderstandings and disagreements consistently arise from a difference in semantics or a lack of context.

So, how do we pin down our own biases? One solution is to have open, honest conversations with people who genuinely care about your well-being. These discussions can clear up confusion and help you cut through the noise. I fall victim to many social and psychological biases all the time, even with a lot of education in this space, so please give yourself some grace. We all choose behaviors that don't always make the most sense logically. This is perfectly acceptable as long as we are creating space for awareness and how biases can limit our pursuit of health and pursuit of reliable nutrition perspectives. The key is getting better at being skeptical and recognizing these shortcomings, because once you understand them, you can better avoid being misled by harmful nutrition advice.

Knowing why we fall for nutrition myths is just as important as debunking the myths themselves. While this book doesn't cover a majority of the potential psychological biases we face, it's crucial to approach health claims with a healthy dose of skepticism. Prioritize building sustainable, healthy habits, and you'll be less susceptible to the allure of quick fixes or misleading advice.

RELY ON PLANNING, NOT MOTIVATION

Motivation to change your nutrition habits or overcome nonsensical health advice can kickstart your efforts, but it's nothing compared to having a plan of action. Motivation often relies on fleeting feelings that come and go, but a solid plan, however, will guide you through moments where you will naturally dip in desire. To build an effective plan for a better nutrition identity you need to:

Determine Macro and Micro Needs – Start by understanding your macronutrient (proteins, fats, carbs) and micronutrient (vitamins, minerals) requirements. Tools like the Cronometer app can help track these needs.

Identify Missing or Overused Foods – Audit your current diet to find gaps. Are you eating enough fiber? Too much added sugar? Take on one of these gaps at a time.

Create a Daily Food Goal Sheet – Write down your daily goals, such as "Include 25g of fiber" or "Eat two servings of fruit."

CHAPTER 10: FORWARD

Craft a Shopping List and Find Recipes – Plan your weekly meals, then create a shopping list to avoid impulse buys.

Practice at Home and on the Road – Test out new recipes and meal strategies at home first. When traveling, pack healthy snacks and plan ahead to choose fast food that works with your goals or places that you can shop for food.

NUTRITION RESOURCES

Good planning is always made more efficient and effective by utilizing the resources around us. Here are some websites, apps, and books that can improve your basic nutrition planning and food knowledge.

WEBSITES

Use these sites for recipes, tips, and reliable nutrition advice:

EatingWell – Features healthy, easy-to-make recipes.

Verywell Fit – Offers expert advice on fitness and nutrition.

Foodhub – Specializes in recipes for diabetes management.

Delish – Provides fun and indulgent healthy recipes.

APPS

If you know that tracking intake will not become a mental health problem, it might help you get a sense of calorie and nutrient needs by using an app for a period of time.

Here are a few useful ones:

Cronometer – Tracks nutrients and calories with precision.

Carbon Diet App – Offers personalized diet coaching.

MyFitnessPal – Logs food intake and exercise with a large database.

BOOKS

Expand your understanding of nutrition with these insightful reads:

Is Butter a Carb? – Debunks common nutrition myths.

Food Politics – Explores the influence of politics on our diets.

Flexible Dieting – Offers a balanced approach to eating without strict restrictions.

Burn – Explains how metabolism works and impacts weight.

On Food and Cooking – A comprehensive guide to food science and culinary techniques.

Just Eat – Provides a no-nonsense approach to eating healthily.

You Can't Screw This Up – Encourages a flexible, forgiving approach to diet.

Eat, Drink, and Be Healthy – Offers evidence-based guidelines for a balanced diet.

Atomic Habits – Although not nutrition-specific, it gives great insight into creating new habits.

MAKE SMART GOALS

Rather than vague resolutions, create SMART goals. This means creating goals that are Specific, Measurable, Achievable, Relevant, and Time-bound. So, instead of "eat more veggies," try a SMART goal like, "include two servings of steamed vegetables with lunch and dinner, which are prepped on Sundays." This clarity helps you stay focused and track progress. If you have an accountability method, like keeping a food journal or going over the progress with a friend, it can make you even more likely to succeed.

UNDERSTAND YOUR INFLUENCES AND BARRIERS

Awareness of what influences your eating habits can help you take control:

Emotional Eating – Recognize when you're eating to cope with emotions like stress or boredom and find healthier outlets such as exercise or journaling.

Financial Considerations – Budget for nutritious food and learn cost-effective ways to eat healthily, like buying in bulk.

Barrier of Time and Schedule – If mornings are hectic, simplify your breakfast by preparing overnight oats or pre-made smoothies to ensure a nutritious start to your day.

Social Media – Curate your social media to follow accounts that promote realistic, positive health messages rather than unrealistic body images.

SUBTLE CHANGES

Creating subtle changes can encourage healthier choices without the need for willpower. Here are some practical "nudges" you can use, which were adapted from a meta-analysis on healthy eating behaviors:[2]

Cognitive Nudges – Pay attention to nutritional labels or choose foods with clear, easy-to-understand labels like the Traffic Light system, which highlights healthier options.

Visibility Enhancements – Arrange your kitchen so that healthy foods are at eye level and easily accessible. Keep fruits on the counter and store less healthy snacks out of sight.

Affective Nudges – Choose restaurants or meal services that emphasize healthy, delicious options. Use visual cues, like colorful plates or attractive food presentations, to make healthy meals more appealing.

Behavioral Nudges – Opt for convenience by prepping healthy meals in advance or choosing set menus that default to healthier options, like salads or vegetables as sides. Adjust portion sizes to make healthier foods more prominent on your plate.

In the study that applied these different nudges, the research team found the behavioral nudges were particularly effective, potentially reducing calorie intake by up to 320 kcal per day.[3] But leaning into all of these areas can help. By subtly altering your environment and routines, you can make healthier choices easier and more automatic.

APPROACH TO EATING

In today's world, constant stimulation can drown out your body's natural hunger and satiety cues. Here's how to get back in touch:

Physical vs. Emotional Hunger – Learn to distinguish between the two. Physical hunger develops gradually, is felt in the stomach, and is satisfied with a variety of foods. Emotional hunger, on the other hand, comes on suddenly, often leads to cravings for specific comfort foods, and may result in overeating or guilt.

Steps to Manage Emotional Eating:

1. **Identify** – Pinpoint the emotion triggering your urge to eat. Are you stressed, bored, or anxious? Recognizing this is the first step toward change.

2. **Describe** – Articulate the difference between your physical and emotional responses. For example, you might feel tension in your chest when anxious versus a growling stomach when genuinely hungry.

3. **Participate** – Engage in actions that address your emotions directly rather than turning to food. Practice is key, and setbacks are normal. Use tools like deep breathing, going for a walk, or talking to a friend to create new, healthy habits.

NUTRITION REQUIRES PRACTICE

To get to a place that is truly effective requires consistent and often messy efforts over time. Everyone can follow a meal plan for a while, but true mastery lies in navigating unplanned situations, like holidays, vacations, and weekends, without derailing. Intuitive eating, setting realistic boundaries, and maintaining a flexible mindset allows for enjoyment without losing progress. The key is to practice and learn to balance indulgence with consistency.

10 PRACTICAL NUTRITION APPLICATIONS

1. Less Grazing, More Mindful Eating – Mindless snacking and distracted eating can lead to unnecessary calorie intake and poor food choices, diminishing the enjoyment and satisfaction of meals. Instead of grazing out of boredom or habit, ask yourself if you're truly hungry before reaching for a snack. If you do need a snack, choose something nutritious, like fruit, nuts, or yogurt, and take the time to enjoy it without distractions. Similarly, when it's time for meals, practice mindful eating by eliminating distractions such as TV, phones, or work. Focus on the flavors, textures, and aromas of your food, savoring each bite. This approach not only helps you manage your calorie intake and make healthier food choices but also enhances the overall eating experience, allowing you to better tune in to your hunger and fullness cues.

2. Less Skipping, More Balanced Meals – Skipping meals, whether due to a busy schedule or in an attempt to cut calories, can lead to energy dips, poor concentration, and overeating later in the day. Instead of skipping meals, aim to eat regular, balanced meals that include a mix of macronutrients along with plenty of fiber. This helps keep your energy levels stable and your hunger in check. Plan your meals to include a variety of foods that provide sustained energy and nourishment throughout the day. By focusing on consistent, balanced meals, you can better support your body's needs and maintain a healthier lifestyle.

3. Less Boring, More Diverse – A monotonous diet can make eating feel like a chore, leading to boredom and a lack of enthusiasm for meals. To make your diet more exciting and enjoyable, embrace diversity in the foods you eat. Explore a wide array of ingredients. Experiment with different fruits, vegetables, grains, and proteins to add variety to your meals. Try new cuisines, flavors, and cooking techniques to keep your palate engaged. Incorporate seasonal produce, which not only adds freshness but also naturally varies your diet throughout the year. By diversifying your meals, you'll not only improve your nutrition but also find greater satisfaction and enjoyment in the foods you eat.

4. Less About Others, More About Your Own Needs – It's easy to compare yourself to others, but nutrition and health are deeply personal. What works for someone else may not work for you. Focus on understanding your body's signals, honoring your hunger and fullness cues, and tailoring your diet and exercise routine to what makes you feel your best. By concentrating on your unique needs, you can build a healthier, more sustainable lifestyle without the pressure of living up to someone else's standards.

5. Less Wild Claims, More Creative Solutions – The world of nutrition is filled with wild claims and quick fixes, but these are often unsupported by science. Instead of chasing after the latest fad, focus on creative, practical solutions to improve your health. For instance, explore recipes that can help reduce added sugar intake or find fun ways to incorporate more vegetables into your meals. By focusing on realistic, evidence-based approaches, you'll find more satisfaction and success in your health journey.

6. Less Ideas, More Habit Forming – Ideas and goals are important, but they only become powerful when put into action. Instead of being overwhelmed by possibilities, focus on forming small, concrete habits that drive lasting change. Start with one habit and build consistency from there.

7. Less Perfection, More Progress – Perfection is an unattainable goal that can lead to frustration, especially in nutrition and health. Instead of striving for perfection, focus on making consistent progress. It's okay to indulge occasionally or have a less-than-perfect meal. What matters most is your overall pattern of behavior and the progress you're making toward a healthier lifestyle. Celebrate small wins and learn from setbacks to create a more sustainable approach to health.

8. Less About Competition, More About Supporting Your Well-Being – The competitive mindset in health and fitness can be damaging, leading to stress and a negative relationship with food and exercise. Instead of comparing yourself to others, focus on supporting your physical and mental health in a way that's right for you. Prioritize rest, choose enjoyable activities, and practice self-compassion. By shifting your focus from competition to well-being, you'll cultivate a healthier, more balanced approach to life.

9. Less Quantity, More Quality – Eating well isn't about eating more; it's about eating better. Shift your focus from quantity to quality by choosing foods that are rich in nutrients. Opt for whole foods like fruits, vegetables, whole grains, and lean proteins, which provide essential vitamins, minerals, and fiber. By prioritizing quality over quantity, you can nourish your body more effectively and feel more satisfied with your meals.

10. Less Nonsense, More Love for Food – Too often, nutrition advice is framed in terms of restriction and fear. However, a healthy relationship with food should be rooted in love and appreciation. Reconnect with the pleasure of eating by trying new recipes, savoring your favorite meals, and enjoying food in a relaxed setting. When you focus on the love of food rather than fear-based messaging, healthy eating becomes a more enjoyable and natural part of your life.

SENSIBLE **NUTRITION**

While nutrition can be imperfect and messy, it also holds the potential to be a powerful and transformative part of your life. At the beginning of this book, I mentioned that nutrition nonsense is constantly getting in the way of good nutrition habits. This nonsense comes from many places—corporate greed, social inequality, demanding work schedules, the chaos of parenting, laziness, misplaced priorities, relentless marketing, the allure of quick fixes, the pursuit of fame, flawed science, poor education, miscommunication, biases, or the natural pitfalls of our broken human nature. And even though all of these influences can be powerful and overwhelming, there's an opportunity to take a new step forward. Start practicing positive eating habits and allow a more reasonable nutrition outlook to drown out the nonsense.

Instead of getting caught up in these distractions, focus on what food can do for you. It's not just about what's on your plate; it's about how it can bring people together, create moments of joy, and support your health and well-being. Share meals with family or friends, savor the time spent around the table, and let food be a source of connection rather than stress. Prioritize your health by taking small, meaningful steps and letting go of the fear and confusion that often surround nutrition.

Remember, it's not about perfection. It's about making choices that nourish your body and soul, one meal at a time. Start today with one mindful step, and watch how food can transform your life for the better. Ultimately, awareness and discussion are the first steps, but change only happens through action. Confidence comes from trying, not from waiting. Embrace the small steps, the small habits, and the journey itself. Behaviors will drive change, not the other way around. Don't allow another day to go by when you are manipulated by the nonsense of food marketing, false promises, and biased beliefs. Enjoy your food and make sensible decisions that support your own health goals.

REFERENCES

INTRODUCTION

1. G A. Eating disorder statistics. National Association of Anorexia Nervosa and Associated Disorders. Published October 31, 2024. https://anad.org/eating-disorder-statistic.
2. Eating disorders are on the rise. American Society for Nutrition. Published February 8, 2022. https://nutrition.org/eating-disorders-are-on-the-rise/.
3. Arcelus J, Mitchell AJ, Wales J, Nielsen S. Mortality rates in patients with anorexia nervosa and other eating disorders: a meta-analysis of 36 studies. Arch Gen Psychiatry. 2011;68(7):724-731. doi:10.1001/archgenpsychiatry.2011.74.
4. About chronic diseases. Chronic Disease. Published October 4, 2024. https://www.cdc.gov/chronic-disease/about/.
5. Vegan raw food influencer who ate all-fruit diet allegedly dies of malnutrition, infections. Nationalpost. Published August 4, 2023. https://nationalpost.com/news/vegan-raw-food-influencer-who-ate-all-fruit-diet-allegedly-dies-of-malnutrition-infections.
6. Cost B. Vegan raw food diet influencer Zhanna D'Art dies of suspected starvation: report. New York Post. Published July 31, 2023. https://nypost.com/2023/07/31/vegan-influencer-starved-to-death-friends/.
7. Hall H. Australian naturopath Barbara O'Neill banned for her dangerous health advice. Science-Based Medicine. Published October 14, 2019. https://sciencebasedmedicine.org/australian-naturopath-barbara-oneill-banned-for-her-dangerous-health-advice/.

REFERENCES

CHAPTER 1: PANACEA

1. Worldwide Detox Products Industry to 2026: Rising Awareness Regarding the Adverse Effects of Alcohol and Cigarette Consumption is Driving Growth. GlobeNewswire. Published October 18, 2021. https://www.globenewswire.com/news-release/2021/10/18/2315656/28124/en/Worldwide-Detox-Products-Industry-to-2026-Rising-Awareness-Regarding-the-Adverse-Effects-of-Alcohol-and-Cigarette-Consumption-is-Driving-Growth.html.
2. Roehr B. US has highest dissatisfaction with health care. BMJ. 2007;335(7627):956. doi:10.1136/bmj.39388.639028.DB
3. Ducharme J. Exclusive: More Than 70% of Americans Feel Failed by the Health Care System. Time. Published May 16, 2023. https://time.com/6279937/us-health-care-system-attitudes/.
4. Berger M. Penn Nutritionist and Psychologist Explain the Allure of Fad Diets—and Why They Fail. Penn Today. Published March 2, 2022. https://penntoday.upenn.edu/news/Penn-nutritionist-psychologist-allure-fad-diets-and-why-they-fail.
5. Detoxification. Texas A&M University School of Veterinary Medicine. https://vetmed.tamu.edu/peer/detoxification/.
6. Alcohol Metabolism: An Update. National Institute on Alcohol Abuse and Alcoholism. https://www.niaaa.nih.gov/publications/alcohol-metabolism.
7. How Is Alcohol Eliminated From the Body? Duke University. https://sites.duke.edu/apep/module-1-gender-matters/science-content/how-is-alcohol-eliminated-from-the-body/.
8. Woman Almost Died Trying to Cure Cancer With Juice Diet. Peeblesshire News. Published July 31, 2023. https://www.peeblesshirenews.com/news/national/24266499.woman-almost-died-trying-cure-cancer-juice-diet/.
9. Davey M. Jessica Ainscough: Australia's 'Wellness Warrior' Dies of Cancer Aged 30. The Guardian. Published February 15, 2015. https://www.theguardian.com/australia-news/2015/mar/01/jessica-ainscough-australia-wellness-warrior-dies-cancer-aged-30.

REFERENCES

10. Klein AV, Kiat H. Detox diets for toxin elimination and weight management: a critical review of the evidence. J Hum Nutr Diet. 2015;28(6):675-686. doi:10.1111/jhn.12286
11. Wheless JW. History of the Ketogenic Diet. Epilepsia. 2008;49 Suppl 8:3-5. doi:10.1111/j.1528-1167.2008.01821.x.
12. Newton RW. The Treatment of Epilepsy, 2nd Edition. Arch Dis Child. 2006;91(5):452. doi:10.1136/adc.2004.060517.
13. Mahdi GS. The Atkins Diet Controversy. Ann Saudi Med. 2006;26(3):244-245. doi:10.5144/0256-4947.2006.244.
14. Yang MU, Van Itallie TB. Composition of Weight Lost During Short-Term Weight Reduction. Metabolic Responses of Obese Subjects to Starvation and Low-Calorie Ketogenic and Nonketogenic Diets. J Clin Invest. 1976;58(3):722-730. doi:10.1172/JCI108519.
15. Hall KD, Guo J, Courville AB, et al. Effect of a Plant-Based, Low-Fat Diet Versus an Animal-Based, Ketogenic Diet on Ad Libitum Energy Intake. Nat Med. 2021;27(2):344-353. doi:10.1038/s41591-020-01209-1.
16. Kinsell LW, Gunning B, Michaels GD, Richardson J, Cox SE, Lemon C. Calories Do Count. Metabolism. 1964;13:195-204. doi:10.1016/0026-0495(64)90098-8.
17. Hall KD, Guo J. Obesity Energetics: Body Weight Regulation and the Effects of Diet Composition. Gastroenterology. 2017;152(7):1718-1727.e3. doi:10.1053/j.gastro.2017.01.052.
18. Hosie R. Bodybuilder Got Ripped Eating Only Potatoes. Business Insider. Published May 11, 2024. https://www.businessinsider.com/bodybuilder-got-ripped-built-muscle-eating-potato-carbs-mark-taylor-2024-4?amp.
19. Fenton TR, Fenton CJ. Evidence Does Not Support the Alkaline Diet. Osteoporos Int. 2016;27(7):2387-2388. doi:10.1007/s00198-016-3504-z.
20. Fenton TR, Tough SC, Lyon AW, Eliasziw M, Hanley DA. Causal Assessment of Dietary Acid Load and Bone Disease: A Systematic Review and Meta-Analysis Applying Hill's Epidemiologic Criteria for Causality. Nutr J. 2011;10:41. Published April 30, 2011. doi:10.1186/1475-2891-10-41.

REFERENCES

21. Fenton TR, Huang T. Systematic Review of the Association Between Dietary Acid Load, Alkaline Water and Cancer. BMJ Open. 2016;6(6)
. Published June 13, 2016. doi:10.1136/bmjopen-2015-010438.
22. Figueroa T. Jury Awards $105M in Suit Against pH Miracle Author. San Diego Union Tribune. Published November 2, 2018. https://www.sandiegouniontribune.com/2018/11/02/jury-awards-105m-in-suit-against-ph-miracle-author/#:~:text=A%20San%20Diego%20jury%20sided,to%20forego%20traditional%20medical%20treatment.
23. Petre A. The Autoimmune Protocol Diet (AIP Diet). Healthline. Published April 25, 2019. https://www.healthline.com/nutrition/aip-diet-autoimmune-protocol-diet#faq.
24. Autoimmune Diseases. National Institute of Environmental Health Sciences. Updated August 25, 2022. https://www.niehs.nih.gov/health/topics/conditions/autoimmune#:~:text=Scientists%20know%20about%20more%20than,before%20getting%20a%20proper%20diagnosis.
25. Bagur MJ, Murcia MA, Jiménez-Monreal AM, et al. Influence of Diet in Multiple Sclerosis: A Systematic Review. Adv Nutr. 2017;8(3):463-472. Published May 15, 2017. doi:10.3945/an.116.014191.
26. Gu L, Fu R, Hong J, Ni H, Yu K, Lou H. Effects of Intermittent Fasting in Humans Compared to a Non-intervention Diet and Caloric Restriction: A Meta-Analysis of Randomized Controlled Trials. Front Nutr. 2022;9:871682. Published May 2, 2022. doi:10.3389/fnut.2022.871682.
27. Ezzati A, Rosenkranz SK, Phelan J, Logan C. The Effects of Isocaloric Intermittent Fasting vs Daily Caloric Restriction on Weight Loss and Metabolic Risk Factors for Noncommunicable Chronic Diseases: A Systematic Review of Randomized Controlled or Comparative Trials. J Acad Nutr Diet. 2023;123(2):318-329.e1. doi:10.1016/j.jand.2022.09.013.

REFERENCES

28. Maruthur NM, Pilla SJ, White K, et al. Effect of Isocaloric, Time-Restricted Eating on Body Weight in Adults With Obesity: A Randomized Controlled Trial. Ann Intern Med. 2024;177(5):549-558. doi:10.7326/M23-3132.
29. Wei X, Cooper A, Lee I, et al. Intermittent Energy Restriction for Weight Loss: A Systematic Review of Cardiometabolic, Inflammatory and Appetite Outcomes. Biol Res Nurs. 2022;24(3):410-428. doi:10.1177/10998004221078079.
30. Seimon RV, Roekenes JA, Zibellini J, et al. Do Intermittent Diets Provide Physiological Benefits Over Continuous Diets for Weight Loss? A Systematic Review of Clinical Trials. Mol Cell Endocrinol. 2015;418 Pt 2:153-172. doi:10.1016/j.mce.2015.09.014.
31. Headland M, Clifton PM, Carter S, Keogh JB. Weight-Loss Outcomes: A Systematic Review and Meta-Analysis of Intermittent Energy Restriction Trials Lasting a Minimum of 6 Months. Nutrients. 2016;8(6):354. Published June 8, 2016. doi:10.3390/nu8060354.
32. Varady KA, Oddo VM. Untangling the Benefits of Time-Restricted Eating: Is It the Calories or the Time Restriction? Ann Intern Med. 2024;177(5):672-673. doi:10.7326/M24-0695.
33. Finkbeiner S. The Autophagy Lysosomal Pathway and Neurodegeneration. Cold Spring Harb Perspect Biol. 2020;12(3).Published March 2, 2020. doi:10.1101/cshperspect.a033993.
34. Templeman I, Smith HA, Chowdhury E, et al. A Randomized Controlled Trial to Isolate the Effects of Fasting and Energy Restriction on Weight Loss and Metabolic Health in Lean Adults. Sci Transl Med. 2021;13(598) . doi:10.1126/scitranslmed.abd8034.
35. Multivitamin/Mineral Supplements. Office of Dietary Supplements, National Institutes of Health. Updated September 2, 2022. https://ods.od.nih.gov/factsheets/MVMS-HealthProfessional/.
36. Ogilvie A. How Much Do Americans Spend on Health and Fitness? MyProtein USA. Published 2019. https://us.myprotein.com/thezone/training/much-americans-spend-health-fitness-survey-results-revealed/.

REFERENCES

37. How Much Do Americans Spend on Health and Fitness? ATH Sport. Updated December 4, 2023. https://www.ath-sport.co/blogs/learn/how-much-do-americans-spend-on-their-health-and-fitness.
38. Wunsch NG. U.S. Consumers' Vitamins and Supplements Spend by Generation. Statista. Published 2019. https://www.statista.com/statistics/1086289/us-consumers-vitamins-and-supplements-spend-by-generation/.
39. Putterman S. Biden's Prescription Drug Price Reforms: Fact Check. KFF Health News. Published March 6, 2024. https://kffhealthnews.org/news/article/fact-check-biden-prescription-drug-prices-nation-comparison/#:~:text=The%20Peterson%2DKFF%20report%2C%20using,%2Dof%2Dpocket%20consumer%20costs.
40. Global Wellness Institute. Global Wellness Economy: Industry Overview 2023. Global Wellness Institute. Published November 9, 2023. https://globalwellnessinstitute.org/wp-content/uploads/2023/11/GWI-WE-Monitor-2023_FINAL.pdf.
41. Rappaport S. The Global Wellness Industry is Now Worth $5.6 Trillion. Bloomberg. Published November 9, 2023. https://www.bloomberg.com/news/articles/2023-11-09/the-global-wellness-industry-is-now-worth-5-6-trillion.
42. Mikulic M. Pharmaceutical Market Worldwide Revenue. Statista. Published May 22, 2024. https://www.statista.com/statistics/263102/pharmaceutical-market-worldwide-revenue-since-2001/#:~:text=The%20global%20pharmaceutical%20market%20has,around%201.6%20trillion%20U.S.%20dollars.
43. The dangers of dietary and nutritional supplements investigated: What you don't know about these 12 ingredients could hurt you. Consumer Reports. Published September, 2010. https://www.consumerreports.org/cro/2012/05/dangerous-supplements/index.htm.
44. Esch M. Study: Many herbal supplements aren't what the label says. Associated Press. Published 2015. https://apnews.com/general-news-120c82596385478ea56aece0499f4447.

REFERENCES

45. Eichner AK, Coyles J, Fedoruk M, et al. Essential Features of Third-Party Certification Programs for Dietary Supplements: A Consensus Statement. Curr Sports Med Rep. 2019;18(5):178-182. doi:10.1249/JSR.0000000000000595
46. Navarro VJ, Khan I, Björnsson E, Seeff LB, Serrano J, Hoofnagle JH. Liver Injury from Herbal and Dietary Supplements. Hepatology. 2017;65(1):363-373. doi:10.1002/hep.28813.
47. Toxic hepatitis - Symptoms and causes. Mayo Clinic. Published June 4, 2022. https://www.mayoclinic.org/diseases-conditions/toxic-hepatitis/symptoms-causes/syc-20352202#:~:text=Herbs%20and%20supplements.,candy%20and%20take%20large%20doses.
48. Institute of Medicine (US) and National Research Council (US) Committee on the Framework for Evaluating the Safety of Dietary Supplements. Dietary Supplements: A Framework for Evaluating Safety. Washington (DC): National Academies Press (US); 2005.
49. U.S. Food and Drug Administration. Facts About Dietary Supplements. FDA. Updated 2023. https://www.fda.gov/news-events/rumor-control/facts-about-dietary-supplements.
50. Blumberg JB, Frei BB, Fulgoni VL, Weaver CM, Zeisel SH. Impact of Frequency of Multi-Vitamin/Multi-Mineral Supplement Intake on Nutritional Adequacy and Nutrient Deficiencies in U.S. Adults. Nutrients. 2017;9(8):849. Published 2017 Aug 9. doi:10.3390/nu9080849
51. Wallace TC, Frankenfeld CL, Frei B, et al. Multivitamin/Multimineral Supplement Use is Associated with Increased Micronutrient Intakes and Biomarkers and Decreased Prevalence of Inadequacies and Deficiencies in Middle-Aged and Older Adults in the United States. J Nutr Gerontol Geriatr. 2019;38(4):307-328. doi:10.1080/21551197.2019.1656135
52. O'Connor EA, Evans CV, Ivlev I, et al. Vitamin and Mineral Supplements for the Primary Prevention of Cardiovascular Disease and Cancer: Updated Evidence Report and Systematic Review for the US Preventive Services Task Force. JAMA. 2022;327(23):2334-2347. doi:10.1001/jama.2021.15650

REFERENCES

53. Macpherson H, Pipingas A, Pase MP. Multivitamin-multimineral supplementation and mortality: a meta-analysis of randomized controlled trials. Am J Clin Nutr. 2013;97(2):437-444. doi:10.3945/ajcn.112.049304
54. National Institutes of Health (NIH). For healthy adults, taking multivitamins daily is not associated with a lower risk of death. NIH. Published October 10, 2020. https://www.nih.gov/news-events/news-releases/healthy-adults-taking-multivitamins-daily-not-associated-lower-risk-death#:~:text=The%20analysis%20showed%20that%20people,heart%20disease%2C%20or%20cerebrovascular%20diseases.
55. National Institutes of Health Office of Dietary Supplements. Vitamin C - Consumer. NIH. Updated September 16, 2022. https://ods.od.nih.gov/factsheets/VitaminC-Consumer/.
56. Douglas RM, Hemilä H, Chalker E, Treacy B. Vitamin C for preventing and treating the common cold. Cochrane Database Syst Rev. 2007;(3):CD000980. Published 2007 Jul 18. doi:10.1002/14651858.CD000980.pub3
57. Cerullo G, Negro M, Parimbelli M, et al. The Long History of Vitamin C: From Prevention of the Common Cold to Potential Aid in the Treatment of COVID-19. Front Immunol. 2020;11:574029. Published 2020 Oct 28. doi:10.3389/fimmu.2020.574029
58. Crawford C, Avula B, Lindsey AT, et al. Analysis of Select Dietary Supplement Products Marketed to Support or Boost the Immune System. JAMA Netw Open. 2022;5(8):e2226040. Published 2022 Aug 1. doi:10.1001/jamanetworkopen.2022.26040
59. Can You Really Boost Your Immune System? Cedars-Sinai. Published June 1, 2020. https://www.cedars-sinai.org/blog/boosting-your-immune-system.html.
60. Bekar O, Yilmaz Y, Gulten M. Kefir improves the efficacy and tolerability of triple therapy in eradicating Helicobacter pylori. J Med Food. 2011;14(4):344-347. doi:10.1089/jmf.2010.0099
61. Na X, Kelly C. Probiotics in clostridium difficile Infection. J Clin Gastroenterol. 2011;45 Suppl(Suppl):S154-S158. doi:10.1097/MCG.0b013e31822ec787

REFERENCES

62. So D, Quigley EMM, Whelan K. Probiotics in irritable bowel syndrome and inflammatory bowel disease: review of mechanisms and effectiveness. Curr Opin Gastroenterol. 2023;39(2):103-109. doi:10.1097/MOG.0000000000000902
63. Suez J, Zmora N, Zilberman-Schapira G, et al. Post-Antibiotic Gut Mucosal Microbiome Reconstitution Is Impaired by Probiotics and Improved by Autologous FMT. Cell. 2018;174(6):1406-1423.e16. doi:10.1016/j.cell.2018.08.047
64. Hersh AL, King LM, Shapiro DJ, Hicks LA, Fleming-Dutra KE. Unnecessary Antibiotic Prescribing in US Ambulatory Care Settings, 2010-2015. Clin Infect Dis. 2021;72(1):133-137. doi:10.1093/cid/ciaa667
65. National Institutes of Health Office of Dietary Supplements. Probiotics - Health Professional. Updated 2023. NIH. https://ods.od.nih.gov/factsheets/Probiotics-HealthProfessional/.
66. Maddox W. Woman's Death After IV Therapy Leads to License Suspension for Frisco Anesthesiologist. D Magazine. Published 2023. https://www.dmagazine.com/healthcare-business/2023/10/womans-death-after-iv-therapy-leads-to-license-suspension-for-frisco-anesthesiologist/.
67. Edwards E, Kopf M. Warnings grow about risky IV drips and injections at unregulated med spas. NBC News. Published 2024. https://www.nbcnews.com/health/health-news/warnings-grow-risky-iv-drips-injections-unregulated-med-spas-rcna131495.
68. Mitchell A. My body was eating itself alive after getting fat-dissolving injections at a luxury spa. New York Post. Published October 23, 2023. https://nypost.com/2023/10/23/lifestyle/my-body-was-eating-itself-alive-after-fat-dissolving-injections/.
69. Palacios AM, Cardel MI, Parker E, et al. Effectiveness of lactation cookies on human milk production rates: a randomized controlled trial. Am J Clin Nutr. 2023;117(5):1035-1042. doi:10.1016/j.ajcnut.2023.03.010
70. Jumpertz R, Venti CA, Le DS, et al. Food label accuracy of common snack foods. Obesity (Silver Spring). 2013;21(1):164-169. doi:10.1002/oby.20185

REFERENCES

71. Shcherbina A, Mattsson CM, Waggott D, et al. Accuracy in Wrist-Worn, Sensor-Based Measurements of Heart Rate and Energy Expenditure in a Diverse Cohort. J Pers Med. 2017;7(2):3. Published 2017 May 24. doi:10.3390/jpm7020003
72. Dusheck J. Fitness trackers accurately measure heart rate but not calories burned. Stanford Medicine. Published May 24, 2017. https://med.stanford.edu/news/all-news/2017/05/fitness-trackers-accurately-measure-heart-rate-but-not-calories-burned.html.
73. Gebauer SK, Novotny JA, Bornhorst GM, Baer DJ. Food processing and structure impact the metabolizable energy of almonds. Food Funct. 2016;7(10):4231-4238. doi:10.1039/c6fo01076h
74. Stapel SO, Asero R, Ballmer-Weber BK, et al. Testing for IgG4 against foods is not recommended as a diagnostic tool: EAACI Task Force Report. Allergy. 2008;63(7):793-796. doi:10.1111/j.1398-9995.2008.01705.x
75. Burks AW, Tang M, Sicherer S, et al. ICON: food allergy. J Allergy Clin Immunol. 2012;129(4):906-920. doi:10.1016/j.jaci.2012.02.001
76. Mufson S, Branigin W. European Union Urges Testing of US Wheat Imports for Unapproved Strain. Washington Post. https://www.washingtonpost.com/business/economy/european-union-urges-testing-of-us-wheat-imports-for-unapproved-strain/2013/05/31/eaaefcdc-c9fc-11e2-8da7-d274bc611a47_story.html. Published May 31, 2013.
77. Mönnikes H, Tebbe JJ, Hildebrandt M, et al. Role of stress in functional gastrointestinal disorders. Evidence for stress-induced alterations in gastrointestinal motility and sensitivity. Dig Dis. 2001;19(3):201-211. doi:10.1159/000050681
78. Howard R, Guo J, Hall KD. Imprecision nutrition? Different simultaneous continuous glucose monitors provide discordant meal rankings for incremental postprandial glucose in subjects without diabetes. Am J Clin Nutr. 2020;112(4):1114-1119. doi:10.1093/ajcn/nqaa198

REFERENCES

79. Glucose Two-Hour Postprandial Glucose. University of Rochester Medical Center. Published 2021. https://www.urmc.rochester.edu/encyclopedia/content.aspx?contenttypeid=167&contentid=glucose_two_hour_postprandial.
80. USDA Agricultural Research Service. Grapes, red or green (European type, such as Thompson seedless), raw. FoodData Central. Published 2019. https://fdc.nal.usda.gov/fdc-app.html#/food-details/174683/nutrients.
81. Recipal. Oreo Cookies - Nutrition Facts. Recipal. https://www.recipal.com/ingredients/7622-nutrition-facts-calories-protein-carbs-fat-oreo-cookies.
82. Dohadwala MM, Vita JA. Grapes and cardiovascular disease. J Nutr. 2009;139(9):1788S-93S. doi:10.3945/jn.109.107474
83. Yang J, Xiao YY. Grape phytochemicals and associated health benefits. Crit Rev Food Sci Nutr. 2013;53(11):1202-1225. doi:10.1080/10408398.2012.692408
84. Schultes B, Panknin AK, Hallschmid M, et al. Glycemic increase induced by intravenous glucose infusion fails to affect hunger, appetite, or satiety following breakfast in healthy men. Appetite. 2016;105:562-566. doi:10.1016/j.appet.2016.06.032
85. Corpeleijn E. Commentary: Does Hunger Manipulate Glucose Levels, or Do Glucose Levels Make You Eat? University of Chicago Press Journals. https://www.journals.uchicago.edu/doi/abs/10.1086/684460?journalCode=jacr.
86. Hosie R. A fat-loss coach lost 12 pounds while spiking his blood sugar to prove you don't need to be scared of fruit and oatmeal. Business Insider. Published October 10, 2023. https://www.businessinsider.com/man-weight-loss-12-pounds-spiking-increasing-blood-sugar-levels-2023-10#:~:text=To%20allay%20their%20fears%2C%20he,high%20in%20carbohydrates%20every%20day.
87. Muller E, Algavi YM, Borenstein E. A meta-analysis study of the robustness and universality of gut microbiome-metabolome associations. Microbiome. 2021;9(1):203. Published 2021 Oct 12. doi:10.1186/s40168-021-01149-z

REFERENCES

88. Staley, C., Kaiser, T. & Khoruts, A. Clinician Guide to Microbiome Testing. Dig Dis Sci 63, 3167–3177 (2018). https://doi.org/10.1007/s10620-018-5299-6.
89. Shalon D, Culver RN, Grembi JA, et al. Profiling the human intestinal environment under physiological conditions. Nature. 2023;617(7961):581-591. doi:10.1038/s41586-023-05989-7
90. Ahn, Ji-Seon, Lkhagva, Enkhchimeg, Jung, Sunjun, Kim, Hyeon-Jin, Chung, Hea-Jong, Hong, Seong-Tshool, Fecal Microbiome Does Not Represent Whole Gut Microbiome, Cellular Microbiology, 2023, 6868417, 14 pages, 2023. https://doi.org/10.1155/2023/6868417
91. Damisch L, Stoberock B, Mussweiler T. Keep your fingers crossed!: how superstition improves performance. Psychol Sci. 2010;21(7):1014-1020. doi:10.1177/0956797610372631
92. The Truth About Toxins. Rush University Medical Center. Published 2021. https://www.rush.edu/news/truth-about-toxins.
93. Hall H. Rope Worms: C'est la Merde. Science-Based Medicine. Published May 27, 2014. https://sciencebasedmedicine.org/rope-worms-cest-la-merde/.
94. Pélissier L, Bagot S, Miles-Chan JL, et al. Is dieting a risk for higher weight gain in normal-weight individual? A systematic review and meta-analysis. Br J Nutr. 2023;130(7):1190-1212. doi:10.1017/S0007114523000132
95. Siahpush M, Tibbits M, Shaikh RA, Singh GK, Sikora Kessler A, Huang TT. Dieting Increases the Likelihood of Subsequent Obesity and BMI Gain: Results from a Prospective Study of an Australian National Sample. Int J Behav Med. 2015;22(5):662-671. doi:10.1007/s12529-015-9463-5
96. Ramirez J, Guarner F, Bustos Fernandez L, Maruy A, Sdepanian VL, Cohen H. Antibiotics as Major Disruptors of Gut Microbiota. Front Cell Infect Microbiol. 2020;10:572912. Published 2020 Nov 24. doi:10.3389/fcimb.2020.572912
97. Lange K, Buerger M, Stallmach A, Bruns T. Effects of Antibiotics on Gut Microbiota. Dig Dis. 2016;34(3):260-268. doi:10.1159/000443360

REFERENCES

98. Does Diarrhea Clean You Out? Cary Gastroenterology Associates. Published June 27, 2023. https://www.carygastro.com/blog/does-diarrhea-clean-you-out.
99. Downs M. Why Do We Keep Falling for Fad Diets? WebMD. Published 2005. https://www.webmd.com/diet/features/why-do-we-keep-falling-for-fad-diets.
100. Eurich DT, Majumdar SR. Statins and sepsis - scientifically interesting but clinically inconsequential. J Gen Intern Med. 2012;27(3):268-269. doi:10.1007/s11606-011-1939-7

IMAGE #1:

Neal Smoller. The 14 Mega-Corporations That Own Your Supplement Brand. Dr. Neal Smoller website. Published August 12, 2021. https://drnealsmoller.com/rant/the-14-mega-corporations-that-own-your-supplement-brand/

REFERENCES

CHAPTER 2: ORIGINS

1. Paleo food market: Global industry analysis, 2017–2032. Future Market Insights. Published 2023. https://www.futuremarketinsights.com/reports/paleo-food-market.
2. Paleolithic Period. In: Encyclopædia Britannica. https://www.britannica.com/event/Paleolithic-Period.
3. Zuk M. Paleofantasy: What Evolution Really Tells Us About Sex, Diet, and How We Live. New York, NY: W.W. Norton & Company; 2013.
4. The Paleolithic diet: Is it the diet of our ancestors? National Center for Biotechnology Information. Published 2018. https://www.ncbi.nlm.nih.gov/books/NBK482457/#:~:text=The%20concept%20of%20the%20Paleolithic,by%20Loren%20Cordain%20in%202002.
5. Paleo diet: What it is and why it's not for everyone. UC Davis Health. Published April 6, 2022. https://health.ucdavis.edu/blog/good-food/paleo-diet-what-it-is-and-why-its-not-for-everyone/2022/04.
6. What is the paleo diet? The Paleo Diet. Published 2024. https://thepaleodiet.com/try-the-paleo-diet/what-is-the-paleo-diet/.
7. Starkovich BM, Conard NJ. Bone taphonomy of the Schöningen "Spear Horizon South" and its implications for site formation and hominin meat provisioning. J Hum Evol. 2015;89:154-171. doi:10.1016/j.jhevol.2015.09.015
8. Singh A, Singh D. The Paleolithic Diet. Cureus. 2023;15(1):e34214. Published 2023 Jan 25. doi:10.7759/cureus.34214
9. Legumes: Family Fabaceae (Leguminosae). United States Department of Agriculture Forest Service. Published 2024. https://www.fs.usda.gov/wildflowers/ethnobotany/food/legumes.shtml.
10. Huebbe P, Rimbach G. Historical Reflection of Food Processing and the Role of Legumes as Part of a Healthy Balanced Diet. Foods. 2020;9(8):1056. Published 2020 Aug 4. doi:10.3390/foods9081056

REFERENCES

11. Henry AG, Brooks AS, Piperno DR. Microfossils in calculus demonstrate consumption of plants and cooked foods in Neanderthal diets (Shanidar III, Iraq; Spy I and II, Belgium). Proc Natl Acad Sci U S A. 2011;108(2):486-491. doi:10.1073/pnas.1016868108
12. Lev, Efraim & Kislev, Mordechai & Bar-Yosef, Ofer. (2005). Mousterian vegetal food in Kebara Cave, Mt. Carmel. Journal of Archaeological Science. 32. 475-484. 10.1016/j.jas.2004.11.006.
13. Humphrey LT, De Groote I, Morales J, et al. Earliest evidence for caries and exploitation of starchy plant foods in Pleistocene hunter-gatherers from Morocco. Proc Natl Acad Sci U S A. 2014;111(3):954-959. doi:10.1073/pnas.1318176111
14. Ambika, Aski MS, Gayacharan, et al. Unraveling Origin, History, Genetics, and Strategies for Accelerated Domestication and Diversification of Food Legumes. Front Genet. 2022;13:932430. Published 2022 Jul 22. doi:10.3389/fgene.2022.932430
15. Igolkina, Anna & Noujdina, Nina & ra-ra, kwa-kwa & Wettberg, Eric & Longcore, Travis & Nuzhdin, Sergey. (2021). Historical trade routes for diversification of domesticated chickpea inferred from landrace genomics. 10.1101/2021.01.27.428389.
16. Agricultural revolution. In: Encyclopædia Britannica. https://www.britannica.com/topic/agricultural-revolution.
17. Mariotti Lippi M, Foggi B, Aranguren B, Ronchitelli A, Revedin A. Multistep food plant processing at Grotta Paglicci (Southern Italy) around 32,600 cal B.P. Proc Natl Acad Sci U S A. 2015;112(39):12075-12080. doi:10.1073/pnas.1505213112
18. Revedin A, Aranguren B, Becattini R, et al. Thirty thousand-year-old evidence of plant food processing. Proc Natl Acad Sci U S A. 2010;107(44):18815-18819. doi:10.1073/pnas.1006993107
19. Grain. National Geographic Resource Library. Published 2023. https://education.nationalgeographic.org/resource/grain/.
20. Mercader J. Mozambican grass seed consumption during the Middle Stone Age. Science. 2009;326(5960):1680-1683. doi:10.1126/science.1173966

21. Warinner C, Hendy J, Speller C, et al. Direct evidence of milk consumption from ancient human dental calculus. Sci Rep. 2014;4:7104. Published 2014 Nov 27. doi:10.1038/srep07104
22. Forsgård RA. Lactose digestion in humans: intestinal lactase appears to be constitutive whereas the colonic microbiome is adaptable. Am J Clin Nutr. 2019;110(2):273-279. doi:10.1093/ajcn/nqz104
23. InformedHealth.org [Internet]. Cologne, Germany: Institute for Quality and Efficiency in Health Care (IQWiG); 2006-. Lactose intolerance: Learn More – What can lactose-intolerant people eat? [Updated 2022 Jan 25]. Available from: https://www.ncbi.nlm.nih.gov/books/NBK534631/
24. Visioli F, Strata A. Milk, dairy products, and their functional effects in humans: a narrative review of recent evidence. Adv Nutr. 2014;5(2):131-143. Published 2014 Mar 1. doi:10.3945/an.113.005025
25. Development of agriculture. National Geographic Resource Library. Published 2023. https://education.nationalgeographic.org/resource/development-agriculture/.
26. Gibbons A. Humans were drinking milk before they could digest it. Science. 2019. https://www.science.org/content/article/humans-were-drinking-milk-they-could-digest-it#:~:text=Now%2C%20scientists%20have%20found%20some,tools%20to%20properly%20digest%20it.
27. Salt: A World History. In: History.com. Off the spice rack: The story of salt. Published 2018. https://www.history.com/news/off-the-spice-rack-the-story-of-salt.
28. Kurlansky M. Salt: A World History. New York, NY: Walker & Company; 2002.
29. Roberts WC. Facts and ideas from anywhere. Proc (Bayl Univ Med Cent). 2001;14(3):314-322. doi:10.1080/08998280.2001.11927784
30. Frassetto L, Morris RC Jr, Sellmeyer DE, Todd K, Sebastian A. Diet, evolution and aging--the pathophysiologic effects of the post-agricultural inversion of the potassium-to-sodium and base-

to-chloride ratios in the human diet. Eur J Nutr. 2001;40(5):200-213. doi:10.1007/s394-001-8347-4
31. Shivay YS. Ecosystems and history of evolution and spread of sugar-producing plants in the world: An overview. Resgate. 2020;1:1-25. https://www.researchgate.net/profile/Yashbir-Shivay/publication/344089098_Ecosystems_and_History_of_Evolution_and_Spread_of_Sugar_Producing_Plants_in_the_World-an_Overview/links/5fc51f3b299bf1a422c308d6/Ecosystems-and-History-of-Evolution-and-Spread-of-Sugar-Producing-Plants-in-the-World-an-Overview.pdf.
32. Monteiro CA, Cannon G, Levy RB, et al. Ultra-processed foods: what they are and how to identify them. Public Health Nutr. 2019;22(5):936-941. doi:10.1017/S1368980018003762
33. Monteiro CA. Nutrition and health. The issue is not food, nor nutrients, so much as processing. Public Health Nutr. 2009;12(5):729-731. doi:10.1017/S1368980009005291
34. Dos Santos EM, Moreira ASB, Huguenin GVB, Tibiriça E, De Lorenzo A. Effects of Whey Protein Isolate on Body Composition, Muscle Mass, and Strength of Chronic Heart Failure Patients: A Randomized Clinical Trial. Nutrients. 2023;15(10):2320. Published 2023 May 16. doi:10.3390/nu15102320
35. Ambulkar P, Hande P, Tambe B, et al. Efficacy and safety assessment of protein supplement - micronutrient fortification in promoting health and wellbeing in healthy adults - a randomized placebo-controlled trial. Transl Clin Pharmacol. 2023;31(1):13-27. doi:10.12793/tcp.2023.31.e1
36. Malik VS, Popkin BM, Bray GA, Després JP, Willett WC, Hu FB. Sugar-sweetened beverages and risk of metabolic syndrome and type 2 diabetes: a meta-analysis. Diabetes Care. 2010;33(11):2477-2483. doi:10.2337/dc10-1079
37. Lane MM, Davis JA, Beattie S, et al. Ultraprocessed food and chronic noncommunicable diseases: A systematic review and meta-analysis of 43 observational studies. Obes Rev. 2021;22(3):e13146. doi:10.1111/obr.13146

REFERENCES

38. Lane MM, Gamage E, Du S, et al. Ultra-processed food exposure and adverse health outcomes: umbrella review of epidemiological meta-analyses. BMJ. 2024;384:e077310. Published 2024 Feb 28. doi:10.1136/bmj-2023-077310
39. Gibbons A. The evolution of diet. National Geographic. Published 2014. https://www.nationalgeographic.com/foodfeatures/evolution-of-diet/.
40. Gupta S. The evolution of our diet and lifestyle. Chasing Life [podcast]. CNN Audio. Released September 4, 2024. https://www.cnn.com/audio/podcasts/chasing-life/episodes/dda466f2-8efa-11ee-ae9c-0bff38544eed.
41. Pontzer H. Burn: New Research Blows the Lid Off How We Really Burn Calories, Lose Weight, and Stay Healthy. New York, NY: Avery; 2021.
42. Luca F, Perry GH, Di Rienzo A. Evolutionary adaptations to dietary changes. Annu Rev Nutr. 2010;30:291-314. doi:10.1146/annurev-nutr-080508-141048
43. Fu J, Zheng Y, Gao Y, Xu W. Dietary Fiber Intake and Gut Microbiota in Human Health. Microorganisms. 2022;10(12):2507. Published 2022 Dec 18. doi:10.3390/microorganisms10122507
44. Are humans omnivores? Biology Online. Published 2023. https://www.biologyonline.com/articles/humans-omnivores.
45. Nestle, M. (2000), Paleolithic diets: a sceptical view. Nutrition Bulletin, 25: 43-47. https://doi.org/10.1046/j.1467-3010.2000.00019.x
46. Milton K. Hunter-gatherer diets-a different perspective. Am J Clin Nutr. 2000;71(3):665-667. doi:10.1093/ajcn/71.3.665
47. Cordain L. Why dairy isn't paleo. The Paleo Diet. https://thepaleodiet.com/why-dairy-isnt-paleo/. Published June 19, 2019.
48. McClellan M. Are ancient grains gluten-free and healthy? The Paleo Diet. https://thepaleodiet.com/are-ancient-grains-gluten-free-and-healthy/. Published February 10, 2021.
49. Cordain L. Are beans healthy? Why the paleo diet bans beans. The Paleo Diet. Published July 1, 2021. https://thepaleodiet.com/are-beans-healthy-why-the-paleo-diet-bans-beans/.

50. USDA FoodData Central. Peas, green, raw. U.S. Department of Agriculture. Published April 1, 2019. https://fdc.nal.usda.gov/fdc-app.html#/food-details/170419/nutrients.
51. USDA FoodData Central. Milk, whole, 3.25% milkfat. U.S. Department of Agriculture. https://fdc.nal.usda.gov/fdc-app.html#/food-details/1097512/nutrients. Published April 1, 2019.
52. USDA FoodData Central. Oats, raw. U.S. Department of Agriculture. Published April 1, 2019. https://fdc.nal.usda.gov/fdc-app.html#/food-details/1101825/nutrients.
53. Costabile A, Klinder A, Fava F, et al. Whole-grain wheat breakfast cereal has a prebiotic effect on the human gut microbiota: a double-blind, placebo-controlled, crossover study. Br J Nutr. 2008;99(1):110-120. doi:10.1017/S0007114507793923
54. Petroski W, Minich DM. Is There Such a Thing as "Anti-Nutrients"? A Narrative Review of Perceived Problematic Plant Compounds. Nutrients. 2020;12(10):2929. Published 2020 Sep 24. doi:10.3390/nu12102929
55. López Moreno, Miguel & Garcés-Rimón, Marta & Miguel, Marta. (2022). Antinutrients: Lectins, goitrogens, phytates and oxalates, friends or foe?. Journal of Functional Foods. 89. 104938. 10.1016/j.jff.2022.104938.
56. Dahl WJ, Foster LM, Tyler RT. Review of the health benefits of peas (Pisum sativum L.). Br J Nutr. 2012;108 Suppl 1:S3-S10. doi:10.1017/S0007114512000852
57. Venn BJ, Mann JI. Cereal grains, legumes and diabetes. Eur J Clin Nutr. 2004;58(11):1443-1461. doi:10.1038/sj.ejcn.1601995
58. Jukanti AK, Gaur PM, Gowda CL, Chibbar RN. Nutritional quality and health benefits of chickpea (Cicer arietinum L.): a review. Br J Nutr. 2012;108 Suppl 1:S11-S26. doi:10.1017/S0007114512000797
59. Zhang J, Li L, Song P, et al. Randomized controlled trial of oatmeal consumption versus noodle consumption on blood lipids of urban Chinese adults with hypercholesterolemia. Nutr J.

2012;11:54. Published 2012 Aug 6. doi:10.1186/1475-2891-11-54

60. Whitehead A, Beck EJ, Tosh S, Wolever TM. Cholesterol-lowering effects of oat β-glucan: a meta-analysis of randomized controlled trials. Am J Clin Nutr. 2014;100(6):1413-1421. doi:10.3945/ajcn.114.086108

61. Hajihashemi P, Haghighatdoost F. Effects of Whole-Grain Consumption on Selected Biomarkers of Systematic Inflammation: A Systematic Review and Meta-analysis of Randomized Controlled Trials. J Am Coll Nutr. 2019;38(3):275-285. doi:10.1080/07315724.2018.1490935

62. Aune D, Keum N, Giovannucci E, et al. Whole grain consumption and risk of cardiovascular disease, cancer, and all cause and cause specific mortality: systematic review and dose-response meta-analysis of prospective studies. BMJ. 2016;353:i2716. Published 2016 Jun 14. doi:10.1136/bmj.i2716

63. Jensen MK, Koh-Banerjee P, Franz M, Sampson L, Grønbaek M, Rimm EB. Whole grains, bran, and germ in relation to homocysteine and markers of glycemic control, lipids, and inflammation 1 [published correction appears in Am J Clin Nutr. 2006 Jun;83(6):1443]. Am J Clin Nutr. 2006;83(2):275-283. doi:10.1093/ajcn/83.2.275

64. Aune D, Chan DS, Lau R, et al. Dietary fibre, whole grains, and risk of colorectal cancer: systematic review and dose-response meta-analysis of prospective studies. BMJ. 2011;343:d6617. Published 2011 Nov 10. doi:10.1136/bmj.d6617

65. Flight I, Clifton P. Cereal grains and legumes in the prevention of coronary heart disease and stroke: a review of the literature. Eur J Clin Nutr. 2006;60(10):1145-1159. doi:10.1038/sj.ejcn.1602435

66. Viguiliouk E, Blanco Mejia S, Kendall CW, Sievenpiper JL. Can pulses play a role in improving cardiometabolic health? Evidence from systematic reviews and meta-analyses. Ann N Y Acad Sci. 2017;1392(1):43-57. doi:10.1111/nyas.13312

67. Williamson, O. M. Logical Fallacies. https://utminers.utep.edu/omwilliamson/engl1311/fallacies.htm

68. Beckman JA, Shibao CA. Trimethylamine-N-Oxide, More Red Meat for the Vascular Scientists. Hypertension. 2020;76(1):40-41. doi:10.1161/HYPERTENSIONAHA.120.14857
69. Wang, Z., Klipfell, E., Bennett, B. et al. Gut flora metabolism of phosphatidylcholine promotes cardiovascular disease. Nature 472, 57–63 (2011). https://doi.org/10.1038/nature09922
70. Tang WH, Hazen SL. The contributory role of gut microbiota in cardiovascular disease. J Clin Invest. 2014;124(10):4204-4211. doi:10.1172/JCI72331
71. Ulven SM, Holven KB, Gil A, Rangel-Huerta OD. Milk and Dairy Product Consumption and Inflammatory Biomarkers: An Updated Systematic Review of Randomized Clinical Trials. Adv Nutr. 2019;10(suppl_2):S239-S250. doi:10.1093/advances/nmy072
72. Caroli A, Poli A, Ricotta D, Banfi G, Cocchi D. Invited review: Dairy intake and bone health: a viewpoint from the state of the art. J Dairy Sci. 2011;94(11):5249-5262. doi:10.3168/jds.2011-4578
73. Heaney RP. Dairy and bone health. J Am Coll Nutr. 2009;28 Suppl 1:82S-90S. doi:10.1080/07315724.2009.10719808
74. Rizzoli R. Dairy products and bone health. Aging Clin Exp Res. 2022;34(1):9-24. doi:10.1007/s40520-021-01970-4
75. Rozenberg S, Body JJ, Bruyère O, et al. Effects of Dairy Products Consumption on Health: Benefits and Beliefs--A Commentary from the Belgian Bone Club and the European Society for Clinical and Economic Aspects of Osteoporosis, Osteoarthritis and Musculoskeletal Diseases. Calcif Tissue Int. 2016;98(1):1-17. doi:10.1007/s00223-015-0062-x
76. StateFoodSafety. Toxic Beans: The Danger of Undercooked Beans. https://www.statefoodsafety.com/Resources/Resources/toxic-beans#:~:text=As%20it%20turns%20out%2C%20the,most%20folks%20to%20the%20bathroom.
77. Armelagos GJ. Brain evolution, the determinates of food choice, and the omnivore's dilemma. Crit Rev Food Sci Nutr. 2014;54(10):1330-1341. doi:10.1080/10408398.2011.635817

78. McGlade, M. Debunking the Paleo Diet: Manuscript. Western Oregon University. https://people.wou.edu/~mcgladm/Geography%20107%20Cultural%20Geography/unit%203%20human%20diet/optional/Debunking%20Paleo%20Diet%20manuscript.pdf
79. Menzel P, D'Aluisio F. What the World Eats. National Geographic. https://www.nationalgeographic.com/what-the-world-eats/
80. Trinkaus E. Late Pleistocene adult mortality patterns and modern human establishment. Proc Natl Acad Sci U S A. 2011;108(4):1267-1271. doi:10.1073/pnas.1018700108

IMAGE #1:
Monteiro CA, Cannon G, Levy RB, et al. Spectrum of processing of foods based on the NOVA classification. In: The UN Decade of Nutrition: The NOVA Food Classification and the Trouble with Ultra-Processing. ResearchGate. Published 2021. https://www.researchgate.net/figure/Spectrum-of-processing-of-foods-based-on-the-NOVA-classification-The-figure-provides_fig1_355481122

IMAGE #2:
Goldman L. Three Stages of Health Encounters Over 8000 Human Generations and How They Inform Future Public Health. Am J Public Health. 2018;108(1):60-62. doi:10.2105/AJPH.2017.304164

REFERENCES

CHAPTER 3: MARKETING

1. Rudd Center for Food Policy and Health. Food marketing. University of Connecticut. https://uconnruddcenter.org/research/food-marketing/#:~:text=Food%20Marketing.%20Food%2C%20beverage%20and%20restaurant%20companies,budget%20for%20all%20chronic%20disease%20prevention%20and.
2. Popcorn Board. Popcorn myths. https://www.popcorn.org/All-About-Popcorn/Popcorn-Myths.
3. American Cancer Society. Understanding food labels. https://www.cancer.org/cancer/risk-prevention/diet-physical-activity/eat-healthy/understanding-food-labels.html.
4. University of Houston. Food marketers exploit consumer confusion over health benefits of added fiber. ScienceDaily. Published June 13, 2014. https://www.sciencedaily.com/releases/2014/06/140613130717.htm#:~:text=Food%20marketers%20are%20exploiting%20consumer,a%20False%20Sense%20of%20Health.%22.
5. Tufts University. Beware of health washing. Tufts University Health & Nutrition Letter. https://www.nutritionletter.tufts.edu/healthy-eating/beware-of-health-washing/.
6. Heiss R, Naderer B, Matthes J. Healthwashing in high-sugar food advertising: the effect of prior information on healthwashing perceptions in Austria. Health Promot Int. 2021;36(4):1029-1038. doi:10.1093/heapro/daaa086.
7. National Institute on Aging. How to read food and beverage labels. https://www.nia.nih.gov/health/healthy-eating-nutrition-and-diet/how-read-food-and-beverage-labels#:~:text=This%20information%20lists%20each%20ingredient,the%20least%20is%20listed%20last.
8. Magnuson EA, Chan PS. Added Sugar Labeling. Circulation. 2019;139(23):2625-2627. doi:10.1161/CIRCULATIONAHA.119.040325
9. Camire ME, Kubow S, Donnelly DJ. Potatoes and human health. Crit Rev Food Sci Nutr. 2009;49(10):823-840. doi:10.1080/10408390903041996

REFERENCES

10. Laveriano-Santos EP, López-Yerena A, Jaime-Rodríguez C, et al. Sweet Potato Is Not Simply an Abundant Food Crop: A Comprehensive Review of Its Phytochemical Constituents, Biological Activities, and the Effects of Processing. Antioxidants (Basel). 2022;11(9):1648. Published 2022 Aug 25. doi:10.3390/antiox11091648
11. Durbin DA. Poppi Prebiotic Soda Faces Lawsuit Over Gut Health Claims. AP News. Published June 3, 2024. https://apnews.com/article/poppi-prebiotic-lawsuit-gut-health-30331ef5875e5b82caadef5090ba1195
12. Holscher HD. Dietary fiber and prebiotics and the gastrointestinal microbiota. Gut Microbes. 2017;8(2):172-184. doi:10.1080/19490976.2017.1290756
13. UConn Rudd Center for Food Policy & Health. Packaging, Promotions & Claims. https://uconnruddcenter.org/research/food-marketing/packaging-promotions-claims/.
14. Smith R, Kelly B, Yeatman H, Boyland E. Food Marketing Influences Children's Attitudes, Preferences and Consumption: A Systematic Critical Review. Nutrients. 2019;11(4):875. Published 2019 Apr 18. doi:10.3390/nu11040875
15. Smith R, Kelly B, Yeatman H, Boyland E. Food Marketing Influences Children's Attitudes, Preferences and Consumption: A Systematic Critical Review. Nutrients. 2019;11(4):875. Published 2019 Apr 18. doi:10.3390/nu11040875
16. Houghtaling B, Holston D, Szocs C, Penn J, Qi D, Hedrick V. A rapid review of stocking and marketing practices used to sell sugar-sweetened beverages in U.S. food stores. Obes Rev. 2021;22(4):e13179. doi:10.1111/obr.13179
17. Standing Committee on Childhood Obesity Prevention; Food and Nutrition Board; Institute of Medicine. Challenges and Opportunities for Change in Food Marketing to Children and Youth: Workshop Summary. Washington (DC): National Academies Press (US); May 14, 2013.
18. Ortiz-Ospina E, Giattino C, Roser M. Time Use. Our World in Data. https://ourworldindata.org/time-use.

REFERENCES

19. Diamond A. A Crispy, Salty American History of Fast Food. Smithsonian Magazine. https://www.smithsonianmag.com/history/crispy-salty-american-history-fast-food-180972459/.
20. Grossman M, Kelly I, Chou SY. Fast-Food Advertising on Television and Its Influence on Childhood Obesity. J Law Econ. 2008;51:599-618. doi:10.1086/590132.
21. Kim A, Dennis A. Says Who? The Effects of Presentation Format and Source Rating on Fake News in Social Media. MIS Q. 2019;43:1025-1039. doi:10.25300/MISQ/2019/15188.
22. Kabata P, Winniczuk-Kabata D, Kabata PM, Jaśkiewicz J, Połom K. Can Social Media Profiles Be a Reliable Source of Information on Nutrition and Dietetics?. Healthcare (Basel). 2022;10(2):397. Published 2022 Feb 20. doi:10.3390/healthcare10020397
23. Denniss E, Lindberg R, McNaughton SA. Quality and accuracy of online nutrition-related information: a systematic review of content analysis studies. Public Health Nutr. 2023;26(7):1345-1357. doi:10.1017/S1368980023000873
24. Dimitroyannis R, Fenton D, Cho S, Nordgren R, Pinto JM, Roxbury CR. A Social Media Quality Review of Popular Sinusitis Videos on TikTok. Otolaryngol Head Neck Surg. 2024;170(5):1456-1466. doi:10.1002/ohn.688
25. Kreft M, Smith B, Hopwood D, Blaauw R. The use of social media as a source of nutrition information. S Afr J Clin Nutr. 2023;36(4):162-168. doi:10.1080/16070658.2023.2175518.
26. New Statistics Highlight Inaccurate Nutrition Trends on TikTok. PR Newswire. Published April 11, 2024. https://www.prnewswire.com/news-releases/new-statistics-highlight-inaccurate-nutrition-trends-on-tiktok-301795642.html.
27. Lanier J. Ten Arguments for Deleting Your Social Media Accounts Right Now. New York, NY: Henry Holt and Co.; 2018. https://www.amazon.com/Arguments-Deleting-Social-Media-Accounts/dp/125019668X.

REFERENCES

28. Steger M. 6 reasons why eggs are the healthiest food on the planet. Healthline. Published April 19, 2023. https://www.healthline.com/nutrition/6-reasons why-eggs-are-the-healthiest-food-on-the-planet
29. Health benefits of eggs. Australian Eggs. https://www.australianeggs.org.au/nutrition/health-benefits
30. Why you should not eat eggs. FiveSec Blog. Published 2023. https://www.fivesec.co/blog/why-you-should-not-eat-eggs
31. Health concerns with eggs. Physicians Committee for Responsible Medicine. https://www.pcrm.org/good-nutrition/nutrition-information/health-concerns-with-eggs
32. The power of influencers report. Sortlist. Published 2023. https://www.sortlist.com/datahub/reports/the-power-of-influencers/
33. Praderio C. These fake weight-loss photos show just how deceptive before-and-after pictures can be. Business Insider. Published 2017. https://www.businessinsider.com/fake-before-and-after-weight-loss-pictures-2017-2
34. Jiotsa B, Naccache B, Duval M, Rocher B, Grall-Bronnec M. Social media use and body image disorders: association between frequency of comparing one's own physical appearance to that of people being followed on social media and body dissatisfaction and drive for thinness. Int J Environ Res Public Health. 2021;18(6):2880. doi:10.3390/ijerph18062880
35. Reducing social media use significantly improves body image in teens, young adults. American Psychological Association. Published 2023. https://www.apa.org/news/press/releases/2023/02/social-media-body-image
36. Food advertising and marketing to children. American Psychological Association. Published 2010. https://www.apa.org/topics/obesity/food-advertising-children
37. Dodgson L, Hosie R. Fitness influencers are hiding their steroid use, and it's making their followers sick. Business Insider. Published 2021. https://www.businessinsider.com/fitness-influencers-steroids-secret-dangerous-body-dysmorphia

REFERENCES

38. Hearing A. Liver King apologizes after leaked emails show he took steroids to build his body. Fortune. Published December 6, 2022. https://fortune.com/well/2022/12/06/liver-king-leaked-steroids-email-apology-video/
39. Paul Saladino MD. Yes, I was once a raw vegan.... YouTube. Published April 8, 2022. https://www.youtube.com/shorts/gZWC_JxjljM
40. Mark's Daily Apple. Paul Saladino: Is Nose-to-Tail Carnivore the Optimal Human Diet? YouTube. Published July 19, 2019. https://www.youtube.com/watch?v=W_ARV4RN1aw
41. Paul Saladino MD. Why I QUIT keto. YouTube. Published August 29, 2022. https://www.youtube.com/watch?v=XhSWrvtvsag
42. Paul Saladino MD. What I eat in a day. YouTube. Published December 5, 2022. https://www.youtube.com/watch?v=6rvelXwG_Tk
43. Paul Saladino MD. I ate carbs! Does that trigger you? YouTube. Published June 1, 2020. https://www.youtube.com/watch?v=1xdvzYLGIds
44. More Plates More Dates. Why Paul Saladino stopped the carnivore diet after 2 years. YouTube. Published May 5, 2024. https://www.youtube.com/watch?v=stc62YKYlLc
45. Linton D. The wellness Instagrammer who learned to let go. The Guardian. Published March 31, 2024. https://amp.theguardian.com/lifeandstyle/2024/mar/31/the-wellness-instagrammer-who-learned-to-let-go
46. Collier J. Messiah syndrome in nutrition. Substack. Published August 15, 2024. https://jamescollier.substack.com/p/messiah-syndrome-in-nutrition.
47. Scacco J, Muddiman A. The current state of news headlines. Center for Media Engagement. Published May 16, 2019. https://mediaengagement.org/research/the-current-state-of-news-headlines/.
48. Headlines. Coral Gables Museum. https://coralgablesmuseum.org/project/headlines/.

REFERENCES

49. Starr, M. Major study claims to identify the root cause of obesity: fructose. ScienceAlert. https://www.sciencealert.com/major-study-claims-to-identify-the-root-cause-of obesity-fructose.
50. Johnson RJ, Lanaspa MA, Sanchez-Lozada LG, et al. The fructose survival hypothesis for obesity. Philos Trans R Soc Lond B Biol Sci. 2023;378(1885):20220230. doi:10.1098/rstb.2022.0230
51. Mutnick A. Senators scold Dr. Oz for weight-loss scams. USA TODAY. https://www.usatoday.com/story/life/people/2014/06/17/dr-oz-senate-panel-weight-scams/10701067/
52. Firger J. Dr. Oz defends weight-loss advice at Senate hearing on diet scams. CBS News. https://www.cbsnews.com/news/dr-oz-defends-weight-loss-advice-at-senate-hearing-on-diet-scams/
53. Written Testimony of Dr. Mehmet Oz MD. Hearing "Protecting Consumers from false and deceptive advertising of weight-loss products". U.S. Senate Committee Commerce, Science, and Transportation Subcommittee on Consumer Protection, Product Safety, and Insurance. June 17, 2014.
54. Quyen D, Truong A. Evaluation of Recommendations made on The Dr. Oz Show from the first 30 episodes of season 5. University of Arizona. Published May 24, 2017.
55. Sony Pictures Television. Shark Tank US. Sharks Get Into A Heated Argument Over Minus Cal Product. Youtube. Published September 3, 2021. https://www.youtube.com/watch?v=pwf1UmbjQho
56. Weight Loss Supplement Market Trends. Grand View Research website. Published 2024. https://www.grandviewresearch.com/industry-analysis/weight-loss-supplements-market-report#:~:text=Weight%20Loss%20Supplement%20Market%20Trends,13.70%25%20from%202024%20to%202030.
57. 1951: Psychologist Solomon Asch's famous experiments. Swarthmore College. https://www.swarthmore.edu/a-brief-history/1951-psychologist-solomon-aschs-famous-experiments.
58. Asch conformity experiment. Simply Psychology. https://www.simplypsychology.org/asch-conformity.html.

CHAPTER 4: EXPERTISE

1. Vijaykumar S, McNeill A, Simpson J. Associations between conflicting nutrition information, nutrition confusion and backlash among consumers in the UK. Public Health Nutr. 2021;24(5):914-923. doi:10.1017/S1368980021000124
2. Nichols T. The Death of Expertise: The Campaign Against Established Knowledge and Why It Matters. New York, NY: Oxford University Press; 2017.
3. Minor L. Why Medical Schools Need to Focus on Nutrition. Stanford Medicine. Published October 10, 2019. https://med.stanford.edu/school/leadership/dean/precision-health-in-the-news/why-medica-schools-need-focus-nutrition.html.
4. How Much Does Your Doctor Actually Know About Nutrition? American Heart Association website. Published May 3, 2018. https://www.heart.org/en/news/2018/05/03/how-much-does-your-doctor-actually-know-about-nutrition.
5. Marton RM, Wang X, Barabási AL, et al. Science, advocacy, and quackery in nutritional books: an analysis of conflicting advice and purported claims of nutritional best-sellers. Palgrave Commun. 2020;6(43). doi:10.1057/s41599-020-0415-6.
6. Belluz J. The problem with diet books written by doctors. Vox. March 24, 2016. https://www.vox.com/2016/3/24/11296168/down-with-diet-books.
7. Oono F, Adachi R, Yaegashi A, et al. Are popular books about diet and health written based on scientific evidence? A comparison of citations between the USA and Japan. Public Health Nutr. 2023;26(12):2815-2825. doi:10.1017/S1368980023002549
8. Loung CY, Sarfaraz S, Carew AS, MacKay D, Cahill LE. Many authors of publicly available top-selling nutrition books in Canada are without clinical nutrition credentials, do not cite evidence, and promote their own services or products. Appl Physiol Nutr Metab. 2022;47(12):1187-1193. doi:10.1139/apnm-2022-0051

REFERENCES

9. Swartz. The sense and nonsense of the best-selling diet books. CMAJ. 1987;136(5):561-563. https://www.ncbi.nlm.nih.gov/pmc/articles/PMC1863236/.
10. Game Changers. The Game Changers [film]. Directed by Louie Psihoyos. Produced by James Wilks, Joseph Pace, and Louie Psihoyos. Released 2019. https://gamechangersmovie.com.
11. The Game Changers. The Game Changers Full Documentary. YouTube. Published September 16, 2019. https://www.youtube.com/watch?v=YbfXtcaJ7AU.
12. Carlsen MH, Halvorsen BL, Holte K, et al. The total antioxidant content of more than 3100 foods, beverages, spices, herbs and supplements used worldwide. Nutr J. 2010;9:3. Published 2010 Jan 22. doi:10.1186/1475-2891-9-3
13. Li Z, Wong A, Henning SM, et al. Hass avocado modulates postprandial vascular reactivity and postprandial inflammatory responses to a hamburger meal in healthy volunteers. Food Funct. 2013;4(3):384-391. doi:10.1039/c2fo30226h
14. Michael Phelps' 10,000 Calorie Diet. Olympics website. Published June 24, 2021. https://olympics.com/en/news/michael-phelps-10000-calories-diet-what-the-american-swimmer-ate-while-training-.
15. Zaccardi N. Usain Bolt estimates he ate 1,000 chicken McNuggets at Beijing Olympics. NBC Sports. Published November 3, 2013. https://www.nbcsports.com/olympics/news/usain-bolt-chicken-mcnuggets-beijing-olympics.
16. Huberman Lab. About. Huberman Lab website. https://www.hubermanlab.com/.
17. Huberman Lab. Dr. Robert Lustig: How Sugar & Processed Foods Impact Your Health. Huberman Lab podcast. https://www.hubermanlab.com/episode/dr-robert-lustig-how-sugar-processed-foods-impact-your-health.
18. Maersk M, Belza A, Stødkilde-Jørgensen H, et al. Sucrose-sweetened beverages increase fat storage in the liver, muscle, and visceral fat depot: a 6-mo randomized intervention study. Am J Clin Nutr. 2012;95(2):283-289. doi:10.3945/ajcn.111.022533

REFERENCES

19. Nguyen M, Jarvis SE, Tinajero MG, et al. Sugar-sweetened beverage consumption and weight gain in children and adults: a systematic review and meta-analysis of prospective cohort studies and randomized controlled trials. Am J Clin Nutr. 2023;117(1):160-174. doi:10.1016/j.ajcnut.2022.11.008
20. Santos LP, Gigante DP, Delpino FM, Maciel AP, Bielemann RM. Sugar sweetened beverages intake and risk of obesity and cardiometabolic diseases in longitudinal studies: A systematic review and meta-analysis with 1.5 million individuals. Clin Nutr ESPEN. 2022;51:128-142. doi:10.1016/j.clnesp.2022.08.021
21. Andrew Huberman on Supplements, the Covid Lab Leak Theory and more. Gimlet Media. Released 2023. https://gimletmedia.com/shows/science-vs/rnhobned.
22. The Psychology of Celebrity Endorsements: Why We Trust Famous Faces. AAFT. Published July 21, 2023. https://aaft.com/blog/advertising-pr-events/the-psychology-of-celebrity-endorsements-why-we-trust-famous-faces/#:~:text=In%20conclusion%2C%20the%20psychology%20behind,inclination%20to%20trust%20celebrity%20endorsements..
23. Dear Media. Gwyneth Paltrow Wellness Routine Backlash. TikTok. https://www.tiktok.com/@dearmedia/video/7210104654460521774.
24. Court A. Gwyneth Paltrow Faces Backlash Over Daily Wellness Routine. Daily Mail. Published June 16, 2023. https://www.dailymail.co.uk/femail/article-11863081.
25. Saunt R. Rebel Wilson's 600-Calorie Diet Slammed by Dietitian. New York Post. Published March 15, 2023. https://nypost.com/2023/06/16/rebel-wilsons-600-calorie-diet-slammed-by-dietitian-dangerous.
26. Studying for the RD Exam. All Access Dietetics. https://www.allaccessdietetics.com/program-rd-exam-prep/.
27. What's the Difference Between an RD, CNS, and Nutritionist? Skysrooted Nutrition. Published September 21, 2023. https://www.skysrootednutrition.com/blog/whats-the-difference-rd-cns-nutritionist.

REFERENCES

28. Academy of Nutrition and Dietetics. Advanced Degrees in Nutrition and Dietetics: What's Best for You? J Acad Nutr Diet. 2014;114(12):1873-1875. doi:10.1016/j.jand.2014.09.004.
29. BCNS Exam Rates. American Nutrition Association. https://www.theana.org/bcns-exam-rates/.
30. Certified Nutrition Specialist (CNS). NutritionEd. https://www.nutritioned.org/certified-nutrition-specialist/.
31. What's the Difference Between a Dietitian and a Nutritionist? Cleveland Clinic website. Published June 5, 2023. https://health.clevelandclinic.org/dietitian-vs-nutritionist.
32. Aronson V. An Investigation of Bernadean University. Quackwatch. Published 1999. https://quackwatch.org/consumer-education/nonrecorg/aronson/.
33. Diamandis EP. Nobelitis: a common disease among Nobel laureates?. Clin Chem Lab Med. 2013;51(8):1573-1574. doi:10.1515/cclm-2013-0273
34. The Nobel Disease: Why Great Scientists Sometimes Go Crazy. Big Think. Published September 15, 2023. https://bigthink.com/the-past/nobel-disease-great-scientists-go-crazy/.
35. Thielking M. How Linus Pauling duped America into believing vitamin C cures colds. Vox. Published January 15, 2015. https://www.vox.com/2015/1/15/7547741/vitamin-c-myth-pauling.
36. Nelson H. Linus Pauling Stands By His Claim: Second Study Fails to Show Vitamin C Fights Cancer. Los Angeles Times. Published January 17, 1985. https://www.latimes.com/archives/la-xpm-1985-01-17-mn-7720-story.html.
37. Durrani M. Life Beyond the Nobel: Brian Josephson and His Interest in the Mind. Physics World. Published September 29, 2021. https://physicsworld.com/a/life-beyond-the-nobel-brian-josephson-and-his-interest-in-the-mind/.
38. Gorski DH. Luc Montagnier and the Nobel Disease. Science-Based Medicine. Published June 4, 2012. https://sciencebasedmedicine.org/luc-montagnier-and-the-nobel-disease/.

REFERENCES

39. Bahl V. Luc Montagnier, French Nobel Laureate Who Co-Discovered HIV, Dies at 89. France 24. Published October 2, 2022. https://www.france24.com/en/europe/20220210-luc-montagnier-french-nobel-laureate-who-co-discovered-hiv-dies-at-89.
40. Belluz J. DNA scientist James Watson has a remarkably long history of sexist, racist public comments. Vox. Published January 15, 2019. https://www.vox.com/2019/1/15/18182530/james-watson-racist.
41. Harmon A. James Watson Had a Chance to Salvage His Reputation on Race. He Made Things Worse. The New York Times. Published January 1, 2019. https://www.nytimes.com/2019/01/01/science/watson-dna-genetics-race.html.
42. Thomas Delauer. Why Dr. Peter Attia Changed his Mind on Fasting (and 4 other Longevity topics). YouTube. Published March 17, 2010. https://www.youtube.com/watch?v=Tb6gMegtLcg.
43. Science-Based Reviews of Popular Health Books. Red Pen Reviews. https://www.redpenreviews.org/.

IMAGE #1:

Marton RM, Wang X, Barabási AL, et al. Science, advocacy, and quackery in nutritional books: an analysis of conflicting advice and purported claims of nutritional best-sellers. Palgrave Commun. 2020;6(43). doi:10.1057/s41599-020-0415-6.

REFERENCES

CHAPTER 5: SCIENCE

1. Kennedy B, Tyson A. Americans' Trust in Scientists, Positive Views of Science Continue to Decline. Pew Research Center. Published November 14, 2023. https://www.pewresearch.org/science/2023/11/14/americans-trust-in-scientists-positive-views-of-science-continue-to-decline/.
2. Gandhi M, Elfeky O, Ertugrul H, Chela HK, Daglilar E. Scurvy: Rediscovering a Forgotten Disease. Diseases. 2023;11(2):78. Published 2023 May 26. doi:10.3390/diseases11020078
3. Discovering Vitamins. University of Missouri. https://library.missouri.edu/specialcollections/exhibits/show/food/food-and-chemistry/discovering-vitamins.
4. Eschner K. The Father of Modern Chemistry Proved Respiration Occurred by Freezing a Guinea Pig. Smithsonian Magazine. Published August 25, 2017. https://www.smithsonianmag.com/smart-news/father-modern-chemistry-proved-respiration-occurred-freezing-guinea-pig-180964596/.
5. Katch F. Antoine Laurent Lavoisier (1743-1794). Sportscience History Makers. Published January 12, 1998. https://www.sportsci.org/news/history/lavoisier/lavoisier.html
6. Meerman R, Brown AJ. When somebody loses weight, where does the fat go? [published correction appears in BMJ. 2014;349:g7782]. BMJ. 2014;349:g7257. Published 2014 Dec 16. doi:10.1136/bmj.g7257
7. Beriberi. Genetic and Rare Diseases Information Center (GARD). https://rarediseases.info.nih.gov/diseases/9948/beriberi.
8. Pietrzak K. Christiaan Eijkman (1856-1930). J Neurol. 2019;266(11):2893-2895. doi:10.1007/s00415-018-9162-7
9. Thiamin. NIH Office of Dietary Supplements. https://ods.od.nih.gov/factsheets/Thiamin-HealthProfessional/.
10. Vitamin A Discovered. Animal Research Information. https://www.animalresearch.info/en/medical-advances/medical-discovery-timeline/vitamin-discovered/.
11. Semba RD. On the 'discovery' of vitamin A. Ann Nutr Metab. 2012;61(3):192-198. doi:10.1159/000343124

REFERENCES

12. National Institutes of Health (NIH). Vitamin A: Fact Sheet for Consumers. NIH Office of Dietary Supplements. https://ods.od.nih.gov/factsheets/VitaminA-Consumer/.
13. Jones G. 100 YEARS OF VITAMIN D: Historical aspects of vitamin D. Endocr Connect. 2022;11(4):e210594. Published 2022 Apr 22. doi:10.1530/EC-21-0594
14. Vitamin D and Your Health: Breaking Old Rules, Raising New Hopes. Harvard Medical School. https://www.health.harvard.edu/staying-healthy/vitamin-d-and-your-health-breaking-old-rules-raising-new-hopes.
15. Quinn K. Norman E. Borlaug - Extended Biography. World Food Prize Foundation. https://www.worldfoodprize.org/en/dr_norman_e_borlaug/extended_biography/
16. Uman LS. Systematic reviews and meta-analyses. J Can Acad Child Adolesc Psychiatry. 2011;20(1):57-59.
17. He FJ, Li J, Macgregor GA. Effect of longer term modest salt reduction on blood pressure: Cochrane systematic review and meta-analysis of randomised trials. BMJ. 2013;346:f1325. Published 2013 Apr 3. doi:10.1136/bmj.f1325
18. Haidich AB. Meta-analysis in medical research. Hippokratia. 2010;14(Suppl 1):29-37.
19. Wang YJ, Yeh TL, Shih MC, Tu YK, Chien KL. Dietary Sodium Intake and Risk of Cardiovascular Disease: A Systematic Review and Dose-Response Meta-Analysis. Nutrients. 2020;12(10):2934. Published 2020 Sep 25. doi:10.3390/nu12102934
20. Hariton E, Locascio JJ. Randomised controlled trials - the gold standard for effectiveness research: Study design: randomised controlled trials. BJOG. 2018;125(13):1716. doi:10.1111/1471-0528.15199
21. Yu J, Thout SR, Li Q, et al. Effects of a reduced-sodium added-potassium salt substitute on blood pressure in rural Indian hypertensive patients: a randomized, double-blind, controlled trial. Am J Clin Nutr. 2021;114(1):185-193. doi:10.1093/ajcn/nqab054
22. Barrett D, Noble H. What are cohort studies?. Evid Based Nurs. 2019;22(4):95-96. doi:10.1136/ebnurs-2019-103183

REFERENCES

23. Neal B, Wu Y, Feng X, et al. Effect of Salt Substitution on Cardiovascular Events and Death. N Engl J Med. 2021;385(12):1067-1077. doi:10.1056/NEJMoa2105675
24. Setia MS. Methodology Series Module 3: Cross-sectional Studies. Indian J Dermatol. 2016;61(3):261-264. doi:10.4103/0019-5154.182410
25. Sidenur B, Shankar G. A Cross-Sectional Study of Hypertension among 20-40 Years Old Residing in an Urban Area of Bagalkot City, North Karnataka. Indian J Community Med. 2023;48(1):98-102. doi:10.4103/ijcm.ijcm_255_22
26. Tenny S, Kerndt CC, Hoffman MR. Case Control Studies. In: StatPearls. Treasure Island (FL): StatPearls Publishing; March 27, 2023.
27. Case Reports and Case Series. Boston University Medical Campus: Institutional Review Board (IRB). https://www.bumc.bu.edu/irb/submission-requirements/special-submission-requirements/case-reports-and-case-series/#:~:text=A%20case%20report%20is%20a,who%20were%20given%20similar%20treatment.
28. Nissen T, Wynn R. The clinical case report: a review of its merits and limitations. BMC Res Notes. 2014;7:264. Published 2014 Apr 23. doi:10.1186/1756-0500-7-264
29. DASH Eating Plan. National Heart, Lung, and Blood Institute. https://www.nhlbi.nih.gov/education/dash-eating-plan.
30. Bracken MB. Why animal studies are often poor predictors of human reactions to exposure. J R Soc Med. 2009;102(3):120-122. doi:10.1258/jrsm.2008.08k033
31. Fountain JH, Kaur J, Lappin SL. Physiology, Renin Angiotensin System. In: StatPearls. Treasure Island (FL): StatPearls Publishing; March 12, 2023.
32. Weinberger MH, Miller JZ, Luft FC, Grim CE, Fineberg NS. Definitions and characteristics of sodium sensitivity and blood pressure resistance. Hypertension. 1986;8(6 Pt 2):II127-II134. doi:10.1161/01.hyp.8.6_pt_2.ii127

REFERENCES

33. Grillo A, Salvi L, Coruzzi P, Salvi P, Parati G. Sodium Intake and Hypertension. Nutrients. 2019;11(9):1970. Published 2019 Aug 21. doi:10.3390/nu11091970
34. Sackett DL. Evidence-based medicine. Semin Perinatol. 1997;21(1):3-5. doi:10.1016/s0146-0005(97)80013-4
35. Borgida E, Nisbett RE. The differential impact of abstract vs. concrete information on decisions. Journal of Applied Social Psychology. 1977;7(3):258-271. doi:10.1111/j.1559-1816.1977.tb00750.x
36. Freling T, Yang Z, Saini R, Itani O, Abualsamh R. When poignant stories outweigh cold hard facts: A meta-analysis of the anecdotal bias. Organizational Behavior and Human Decision Processes. 2020;160:51-67. doi:10.1016/j.obhdp.2020.01.006
37. Michal AL, Zhong Y, Shah P. When and why do people act on flawed science? Effects of anecdotes and prior beliefs on evidence-based decision-making. Cogn Res Princ Implic. 2021;6(1):28. Published 2021 Apr 6. doi:10.1186/s41235-021-00293-2
38. Inda MC, Muravieva EV, Alberini CM. Memory retrieval and the passage of time: from reconsolidation and strengthening to extinction. J Neurosci. 2011;31(5):1635-1643. doi:10.1523/JNEUROSCI.4736-10.2011
39. Paul M. Your Memory is like the Telephone Game. Northwestern Now. Published 2012. https://news.northwestern.edu/stories/2012/09/your-memory-is-like-the-telephone-game/
40. Cappuccio FP, Campbell NRC, He FJ, et al. Sodium and Health: Old Myths and a Controversy Based on Denial. Curr Nutr Rep. 2022;11(2):172-184. doi:10.1007/s13668-021-00383-z
41. Vitolins MZ, Case TL. What Makes Nutrition Research So Difficult to Conduct and Interpret?. Diabetes Spectr. 2020;33(2):113-117. doi:10.2337/ds19-0077
42. Serra-Garcia M, Gneezy U. Nonreplicable publications are cited more than replicable ones. Sci Adv. 2021;7(21):eabd1705. Published 2021 May 21. doi:10.1126/sciadv.abd1705

REFERENCES

IMAGE #1:

UC Davis Center for Nursing Science. Evidence-Based Practice. Published 2024. https://health.ucdavis.edu/cnr/evidence_based_practice.html

REFERENCES

CHAPTER 6: DUALITY

1. National Weight Control Registry. Research Findings. http://www.nwcr.ws/research/.
2. Consequences of Obesity. Centers for Disease Control and Prevention. Updated May 15, 2023. https://www.cdc.gov/obesity/basics/consequences.html.
3. Managing Overweight and Obesity in Adults: Systematic Evidence Review from the Obesity Expert Panel. National Heart, Lung, and Blood Institute. Published November 2013. https://www.nhlbi.nih.gov/sites/default/files/media/docs/obesity-evidence-review.pdf.
4. Clinical Guidelines on the Identification, Evaluation, and Treatment of Overweight and Obesity in Adults. National Heart, Lung, and Blood Institute. Published September 1998. https://www.nhlbi.nih.gov/files/docs/guidelines/ob_gdlns.pdf.
5. Bhaskaran K, Douglas I, Forbes H, dos-Santos-Silva I, Leon DA, Smeeth L. Body-mass index and risk of 22 specific cancers: a population-based cohort study of 5·24 million UK adults. Lancet. 2014;384(9945):755-765. doi:10.1016/S0140-6736(14)60892-8
6. Kasen S, Cohen P, Chen H, Must A. Obesity and psychopathology in women: a three decade prospective study. Int J Obes (Lond). 2008;32(3):558-566. doi:10.1038/sj.ijo.0803736
7. Luppino FS, de Wit LM, Bouvy PF, et al. Overweight, obesity, and depression: a systematic review and meta-analysis of longitudinal studies. Arch Gen Psychiatry. 2010;67(3):220-229. doi:10.1001/archgenpsychiatry.2010.2
8. Jayedi A, Khan TA, Aune D, Emadi A, Shab-Bidar S. Body fat and risk of all-cause mortality: a systematic review and dose-response meta-analysis of prospective cohort studies. Int J Obes (Lond). 2022;46(9):1573-1581. doi:10.1038/s41366-022-01165-5
9. Matsunaga M, Yatsuya H, Iso H, et al. Impact of Body Mass Index on Obesity-Related Cancer and Cardiovascular Disease Mortality; The Japan Collaborative Cohort Study. J Atheroscler Thromb. 2022;29(10):1547-1562. doi:10.5551/jat.63143

REFERENCES

10. Zhang C, Rexrode KM, van Dam RM, Li TY, Hu FB. Abdominal obesity and the risk of all-cause, cardiovascular, and cancer mortality: sixteen years of follow-up in US women. Circulation. 2008;117(13):1658-1667. doi:10.1161/CIRCULATIONAHA.107.739714
11. Life Insurance for Overweight Individuals. MarketWatch. Published April 11, 2023. https://www.marketwatch.com/guides/life-insurance/life-insurance-overweight/.
12. Keys A, Fidanza F, Karvonen MJ, Kimura N, Taylor HL. Indices of relative weight and obesity. Int J Epidemiol. 2014;43(3):655-665. doi:10.1093/ije/dyu058
13. Body Mass Index (BMI) in Children. Centers for Disease Control and Prevention. Updated September 17, 2020. https://www.cdc.gov/nccdphp/dnpao/growthcharts/training/bmiage/page1.html.
14. Barry VW, Baruth M, Beets MW, Durstine JL, Liu J, Blair SN. Fitness vs. fatness on all-cause mortality: a meta-analysis. Prog Cardiovasc Dis. 2014;56(4):382-390. doi:10.1016/j.pcad.2013.09.002
15. McAuley PA, Blaha MJ, Keteyian SJ, et al. Fitness, Fatness, and Mortality: The FIT (Henry Ford Exercise Testing) Project. Am J Med. 2016;129(9):960-965.e1. doi:10.1016/j.amjmed.2016.04.007
16. Vogel L. Fat shaming is making people sicker and heavier. CMAJ. 2019;191(23):E649. doi:10.1503/cmaj.109-5758
17. Tackling Obesities: Future Choices – Project Report. Government Office for Science. Published October 17, 2007. https://assets.publishing.service.gov.uk/media/5a759da7e5274a4368298a4f/07-1184x-tackling-obesities-future-choices-report.pdf.
18. Khera AV, Chaffin M, Wade KH, et al. Polygenic Prediction of Weight and Obesity Trajectories from Birth to Adulthood. Cell. 2019;177(3):587-596.e9. doi:10.1016/j.cell.2019.03.028
19. Aukan MI, Coutinho S, Pedersen SA, Simpson MR, Martins C. Differences in gastrointestinal hormones and appetite ratings between individuals with and without obesity-A systematic review

and meta-analysis. Obes Rev. 2023;24(2):e13531. doi:10.1111/obr.13531
20. Stunkard AJ, Foch TT, Hrubec Z. A twin study of human obesity. JAMA. 1986;256(1):51-54.
21. Schrempft S, van Jaarsveld CHM, Fisher A, et al. Variation in the Heritability of Child Body Mass Index by Obesogenic Home Environment. JAMA Pediatr. 2018;172(12):1153-1160. doi:10.1001/jamapediatrics.2018.1508
22. Lerma-Cabrera JM, Carvajal F, Lopez-Legarrea P. Food addiction as a new piece of the obesity framework. Nutr J. 2016;15:5. Published 2016 Jan 13. doi:10.1186/s12937-016-0124-6
23. Stice E, Spoor S, Ng J, Zald DH. Relation of obesity to consummatory and anticipatory food reward. Physiol Behav. 2009;97(5):551-560. doi:10.1016/j.physbeh.2009.03.020
24. Noll JG, Zeller MH, Trickett PK, Putnam FW. Obesity risk for female victims of childhood sexual abuse: a prospective study. Pediatrics. 2007;120(1):e61-e67. doi:10.1542/peds.2006-3058
25. Wiss DA, Brewerton TD. Adverse Childhood Experiences and Adult Obesity: A Systematic Review of Plausible Mechanisms and Meta-Analysis of Cross-Sectional Studies. Physiol Behav. 2020;223:112964. doi:10.1016/j.physbeh.2020.112964
26. Kramer EB, Pietri ES, Bryan AD. Reducing anti-fat bias toward the self and others: a randomized controlled trial. J Eat Disord. 2024;12(1):46. Published 2024 Apr 18. doi:10.1186/s40337-024-00994-1
27. Teachman BA, Brownell KD. Implicit anti-fat bias among health professionals: is anyone immune?. Int J Obes Relat Metab Disord. 2001;25(10):1525-1531. doi:10.1038/sj.ijo.0801745
28. U.S. Weight Loss Industry Grows to $90 Billion, Fueled by Obesity Drugs Demand. MarketResearch.com Blog. Published March 6, 2024. https://blog.marketresearch.com/u.s.-weight-loss-industry-grows-to-90-billion-fueled-by-obesity-drugs-demand.
29. Park M. Twinkie diet helps nutrition professor lose 27 pounds. CNN. Published November 8, 2010.

REFERENCES

https://www.cnn.com/2010/HEALTH/11/08/twinkie.diet.professor/index.html.

30. Weiss S. How I stay skinny eating Chipotle every day. New York Post. Published 2019. https://nypost.com/2019/07/30/how-i-stay-skinny-eating-chipotle-every-day/.
31. Bilow R. This Man Ate Only Junk Food for 30 Days and Lost 11 Pounds. Bon Appétit. Published December 16, 2015. https://www.bonappetit.com/entertaining-style/trends-news/article/junk-food-diet-jeff-wilser.
32. Propper D. Nashville grandfather reveals whopping weight loss from 100-day McDonald's diet. New York Post. Published June 2, 2023. https://nypost.com/2023/06/02/kevin-maginnis-reveals-weight-loss-from-mcdonalds-only-diet/.
33. Metabolism. Britannica Published September 10, 2024. https://www.britannica.com/science/metabolism.
34. Belluz J. Most of us misunderstand metabolism. Here are 9 facts to clear that up. Vox. Published May 18, 2016. https://www.vox.com/2016/5/18/11685254/metabolism-definition-booster-weight-loss. Pontzer H, Yamada Y, Sagayama H, et al. Daily energy expenditure through the human life course. Science. 2021;373(6556):808-812. doi:10.1126/science.abe5017
35. Wang Z, Ying Z, Bosy-Westphal A, et al. Specific metabolic rates of major organs and tissues across adulthood: evaluation by mechanistic model of resting energy expenditure. Am J Clin Nutr. 2010;92(6):1369-1377. doi:10.3945/ajcn.2010.29885
36. Pontzer H, Durazo-Arvizu R, Dugas LR, et al. Constrained Total Energy Expenditure and Metabolic Adaptation to Physical Activity in Adult Humans. Curr Biol. 2016;26(3):410-417. doi:10.1016/j.cub.2015.12.046
37. Gebauer SK, Novotny JA, Bornhorst GM, Baer DJ. Food processing and structure impact the metabolizable energy of almonds. Food Funct. 2016;7(10):4231-4238. doi:10.1039/c6fo01076h
38. Once again, US and Europe way ahead on daily calorie intake. United Nations News. Published December 12, 2022. https://news.un.org/en/story/2022/12/1131637.

REFERENCES

39. Lichtman SW, Pisarska K, Berman ER, et al. Discrepancy between self-reported and actual caloric intake and exercise in obese subjects. N Engl J Med. 1992;327(27):1893-1898. doi:10.1056/NEJM199212313272701
40. International Expert Committee. International Expert Committee report on the role of the A1C assay in the diagnosis of diabetes. Diabetes Care. 2009;32(7):1327-1334. doi:10.2337/dc09-9033
41. Aubrey A, Godoy M. 75 Percent of Americans Say They Eat Healthy — Despite Evidence to the Contrary. NPR. https://www.npr.org/sections/thesalt/2016/08/03/487640479/75-percent-of-americans-say-they-eat-healthy-despite-evidence-to-the-contrary. Published August 3, 2016.
42. Understanding A1C. American Diabetes Association. https://diabetes.org/about-diabetes/a1c.
43. Uusitupa M, Khan TA, Viguiliouk E, et al. Prevention of Type 2 Diabetes by Lifestyle Changes: A Systematic Review and Meta-Analysis. Nutrients. 2019;11(11):2611. Published 2019 Nov 1. doi:10.3390/nu11112611
44. About Cholesterol. American Heart Association. https://www.heart.org/en/health-topics/cholesterol/about-cholesterol.
45. Howard VJ, Cushman M, Pulley L, et al. The reasons for geographic and racial differences in stroke study: objectives and design. Neuroepidemiology. 2005;25(3):135-143. doi:10.1159/000086678
46. Study Challenges Good Cholesterol's Role in Universally Predicting Heart Disease Risk. National Heart, Lung, and Blood Institute. Published November 21, 2022. https://www.nhlbi.nih.gov/news/2022/study-challenges-good-cholesterols-role-universally-predicting-heart-disease-risk.
47. Connolly L. Lipoprotein(a): A less understood but critical risk factor for heart disease. UC Davis Health. Published February 16, 2023. https://health.ucdavis.edu/news/headlines/lipoproteina-a-less-understood-but-critical-risk-factor-for-heart-disease/2023/02.

REFERENCES

48. Nawaz G, Rogol AD, Jenkins SM. Amenorrhea. In: StatPearls. Treasure Island (FL): StatPearls Publishing; February 25, 2024.
49. Surwit RS, Feinglos MN, McCaskill CC, et al. Metabolic and behavioral effects of a high-sucrose diet during weight loss. Am J Clin Nutr. 1997;65(4):908-915. doi:10.1093/ajcn/65.4.908
50. Doctor Mike. Confronting Dr. Gundry On Lectins | Inflammation & Leaky Gut. YouTube. Published December 27, 2023. https://www.youtube.com/watch?v=ZemkG6Vj7hc.
51. Pfäfflin A, Schleicher E. Inflammation markers in point-of-care testing (POCT). Anal Bioanal Chem. 2009;393(5):1473-1480. doi:10.1007/s00216-008-2561-3
52. Shmerling R. Should You Be Tested for Inflammation? Harvard Health Blog. Published March 29, 2022. https://www.health.harvard.edu/blog/should-you-be-tested-for-inflammation-202203292715.
53. Maximum health benefits already achieved with less than ten thousand steps per day. Radboud University Medical Center. Published August 31, 2023. https://www.radboudumc.nl/en/news-items/2023/maximum-health-benefits-already-achieved-with-less-than-ten-thousand-steps-per-day.
54. Paluch AE, Bajpai S, Bassett DR, et al. Daily steps and all-cause mortality: a meta-analysis of 15 international cohorts. Lancet Public Health. 2022;7(3):e219-e228. doi:10.1016/S2468-2667(21)00302-9
55. Gillett K. How dangerous nutrition advice is fooling millions of followers on social media. The National. Published January 15, 2024. https://www.thenationalnews.com/lifestyle/2024/01/15/social-media-health-fitness-influencers-versus-experts-dr-idz/.

CHAPTER 7: CONVERSATION

1. Nyhan, B., & Reifler, J. (2010). When corrections fail: The persistence of political misperceptions. Political Behavior, 32(2), 303–330. https://doi.org/10.1007/s11109-010-9112-2
2. Nickerson, R. S. (1998). Confirmation bias: A ubiquitous phenomenon in many guises. Review of General Psychology, 2(2), 175–220. https://doi.org/10.1037/1089-2680.2.2.175
3. Turn the Beet Around: Course Correcting on Diet. The Unbiased Science Podcast. Released May 8, 2024. https://www.unbiasedscipod.com/episodes/turn-the-beet-around-course-correcting-on-diet.
4. Mosier, S.L. and Rimal, A.P. (2020), "Where's the meat? An evaluation of diet and partisanship identification", British Food Journal, Vol. 122 No. 3, pp. 896-909. https://doi.org/10.1108/BFJ-03-2019-0193
5. Hodson G. Meat Eating and Political Ideology. Psychology Today. https://www.psychologytoday.com/us/blog/without-prejudice/201809/meat-eating-and-political-ideology. Published September 5, 2018.
6. Hodson G, Earle M. Conservatism predicts lapses from vegetarian/vegan diets to meat consumption (through lower social justice concerns and social support). Appetite. 2018;120:75-81. doi:10.1016/j.appet.2017.08.027
7. Guidetti M, Carraro L, Cavazza N. Dining with liberals and conservatives: The social underpinnings of food neophobia. PLoS One. 2022;17(1):e0262676. Published 2022 Jan 27. doi:10.1371/journal.pone.0262676
8. Saha S. Why don't politicians talk about meat? The political psychology of human-animal relations in elections. Front Psychol. 2023;14:1021013. Published 2023 Jun 23. doi:10.3389/fpsyg.2023.1021013
9. Why the Low-Fat Diet Failed. Tufts Nutrition Letter. Published August 24, 2020. https://www.nutritionletter.tufts.edu/healthy-eating/why-the-low-fat-diet-failed/.

REFERENCES

10. Vosoughi S, Roy D, Aral S. The spread of true and false news online. Science. 2018;359(6380):1146-1151. doi:10.1126/science.aap9559
11. Cinelli, Matteo & Morales, Gianmarco & Galeazzi, Alessandro & Quattrociocchi, Walter & Starnini, Michele. (2020). Echo Chambers on Social Media: A comparative analysis. 10.48550/arXiv.2004.09603.
12. Mosleh M, Martel C, Eckles D, Rand DG. Shared partisanship dramatically increases social tie formation in a Twitter field experiment. Proc Natl Acad Sci U S A. 2021;118(7):e2022761118. doi:10.1073/pnas.2022761118
13. Sasahara, Kazutoshi & Chen, Wen & Peng, Hao & Ciampaglia, Giovanni & Flammini, Alessandro & Menczer, Filippo. (2021). Social influence and unfollowing accelerate the emergence of echo chambers. Journal of Computational Social Science. 4. 1-22. 10.1007/s42001-020-00084-7.
14. Nestle M. Food Politics: How the Food Industry Influences Nutrition and Health. Berkeley: University of California Press; 2007. https://www.amazon.com/Food-Politics-Influences-Nutrition-California/dp/0520254031.
15. Leme ACB, Hou S, Fisberg RM, Fisberg M, Haines J. Adherence to Food-Based Dietary Guidelines: A Systemic Review of High-Income and Low- and Middle-Income Countries. Nutrients. 2021;13(3):1038. Published 2021 Mar 23. doi:10.3390/nu13031038
16. National Academies of Sciences, Engineering, and Medicine; Health and Medicine Division; Food and Nutrition Board; Committee to Review the Process to Update the Dietary Guidelines for Americans. Redesigning the Process for Establishing the Dietary Guidelines for Americans. Washington (DC): National Academies Press (US); November 16, 2017.
17. Crezo A. Simple, Inexpensive Ways to Eat More Fruit and Veggies. Center for Science in the Public Interest. https://www.cspinet.org/cspi-news/simple-inexpensive-ways-eat-more-fruit-and-veggies. Published March 15, 2023.

REFERENCES

18. MyPlate Plan. United States Department of Agriculture. https://www.myplate.gov/myplate-plan.
19. Food-Based Dietary Guidelines. Food and Agriculture Organization of the United Nations. https://www.fao.org/nutrition/education/food-based-dietary-guidelines.
20. Koch W. Dietary Polyphenols-Important Non-Nutrients in the Prevention of Chronic Noncommunicable Diseases. A Systematic Review. Nutrients. 2019;11(5):1039. Published 2019 May 9. doi:10.3390/nu11051039
21. Conrad Z, Kowalski C, Dustin D, et al. Quality of Popular Diet Patterns in the United States: Evaluating the Effect of Substitutions for Foods High in Added Sugar, Sodium, Saturated Fat, and Refined Grains. Curr Dev Nutr. 2022;6(9):nzac119. Published 2022 Sep 12. doi:10.1093/cdn/nzac119
22. Crum AJ, Corbin WR, Brownell KD, Salovey P. Mind over milkshakes: mindsets, not just nutrients, determine ghrelin response. Health Psychol. 2011;30(4):424-431. doi:10.1037/a0023467
23. Enck P, Bingel U, Schedlowski M, Rief W. The placebo response in medicine: minimize, maximize or personalize?. Nat Rev Drug Discov. 2013;12(3):191-204. doi:10.1038/nrd3923
24. Black CJ, Thakur ER, Houghton LA, Quigley EMM, Moayyedi P, Ford AC. Efficacy of psychological therapies for irritable bowel syndrome: systematic review and network meta-analysis. Gut. 2020;69(8):1441-1451. doi:10.1136/gutjnl-2020-321191
25. van Tilburg MA, Palsson OS, Whitehead WE. Which psychological factors exacerbate irritable bowel syndrome? Development of a comprehensive model. J Psychosom Res. 2013;74(6):486-492. doi:10.1016/j.jpsychores.2013.03.004
26. Lackner JM, Jaccard J, Keefer L, et al. Improvement in Gastrointestinal Symptoms After Cognitive Behavior Therapy for Refractory Irritable Bowel Syndrome [published correction appears in Gastroenterology. 2018 Oct;155(4):1281. doi: 10.1053/j.gastro.2018.09.049]. Gastroenterology. 2018;155(1):47-57. doi:10.1053/j.gastro.2018.03.063

REFERENCES

27. Zernicke KA, Campbell TS, Blustein PK, et al. Mindfulness-based stress reduction for the treatment of irritable bowel syndrome symptoms: a randomized wait-list controlled trial. Int J Behav Med. 2013;20(3):385-396. doi:10.1007/s12529-012-9241-6
28. Mayer EA. Gut feelings: the emerging biology of gut-brain communication. Nat Rev Neurosci. 2011;12(8):453-466. Published 2011 Jul 13. doi:10.1038/nrn3071
29. Bizzaro N, Tozzoli R, Villalta D, Fabris M, Tonutti E. Cutting-edge issues in celiac disease and in gluten intolerance. Clin Rev Allergy Immunol. 2012;42(3):279-287. doi:10.1007/s12016-010-8223-1
30. Bucci C, Zingone F, Russo I, et al. Gliadin does not induce mucosal inflammation or basophil activation in patients with nonceliac gluten sensitivity. Clin Gastroenterol Hepatol. 2013;11(10):1294-1299.e1. doi:10.1016/j.cgh.2013.04.022
31. Henriques HKF, Fonseca LM, de Andrade KS, et al. Gluten-Free Diet Reduces Diet Quality and Increases Inflammatory Potential in Non-Celiac Healthy Women. J Am Nutr Assoc. 2022;41(8):771-779. doi:10.1080/07315724.2021.1962769
32. Jenkins DJ, Kendall CW, Vidgen E, et al. High-protein diets in hyperlipidemia: effect of wheat gluten on serum lipids, uric acid, and renal function. Am J Clin Nutr. 2001;74(1):57-63. doi:10.1093/ajcn/74.1.57
33. Wang Y, Cao Y, Lebwohl B, et al. Gluten Intake and Risk of Digestive System Cancers in 3 Large Prospective Cohort Studies. Clin Gastroenterol Hepatol. 2022;20(9):1986-1996.e11. doi:10.1016/j.cgh.2021.11.016
34. Molina-Infante J, Carroccio A. Suspected Nonceliac Gluten Sensitivity Confirmed in Few Patients After Gluten Challenge in Double-Blind, Placebo-Controlled Trials. Clin Gastroenterol Hepatol. 2017;15(3):339-348. doi:10.1016/j.cgh.2016.08.007
35. Skodje GI, Sarna VK, Minelle IH, et al. Fructan, Rather Than Gluten, Induces Symptoms in Patients With Self-Reported Non-Celiac Gluten Sensitivity. Gastroenterology. 2018;154(3):529-539.e2. doi:10.1053/j.gastro.2017.10.040

REFERENCES

36. Benedetti F, Amanzio M, Casadio C, Oliaro A, Maggi G. Blockade of nocebo hyperalgesia by the cholecystokinin antagonist proglumide. Pain. 1997;71(2):135-140. doi:10.1016/s0304-3959(97)03346-0
37. DiGiacomo DV, Tennyson CA, Green PH, Demmer RT. Prevalence of gluten-free diet adherence among individuals without celiac disease in the USA: results from the Continuous National Health and Nutrition Examination Survey 2009-2010. Scand J Gastroenterol. 2013;48(8):921-925. doi:10.3109/00365521.2013.809598
38. Vici G, Belli L, Biondi M, Polzonetti V. Gluten free diet and nutrient deficiencies: A review. Clin Nutr. 2016;35(6):1236-1241. doi:10.1016/j.clnu.2016.05.002
39. Miranda J, Lasa A, Bustamante MA, Churruca I, Simon E. Nutritional differences between a gluten-free diet and a diet containing equivalent products with gluten [published correction appears in Plant Foods Hum Nutr. 2014 Sep;69(3):290]. Plant Foods Hum Nutr. 2014;69(2):182-187. doi:10.1007/s11130-014-0410-4
40. Fry L, Madden AM, Fallaize R. An investigation into the nutritional composition and cost of gluten-free versus regular food products in the UK. J Hum Nutr Diet. 2018;31(1):108-120. doi:10.1111/jhn.12502
41. Chew S. Myth: We Only Use 10% of Our Brains. Association for Psychological Science. Published July 29, 2011. https://www.psychologicalscience.org/uncategorized/myth-we-only-use-10-of-our-brains.html.

IMAGE #1:
Food and Agriculture Organization of the United Nations. Spain: previous versions of food-based dietary guidelines. Published 2024. https://www.fao.org/nutrition/education/food-dietary-guidelines/regions/spain/previous-versions/en/

IMAGE #2:
Food and Agriculture Organization of the United Nations. Japan: food-based dietary guidelines. Published 2024. https://www.fao.org/nutrition/education/food-dietary-guidelines/regions/countries/japan/en/

REFERENCES

CHAPTER 8: UNIQUE

1. Zeevi D, Korem T, Zmora N, et al. Personalized Nutrition by Prediction of Glycemic Responses. Cell. 2015;163(5):1079-1094. doi:10.1016/j.cell.2015.11.001
2. De Cosmi V, Scaglioni S, Agostoni C. Early Taste Experiences and Later Food Choices. Nutrients. 2017;9(2):107. Published 2017 Feb 4. doi:10.3390/nu9020107
3. Scaglioni S, De Cosmi V, Ciappolino V, Parazzini F, Brambilla P, Agostoni C. Factors Influencing Children's Eating Behaviours. Nutrients. 2018;10(6):706. Published 2018 May 31. doi:10.3390/nu10060706
4. Fildes A, van Jaarsveld CHM, Wardle J, Cooke L. Parent-administered exposure to increase children's vegetable acceptance: a randomized controlled trial. J Acad Nutr Diet. 2014;114(6):881-888. doi:10.1016/j.jand.2013.07.040
5. Spill M, Callahan E, Johns K, et al. Repeated Exposure to Foods and Early Food Acceptance: A Systematic Review. Alexandria (VA): USDA Nutrition Evidence Systematic Review; April 2019.
6. Martinez O, Schmid A. Culture and Childhood Experiences' Effect on Food. Achona Online. Published March 15, 2021. https://achonaonline.com/culture/2021/03/culture-and-childhood-experiences-affect-on-food/.
7. Prescott, J. (2024). Development of Food Preferences. In: Meiselman, H.L. (eds) Handbook of Eating and Drinking. Springer, Cham. https://doi.org/10.1007/978-3-319-75388-1_24-3
8. Mahmood L, Flores-Barrantes P, Moreno LA, Manios Y, Gonzalez-Gil EM. The Influence of Parental Dietary Behaviors and Practices on Children's Eating Habits. Nutrients. 2021;13(4):1138. Published 2021 Mar 30. doi:10.3390/nu13041138
9. Scaglioni S, Arrizza C, Vecchi F, Tedeschi S. Determinants of children's eating behavior. Am J Clin Nutr. 2011;94(6 Suppl):2006S-2011S. doi:10.3945/ajcn.110.001685

REFERENCES

10. Sodium Reduction in the Food Supply. U.S. Food & Drug Administration. https://www.fda.gov/food/food-labeling-nutrition/sodium-reduction-food-supply.
11. van Spronsen FJ, Blau N, Harding C, Burlina A, Longo N, Bosch AM. Phenylketonuria. Nat Rev Dis Primers. 2021;7(1):36. Published 2021 May 20. doi:10.1038/s41572-021-00267-0
12. Patel N, Shackelford KB. Irritable Bowel Syndrome. In: StatPearls. Treasure Island (FL): StatPearls Publishing; October 30, 2022.
13. Fenando A, Rednam M, Gujarathi R, Widrich J. Gout. In: StatPearls. Treasure Island (FL): StatPearls Publishing; February 12, 2024.
14. 37 Million American Adults Now Estimated to Have Chronic Kidney Disease. National Kidney Foundation. Published January 6, 2023. https://www.kidney.org/press-room/37-million-american-adults-now-estimated-to-have-chronic-kidney-disease.
15. Food Elimination Diet for Eosinophilic Esophagitis (EoE). UW Health. https://patient.uwhealth.org/healthfacts/553.
16. Bachmanov AA, Bosak NP, Floriano WB, Inoue M, Li X, Lin C, Murovets VO, Reed DR, Zolotarev VA, Beauchamp GK. Genetics of sweet taste preferences. Flavour Fragr J. 2011 Jul;26(4):286-294. doi: 10.1002/ffj.2074. PMID: 21743773; PMCID: PMC3130742.
17. Wiss DA, Avena N, Rada P. Sugar Addiction: From Evolution to Revolution. Front Psychiatry. 2018;9:545. Published 2018 Nov 7. doi:10.3389/fpsyt.2018.00545
18. Han P, Mohebbi M, Seo HS, Hummel T. Sensitivity to sweetness correlates to elevated reward brain responses to sweet and high-fat food odors in young healthy volunteers. Neuroimage. 2020;208:116413. doi:10.1016/j.neuroimage.2019.116413
19. Maron D. Crave Sugar? Maybe It's in Your Genes. Scientific American. Published March 23, 2018. https://www.scientificamerican.com/article/crave-sugar-maybe-its-in-your-genes/.

REFERENCES

20. Obradovic M, Sudar-Milovanovic E, Soskic S, et al. Leptin and Obesity: Role and Clinical Implication. Front Endocrinol (Lausanne). 2021;12:585887. Published 2021 May 18. doi:10.3389/fendo.2021.585887
21. Perakakis N, Farr OM, Mantzoros CS. Leptin in Leanness and Obesity: JACC State-of-the-Art Review. J Am Coll Cardiol. 2021;77(6):745-760. doi:10.1016/j.jacc.2020.11.069
22. Khera R, Murad MH, Chandar AK, et al. Association of Pharmacological Treatments for Obesity With Weight Loss and Adverse Events: A Systematic Review and Meta-analysis [published correction appears in JAMA. 2016 Sep 6;316(9):995. doi: 10.1001/jama.2016.11657]. JAMA. 2016;315(22):2424-2434. doi:10.1001/jama.2016.7602
23. Ghusn W, De la Rosa A, Sacoto D, et al. Weight Loss Outcomes Associated With Semaglutide Treatment for Patients With Overweight or Obesity. JAMA Netw Open. 2022;5(9):e2231982. Published 2022 Sep 1. doi:10.1001/jamanetworkopen.2022.31982
24. Castro R. GLP-1 agonists: Diabetes drugs and weight loss. Mayo Clinic. Published 2022. https://www.mayoclinic.org/diseases-conditions/type-2-diabetes/expert-answers/byetta/faq-20057955
25. Dina C, Meyre D, Gallina S, et al. Variation in FTO contributes to childhood obesity and severe adult obesity. Nat Genet. 2007;39(6):724-726. doi:10.1038/ng2048
26. Estimating Energy Expenditure. Nutrition and Fitness: A Guide to a Healthy Lifestyle. https://pressbooks.calstate.edu/nutritionandfitness/chapter/estimating-energy-expenditure/.
27. Wang Z, Ying Z, Bosy-Westphal A, et al. Specific metabolic rates of major organs and tissues across adulthood: evaluation by mechanistic model of resting energy expenditure. Am J Clin Nutr. 2010;92(6):1369-1377. doi:10.3945/ajcn.2010.29885
28. Després JP. Body fat distribution and risk of cardiovascular disease: an update. Circulation. 2012;126(10):1301-1313. doi:10.1161/CIRCULATIONAHA.111.067264
29. Kanaley JA, Weltman JY, Veldhuis JD, Rogol AD, Hartman ML, Weltman A. Human growth hormone response to repeated

REFERENCES

bouts of aerobic exercise. J Appl Physiol (1985). 1997;83(5):1756-1761. doi:10.1152/jappl.1997.83.5.1756

30. St-Onge MP, Ard J, Baskin ML, et al. Meal Timing and Frequency: Implications for Cardiovascular Disease Prevention: A Scientific Statement From the American Heart Association. Circulation. 2017;135(9). https://doi.org/10.1161/CIR.0000000000000476.

31. Alkhulaifi F, Darkoh C. Meal Timing, Meal Frequency and Metabolic Syndrome. Nutrients. 2022;14(9):1719. Published 2022 Apr 21. doi:10.3390/nu14091719

32. Ha K, Song Y. Associations of Meal Timing and Frequency with Obesity and Metabolic Syndrome among Korean Adults. Nutrients. 2019;11(10):2437. Published 2019 Oct 13. doi:10.3390/nu11102437

33. Gillett K. How dangerous nutrition advice is fooling millions of followers on social media. The National. Published January 15, 2024. https://www.thenationalnews.com/lifestyle/2024/01/15/social-media-health-fitness-influencers-versus-experts-dr-idz/.

34. Mitchell WK, Williams J, Atherton P, Larvin M, Lund J, Narici M. Sarcopenia, dynapenia, and the impact of advancing age on human skeletal muscle size and strength; a quantitative review. Front Physiol. 2012;3:260. Published 2012 Jul 11. doi:10.3389/fphys.2012.00260

35. Cappuccio FP, Taggart FM, Kandala NB, et al. Meta-analysis of short sleep duration and obesity in children and adults. Sleep. 2008;31(5):619-626. doi:10.1093/sleep/31.5.619

36. Thomas DT, Erdman KA, Burke LM. American College of Sports Medicine Joint Position Statement. Nutrition and Athletic Performance [published correction appears in Med Sci Sports Exerc. 2017 Jan;49(1):222. doi: 10.1249/MSS.0000000000001162]. Med Sci Sports Exerc. 2016;48(3):543-568. doi:10.1249/MSS.0000000000000852

37. USDA. Key Statistics & Graphics: Food Security in the U.S. U.S. Department of Agriculture Economic Research Service. https://www.ers.usda.gov/topics/food-nutrition-assistance/food-security-in-the-u-s/key-statistics-graphics/.

REFERENCES

38. Dutko P, Ver Ploeg M, Farrigan T. Characteristics and Influential Factors of Food Deserts. U.S. Department of Agriculture Economic Research Service; 2012. https://www.ers.usda.gov/webdocs/publications/45014/30940_err140.pdf.
39. Davis B, Carpenter C. Proximity of fast-food restaurants to schools and adolescent obesity. Am J Public Health. 2009;99(3):505-510. doi:10.2105/AJPH.2008.137638
40. Berchick E, Hood E, Barnett J. Health Insurance Coverage in the United States: 2017. Current Population Reports. https://www.census.gov/content/dam/Census/library/publications/2018/demo/p60-264.pdf.
41. Many Americans Want to Eat a Healthier Diet but Face Barriers, Including High Costs, Study Shows. CBS News Philadelphia. Published April 10, 2023. https://www.cbsnews.com/philadelphia/video/many-americans-want-to-eat-a-healthier-diet-but-face-barriers-including-high-costs-study-shows/.

IMAGE #1:
National Center for Health, Behavioral Health, and Intellectual Disabilities. The social determinants of health. Published 2024. https://www.center4healthandsdc.org/the-social-determinants-of-health.html

IMAGE #2:
NOAH. Social determinants of health. Published 2024. https://noah-helps.org/sdoh/

REFERENCES

CHAPTER 9: FUNDAMENTALS

1. Park K. The Role of Dietary Phytochemicals: Evidence from Epidemiological Studies. Nutrients. 2023;15(6):1371. Published 2023 Mar 12. doi:10.3390/nu15061371
2. Phytonutrients: What They Are and Why You Need Them. Cleveland Clinic. https://health.clevelandclinic.org/phytonutrients.
3. Reed KE, Camargo J, Hamilton-Reeves J, Kurzer M, Messina M. Neither soy nor isoflavone intake affects male reproductive hormones: An expanded and updated meta-analysis of clinical studies. Reprod Toxicol. 2021;100:60-67. doi:10.1016/j.reprotox.2020.12.019
4. Taku K, Umegaki K, Sato Y, Taki Y, Endoh K, Watanabe S. Soy isoflavones lower serum total and LDL cholesterol in humans: a meta-analysis of 11 randomized controlled trials [published correction appears in Am J Clin Nutr. 2007 Sep;86(3):809]. Am J Clin Nutr. 2007;85(4):1148-1156. doi:10.1093/ajcn/85.4.1148
5. Otun J, Sahebkar A, Östlundh L, Atkin SL, Sathyapalan T. Systematic Review and Meta-analysis on the Effect of Soy on Thyroid Function. Sci Rep. 2019;9(1):3964. Published 2019 Mar 8. doi:10.1038/s41598-019-40647-x
6. Nechuta SJ, Caan BJ, Chen WY, et al. Soy food intake after diagnosis of breast cancer and survival: an in-depth analysis of combined evidence from cohort studies of US and Chinese women. Am J Clin Nutr. 2012;96(1):123-132. doi:10.3945/ajcn.112.035972
7. Wei Y, Lv J, Guo Y, et al. Soy intake and breast cancer risk: a prospective study of 300,000 Chinese women and a dose-response meta-analysis. Eur J Epidemiol. 2020;35(6):567-578. doi:10.1007/s10654-019-00585-4
8. Nachvak SM, Moradi S, Anjom-Shoae J, et al. Soy, Soy Isoflavones, and Protein Intake in Relation to Mortality from All Causes, Cancers, and Cardiovascular Diseases: A Systematic Review and Dose-Response Meta-Analysis of Prospective Cohort Studies. J Acad Nutr Diet. 2019;119(9):1483-1500.e17. doi:10.1016/j.jand.2019.04.011

9. Soliman GA. Dietary Fiber, Atherosclerosis, and Cardiovascular Disease. Nutrients. 2019;11(5):1155. Published 2019 May 23. doi:10.3390/nu11051155
10. Fu J, Zheng Y, Gao Y, Xu W. Dietary Fiber Intake and Gut Microbiota in Human Health. Microorganisms. 2022;10(12):2507. Published 2022 Dec 18. doi:10.3390/microorganisms10122507
11. Ma W, Nguyen LH, Song M, et al. Dietary fiber intake, the gut microbiome, and chronic systemic inflammation in a cohort of adult men. Genome Med. 2021;13(1):102. Published 2021 Jun 17. doi:10.1186/s13073-021-00921-y
12. Blaak EE, Canfora EE, Theis S, et al. Short chain fatty acids in human gut and metabolic health. Benef Microbes. 2020;11(5):411-455. doi:10.3920/BM2020.0057
13. Yang Y, Zhao LG, Wu QJ, Ma X, Xiang YB. Association between dietary fiber and lower risk of all-cause mortality: a meta-analysis of cohort studies. Am J Epidemiol. 2015;181(2):83-91. doi:10.1093/aje/kwu257
14. Surwit RS, Feinglos MN, McCaskill CC, et al. Metabolic and behavioral effects of a high-sucrose diet during weight loss. Am J Clin Nutr. 1997;65(4):908-915. doi:10.1093/ajcn/65.4.908
15. Korrapati D, Jeyakumar SM, Katragadda S, et al. Development of Low Glycemic Index Foods and Their Glucose Response in Young Healthy Non-Diabetic Subjects. Prev Nutr Food Sci. 2018;23(3):181-188. doi:10.3746/pnf.2018.23.3.181
16. McDevitt RM, Bott SJ, Harding M, Coward WA, Bluck LJ, Prentice AM. De novo lipogenesis during controlled overfeeding with sucrose or glucose in lean and obese women. Am J Clin Nutr. 2001;74(6):737-746. doi:10.1093/ajcn/74.6.737
17. Fazzino TL, Dorling JL, Apolzan JW, Martin CK. Meal composition during an ad libitum buffet meal and longitudinal predictions of weight and percent body fat change: The role of hyper-palatable, energy dense, and ultra-processed foods. Appetite. 2021;167:105592. doi:10.1016/j.appet.2021.105592
18. Liu D, Deng Y, Sha L, Abul Hashem M, Gai S. Impact of oral processing on texture attributes and taste perception. J Food Sci

REFERENCES

Technol. 2017;54(8):2585-2593. doi:10.1007/s13197-017-2661-1

19. Monteiro CA, Cannon G, Levy RB, et al. Ultra-processed foods: what they are and how to identify them. Public Health Nutr. 2019;22(5):936-941. doi:10.1017/S1368980018003762
20. Markus CR, Rogers PJ, Brouns F, Schepers R. Eating dependence and weight gain; no human evidence for a 'sugar-addiction' model of overweight. Appetite. 2017;114:64-72. doi:10.1016/j.appet.2017.03.024
21. Darcey VL, Guo J, Chi M, et al. Brain dopamine responses to ultra-processed milkshakes are highly variable and not significantly related to adiposity in humans. Preprint. medRxiv. 2024;2024.06.24.24309440. Published 2024 Jun 25. doi:10.1101/2024.06.24.24309440
22. Ranjbar YR, Nasrollahzadeh J. Comparison of the impact of saturated fat from full-fat yogurt or low-fat yogurt and butter on cardiometabolic factors: a randomized cross-over trial. Eur J Nutr. 2024;63(4):1213-1224. doi:10.1007/s00394-024-03352-8
23. Tokede OA, Gaziano JM, Djoussé L. Effects of cocoa products/dark chocolate on serum lipids: a meta-analysis. Eur J Clin Nutr. 2011;65(8):879-886. doi:10.1038/ejcn.2011.64
24. Artificial trans fats banned in U.S. Harvard T.H. Chan School of Public Health. Published June 18, 2018. https://www.hsph.harvard.edu/news/hsph-in-the-news/us-bans-artificial-trans-fats/.
25. Aronson D, Bartha P, Zinder O, et al. Obesity is the major determinant of elevated C-reactive protein in subjects with the metabolic syndrome. Int J Obes Relat Metab Disord. 2004;28(5):674-679. doi:10.1038/sj.ijo.0802609
26. Raeisi-Dehkordi H, Amiri M, Humphries KH, Salehi-Abargouei A. The Effect of Canola Oil on Body Weight and Composition: A Systematic Review and Meta-Analysis of Randomized Controlled Clinical Trials. Adv Nutr. 2019;10(3):419-432. doi:10.1093/advances/nmy108
27. Ringseis R, Piwek N, Eder K. Oxidized fat induces oxidative stress but has no effect on NF-kappaB-mediated proinflamma-

tory gene transcription in porcine intestinal epithelial cells. Inflamm Res. 2007;56(3):118-125. doi:10.1007/s00011-006-6122-y

28. Sayon-Orea C, Carlos S, Martínez-Gonzalez MA. Does cooking with vegetable oils increase the risk of chronic diseases?: a systematic review. Br J Nutr. 2015;113 Suppl 2:S36-S48. doi:10.1017/S0007114514002931

29. Li Y, Hruby A, Bernstein AM, et al. Saturated Fats Compared With Unsaturated Fats and Sources of Carbohydrates in Relation to Risk of Coronary Heart Disease: A Prospective Cohort Study. J Am Coll Cardiol. 2015;66(14):1538-1548. doi:10.1016/j.jacc.2015.07.055

30. Palomäki A, Pohjantähti-Maaroos H, Wallenius M, et al. Effects of dietary cold-pressed turnip rapeseed oil and butter on serum lipids, oxidized LDL and arterial elasticity in men with metabolic syndrome. Lipids Health Dis. 2010;9:137. Published 2010 Dec 1. doi:10.1186/1476-511X-9-137

31. Hodson L, Skeaff CM, Chisholm WA. The effect of replacing dietary saturated fat with polyunsaturated or monounsaturated fat on plasma lipids in free-living young adults. Eur J Clin Nutr. 2001;55(10):908-915. doi:10.1038/sj.ejcn.1601234

32. Masson CJ, Mensink RP. Exchanging saturated fatty acids for (n-6) polyunsaturated fatty acids in a mixed meal may decrease postprandial lipemia and markers of inflammation and endothelial activity in overweight men. J Nutr. 2011;141(5):816-821. doi:10.3945/jn.110.136432

33. Drouin-Chartier JP, Tremblay AJ, Lépine MC, Lemelin V, Lamarche B, Couture P. Substitution of dietary ω-6 polyunsaturated fatty acids for saturated fatty acids decreases LDL apolipoprotein B-100 production rate in men with dyslipidemia associated with insulin resistance: a randomized controlled trial. Am J Clin Nutr. 2018;107(1):26-34. doi:10.1093/ajcn/nqx013

34. Keogh JB, Grieger JA, Noakes M, Clifton PM. Flow-mediated dilatation is impaired by a high-saturated fat diet but not by a high-carbohydrate diet. Arterioscler Thromb Vasc Biol.

2005;25(6):1274-1279. doi:10.1161/01.ATV.0000163185.28245.a1
35. Nydahl M, Gustafsson IB, Ohrvall M, Vessby B. Similar serum lipoprotein cholesterol concentrations in healthy subjects on diets enriched with rapeseed and with sunflower oil. Eur J Clin Nutr. 1994;48(2):128-137.
36. Schwab U, Reynolds AN, Sallinen T, Rivellese AA, Risérus U. Dietary fat intakes and cardiovascular disease risk in adults with type 2 diabetes: a systematic review and meta-analysis. Eur J Nutr. 2021;60(6):3355-3363. doi:10.1007/s00394-021-02507-1
37. Fuehrlein BS, Rutenberg MS, Silver JN, et al. Differential metabolic effects of saturated versus polyunsaturated fats in ketogenic diets. J Clin Endocrinol Metab. 2004;89(4):1641-1645. doi:10.1210/jc.2003-031796
38. Bjermo H, Iggman D, Kullberg J, et al. Effects of n-6 PUFAs compared with SFAs on liver fat, lipoproteins, and inflammation in abdominal obesity: a randomized controlled trial. Am J Clin Nutr. 2012;95(5):1003-1012. doi:10.3945/ajcn.111.030114
39. Rosqvist F, Iggman D, Kullberg J, et al. Overfeeding polyunsaturated and saturated fat causes distinct effects on liver and visceral fat accumulation in humans. Diabetes. 2014;63(7):2356-2368. doi:10.2337/db13-1622
40. Marklund M, Wu JHY, Imamura F, et al. Biomarkers of Dietary Omega-6 Fatty Acids and Incident Cardiovascular Disease and Mortality. Circulation. 2019;139(21):2422-2436. doi:10.1161/CIRCULATIONAHA.118.038908
41. Li J, Guasch-Ferré M, Li Y, Hu FB. Dietary intake and biomarkers of linoleic acid and mortality: systematic review and meta-analysis of prospective cohort studies. Am J Clin Nutr. 2020;112(1):150-167. doi:10.1093/ajcn/nqz349
42. Su H, Liu R, Chang M, Huang J, Wang X. Dietary linoleic acid intake and blood inflammatory markers: a systematic review and meta-analysis of randomized controlled trials. Food Funct. 2017;8(9):3091-3103. doi:10.1039/c7fo00433h
43. Gopinath B, Buyken AE, Flood VM, Empson M, Rochtchina E, Mitchell P. Consumption of polyunsaturated fatty acids, fish, and

nuts and risk of inflammatory disease mortality. Am J Clin Nutr. 2011;93(5):1073-1079. doi:10.3945/ajcn.110.009977

44. Rett BS, Whelan J. Increasing dietary linoleic acid does not increase tissue arachidonic acid content in adults consuming Western-type diets: a systematic review. Nutr Metab (Lond). 2011;8:36. Published 2011 Jun 10. doi:10.1186/1743-7075-8-36

45. Zhao G, Etherton TD, Martin KR, West SG, Gillies PJ, Kris-Etherton PM. Dietary alpha-linolenic acid reduces inflammatory and lipid cardiovascular risk factors in hypercholesterolemic men and women. J Nutr. 2004;134(11):2991-2997. doi:10.1093/jn/134.11.2991

46. Halvorsen BL, Blomhoff R. Determination of lipid oxidation products in vegetable oils and marine omega-3 supplements. Food Nutr Res. 2011;55:10.3402/fnr.v55i0.5792. doi:10.3402/fnr.v55i0.5792

47. Zhu Y, Bo Y, Liu Y. Dietary total fat, fatty acids intake, and risk of cardiovascular disease: a dose-response meta-analysis of cohort studies. Lipids Health Dis. 2019;18(1):91. Published 2019 Apr 6. doi:10.1186/s12944-019-1035-2

48. Johnson GH, Fritsche K. Effect of dietary linoleic acid on markers of inflammation in healthy persons: a systematic review of randomized controlled trials. J Acad Nutr Diet. 2012;112(7):1029-1041.e10415. doi:10.1016/j.jand.2012.03.029

49. Valsta LM, Jauhiainen M, Aro A, Katan MB, Mutanen M. Effects of a monounsaturated rapeseed oil and a polyunsaturated sunflower oil diet on lipoprotein levels in humans. Arterioscler Thromb. 1992;12(1):50-57. doi:10.1161/01.atv.12.1.50

50. de Lorgeril M, Renaud S, Mamelle N, et al. Mediterranean alpha-linolenic acid-rich diet in secondary prevention of coronary heart disease [published correction appears in Lancet 1995 Mar 18;345(8951):738]. Lancet. 1994;343(8911):1454-1459. doi:10.1016/s0140-6736(94)92580-1

51. Harris WS, Mozaffarian D, Rimm E, et al. Omega-6 fatty acids and risk for cardiovascular disease: a science advisory from the American Heart Association Nutrition Subcommittee of the

Council on Nutrition, Physical Activity, and Metabolism; Council on Cardiovascular Nursing; and Council on Epidemiology and Prevention. Circulation. 2009;119(6):902-907. doi:10.1161/CIRCULATIONAHA.108.191627
52. Innes JK, Calder PC. Omega-6 fatty acids and inflammation. Prostaglandins Leukot Essent Fatty Acids. 2018;132:41-48. doi:10.1016/j.plefa.2018.03.004
53. Messina M, Shearer G, Petersen K. Soybean oil lowers circulating cholesterol levels and coronary heart disease risk, and has no effect on markers of inflammation and oxidation. Nutrition. 2021;89:111343. doi:10.1016/j.nut.2021.111343
54. Fritsche KL. Linoleic acid, vegetable oils & inflammation. Mo Med. 2014;111(1):41-43.
55. Ajabnoor SM, Thorpe G, Abdelhamid A, Hooper L. Long-term effects of increasing omega-3, omega-6 and total polyunsaturated fats on inflammatory bowel disease and markers of inflammation: a systematic review and meta-analysis of randomized controlled trials. Eur J Nutr. 2021;60(5):2293-2316. doi:10.1007/s00394-020-02413-y
56. Luukkonen PK, Sädevirta S, Zhou Y, et al. Saturated Fat Is More Metabolically Harmful for the Human Liver Than Unsaturated Fat or Simple Sugars. Diabetes Care. 2018;41(8):1732-1739. doi:10.2337/dc18-0071
57. Parry SA, Rosqvist F, Mozes FE, et al. Intrahepatic Fat and Postprandial Glycemia Increase After Consumption of a Diet Enriched in Saturated Fat Compared With Free Sugars. Diabetes Care. 2020;43(5):1134-1141. doi:10.2337/dc19-2331
58. Rosqvist F, Kullberg J, Ståhlman M, et al. Overeating Saturated Fat Promotes Fatty Liver and Ceramides Compared With Polyunsaturated Fat: A Randomized Trial. J Clin Endocrinol Metab. 2019;104(12):6207-6219. doi:10.1210/jc.2019-00160
59. Zong G, Li Y, Wanders AJ, et al. Intake of individual saturated fatty acids and risk of coronary heart disease in US men and women: two prospective longitudinal cohort studies. BMJ. 2016;355:i5796. Published 2016 Nov 23. doi:10.1136/bmj.i5796

60. Nicholls SJ, Lundman P, Harmer JA, et al. Consumption of saturated fat impairs the anti-inflammatory properties of high-density lipoproteins and endothelial function. J Am Coll Cardiol. 2006;48(4):715-720. doi:10.1016/j.jacc.2006.04.080
61. González F, Considine RV, Abdelhadi OA, Xue J, Acton AJ. Saturated fat ingestion stimulates proatherogenic inflammation in polycystic ovary syndrome. Am J Physiol Endocrinol Metab. 2021;321(5):E689-E701. doi:10.1152/ajpendo.00213.2021
62. Mu L, Mukamal KJ, Naqvi AZ. Erythrocyte saturated fatty acids and systemic inflammation in adults. Nutrition. 2014;30(11-12):1404-1408. doi:10.1016/j.nut.2014.04.020
63. Hooper L, Martin N, Jimoh OF, Kirk C, Foster E, Abdelhamid AS. Reduction in saturated fat intake for cardiovascular disease. Cochrane Database Syst Rev. 2020;5(5):CD011737. Published 2020 May 19. doi:10.1002/14651858.CD011737.pub2
64. Ference BA, Ginsberg HN, Graham I, et al. Low-density lipoproteins cause atherosclerotic cardiovascular disease. 1. Evidence from genetic, epidemiologic, and clinical studies. A consensus statement from the European Atherosclerosis Society Consensus Panel. Eur Heart J. 2017;38(32):2459-2472. doi:10.1093/eurheartj/ehx144
65. Sniderman AD, Thanassoulis G, Glavinovic T, et al. Apolipoprotein B Particles and Cardiovascular Disease: A Narrative Review. JAMA Cardiol. 2019;4(12):1287-1295. doi:10.1001/jamacardio.2019.3780
66. Nielsen LB. Transfer of low density lipoprotein into the arterial wall and risk of atherosclerosis. Atherosclerosis. 1996;123(1-2):1-15. doi:10.1016/0021-9150(96)05802-9
67. Ference BA, Yoo W, Alesh I, et al. Effect of long-term exposure to lower low-density lipoprotein cholesterol beginning early in life on the risk of coronary heart disease: a Mendelian randomization analysis. J Am Coll Cardiol. 2012;60(25):2631-2639. doi:10.1016/j.jacc.2012.09.017
68. Peters SA, Singhateh Y, Mackay D, Huxley RR, Woodward M. Total cholesterol as a risk factor for coronary heart disease and stroke in women compared with men: A systematic review and

meta-analysis. Atherosclerosis. 2016;248:123-131. doi:10.1016/j.atherosclerosis.2016.03.016

69. Khan SU, Michos ED. Cardiovascular mortality after intensive LDL-Cholesterol lowering: Does baseline LDL-Cholesterol really matter? [published correction appears in Am J Prev Cardiol. 2021 Mar 29;5:100159. doi: 10.1016/j.ajpc.2021.100159]. Am J Prev Cardiol. 2020;1:100013. Published 2020 May 1. doi:10.1016/j.ajpc.2020.100013

70. NihonSan Study. University of Minnesota. http://www.epi.umn.edu/cvdepi/study-synopsis/nihonsan-study/

71. Silverman MG, Ference BA, Im K, et al. Association Between Lowering LDL-C and Cardiovascular Risk Reduction Among Different Therapeutic Interventions: A Systematic Review and Meta-analysis. JAMA. 2016;316(12):1289-1297. doi:10.1001/jama.2016.13985

72. Hall KD, Guo J. Obesity Energetics: Body Weight Regulation and the Effects of Diet Composition. Gastroenterology. 2017;152(7):1718-1727.e3. doi:10.1053/j.gastro.2017.01.052

73. St. Pierre B, Scott-Dixon K. The Surprising Truth About Sugar: Here's Everything You Need to Know About What It Does to Your Body. MeFitProhttps://www.mefitpro.com/blogs/blog/the-surprising-truth-about-sugar-here-s-everything-you-need-to-know-about-what-it-does-to-your-body

74. Gardner CD, Trepanowski JF, Del Gobbo LC, et al. Effect of Low-Fat vs Low-Carbohydrate Diet on 12-Month Weight Loss in Overweight Adults and the Association With Genotype Pattern or Insulin Secretion: The DIETFITS Randomized Clinical Trial [published correction appears in JAMA. 2018 Apr 3;319(13):1386. doi: 10.1001/jama.2018.2977] [published correction appears in JAMA. 2018 Apr 24;319(16):1728. doi: 10.1001/jama.2018.4854]. JAMA. 2018;319(7):667-679. doi:10.1001/jama.2018.0245

75. Nakamura Y, Watanabe H, Tanaka A, Yasui M, Nishihira J, Murayama N. Effect of Increased Daily Water Intake and Hydration on Health in Japanese Adults. Nutrients. 2020;12(4):1191. Published 2020 Apr 23. doi:10.3390/nu12041191

REFERENCES

76. Popkin BM, D'Anci KE, Rosenberg IH. Water, hydration, and health. Nutr Rev. 2010;68(8):439-458. doi:10.1111/j.1753-4887.2010.00304.x
77. Di Cesare M, Perel P, Taylor S, et al. The Heart of the World. Glob Heart. 2024;19(1):11. Published 2024 Jan 25. doi:10.5334/gh.1288
78. Jahic D, Begic E. Exercise-Associated Muscle Cramp-Doubts About the Cause. Mater Sociomed. 2018;30(1):67-69. doi:10.5455/msm.2018.30.67-69
79. Miller KC, Stone MS, Huxel KC, Edwards JE. Exercise-associated muscle cramps: causes, treatment, and prevention. Sports Health. 2010;2(4):279-283. doi:10.1177/1941738109357299
80. Stofan JR, Zachwieja JJ, Horswill CA, Murray R, Anderson SA, Eichner ER. Sweat and sodium losses in NCAA football players: a precursor to heat cramps?. Int J Sport Nutr Exerc Metab. 2005;15(6):641-652. doi:10.1123/ijsnem.15.6.641
81. Garrison SR, Allan GM, Sekhon RK, Musini VM, Khan KM. Magnesium for skeletal muscle cramps. Cochrane Database Syst Rev. 2012;2012(9):CD009402. Published 2012 Sep 12. doi:10.1002/14651858.CD009402.pub2
82. Fernandez ML, Murillo AG. Is There a Correlation between Dietary and Blood Cholesterol? Evidence from Epidemiological Data and Clinical Interventions. Nutrients. 2022;14(10):2168. Published 2022 May 23. doi:10.3390/nu14102168
83. 4 Protein Mistakes to Avoid. American Heart Association. https://www.heart.org/en/healthy-living/healthy-eating/eat-smart/nutrition-basics/4-protein-mistakes-to-avoid#:~:text=Eggs%20can%20be%20included%20as,as%20a%20high%2Dquality%20protein.
84. Harrold JA, Hill S, Radu C, et al. Non-nutritive sweetened beverages versus water after a 52-week weight management programme: a randomised controlled trial. Int J Obes (Lond). 2024;48(1):83-93. doi:10.1038/s41366-023-01393-3
85. Gibbons C, Beaulieu K, Almiron-Roig E, et al. Acute and two-week effects of neotame, stevia rebaudioside M and sucrose-

sweetened biscuits on postprandial appetite and endocrine response in adults with overweight/obesity-a randomised crossover trial from the SWEET consortium. EBioMedicine. 2024;102:105005. doi:10.1016/j.ebiom.2024.105005

86. Kwok D, Scott C, Strom N, et al. Comparison of a Daily Steviol Glycoside Beverage compared with a Sucrose Beverage for Four Weeks on Gut Microbiome in Healthy Adults. J Nutr. 2024;154(4):1298-1308. doi:10.1016/j.tjnut.2024.01.032
87. Menni C, Jackson MA, Pallister T, Steves CJ, Spector TD, Valdes AM. Gut microbiome diversity and high-fibre intake are related to lower long-term weight gain. Int J Obes (Lond). 2017;41(7):1099-1105. doi:10.1038/ijo.2017.66

REFERENCES

CHAPTER 10: FORWARD

1. How We Change: Intentional Spiritual Formation and Discovering Our True Selves [podcast]. Apple Podcasts. https://podcasts.apple.com/us/podcast/how-we-change-intentional-spiritual-formation-discovering/id1592847144?i=1000556629462
2. Cadario, R., & Chandon, P. (2020). Which healthy eating nudges work best? A meta-analysis of field experiments. Marketing Science, 39(3), 465–486. https://doi.org/10.1287/mksc.2018.1128
3. Which Healthy Eating Nudges Work Best? A Meta-Analysis of Field Experiments. Nutrition Connect. https://nutritionconnect.org/resource-center/which-healthy-eating-nudges-work-best-meta-analysis-field-experiments.

ACKNOWLEDGEMENTS

I wrote this book for a variety of reasons. These are many of the same reasons I pursued a career in nutrition in the first place. As with so many of you, I have witnessed family members go in and out of hospitals and deal with numerous mental and physical health issues. I not only want to be one part of the solution in helping to prevent these challenges for others, but I know how stressful it can be to navigate the health and wellness space in difficult times as well.

Many influential people who inspired this writing include:

- My mom, Phyllis, and my dad, Steve, who raised me to love Jesus and love others.

- My sister, Heather, who shares my most cherished life experiences.

- My wife, Alexis, who was my camp crush.

- My boys, Collin and Max, who bring the most joy.

- THE boys: Justin, Timmy, David, Derek, Boomer, Adam, Benji, and Sean.

- My preceptors for grad school, Scott, Cecilia, Ashley, and Christine. My UNE classmates, instructors, Dr. Boldrin, and Dr. Dodge.

- My favorite former teachers: Mr. J, Mrs. Hoffacker, Mr. Ahn, Mrs. Starr, Mr. Waters, Mr. Tobin.

- To Jon Wallace and Peggy Campbell who showed me how to be a better leader and man of God.

- My SRV coaching family, John, Scott, Tony, Joe, Cindy, Tim, and all of my former players who made me love coaching basketball.

ACKNOWLEDGEMENTS

- Bill Haslim, who officiated an amazing wedding ceremony, continues to offer the best spiritual advice, and was the best boss I will ever have.

- To the Sunol Hills team who does such great work to help those working through the unique challenge of an eating disorder.

- Special thanks to Caleb for the first design on my cover and Miracle who created the final cover and took the time to format my book.

- And all of my former patients and clients who made me better at my job and remind me of just how valuable it can be to serve others in the area of health and nutrition.